Acute Respiratory Distress Syndrome

Acute respiratory distress syndrome is the most lethal form of acute respiratory failure and presents one of the greatest challenges in critical care medicine. Despite its severity and complexity, however, few texts exist that provide a detailed review of how to care for patients who have ARDS. Drs. Russell and Walley have enlisted an expert team of contributors to provide not only the essentials of diagnosis, assessment, and management; they have also taken care to provide just enough pathophysiology to illustrate clearly the science behind the clinical approach.

After giving the history and epidemiology of ARDS, the authors present the essential basic science underlying the causes of this syndrome and explain how to manage patients in its acute and later stages. The thorough clinical portions of the book clearly explain such treatment and management issues as mechanical ventilation and weaning, resolution and repair of lung injury, pneumonia, multiple system organ failure, and cardiovascular and pulmonary physiology and monitoring. An extensive chapter on clinical assessment and total patient care demonstrates the importance of total patient care in ARDS. Superb tables and figures help to make this chapter, and indeed the entire book, indispensible to intensivists, pulmonologists, internists, anesthesiologists, surgeons, and critical care nurses.

Thoroughly referenced and up to date, *Acute Respiratory Distress Syndrome: A Comprehensive Clinical Approach* is the definitive source of information for any physician who treats patients with ARDS.

Dr. James Russell is a practicing intensivist and chair of the Department of Medicine at St. Paul's Hospital, a tertiary teaching hospital of the University of British Columbia. He has twenty years of experience managing critically ill patients in both the United States and Canada and has researched, lectured, and written about ARDS extensively.

Dr. Keith Walley is also a practicing clinical intensivist at St. Paul's Hospital in Vancouver with substantial expertise in both the laboratory and the intensive care unit. He is frequently invited to lecture at key international critical care meetings, including the American Thoracic Society, the Brussels Symposium on Intensive Care, and the Critical Care World Congress.

Acute Respiratory Distress Syndrome

A Comprehensive Clinical Approach

Edited by

JAMES A. RUSSELL
KEITH R. WALLEY

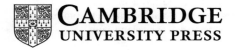

CAMBRIDGE
UNIVERSITY PRESS

PUBLISHED BY THE PRESS SYNDICATE OF THE UNIVERSITY OF CAMBRIDGE
The Pitt Building, Trumpington Street, Cambridge, United Kingdom

CAMBRIDGE UNIVERSITY PRESS
The Edinburgh Building, Cambridge CB2 2RU, UK   http://www.cup.cam.ac.uk
40 West 20th Street, New York, NY 10011-4211, USA   http://www.cup.org
10 Stamford Road, Oakleigh, Melbourne 3166, Australia

First published 1999

Printed in the United States of America

Typeset in Goudy Old Style in QuarkXPress [GH]

A catalog record for this book is available from the British Library

Library of Congress Cataloging-in-Publication Data
Acute respiratory distress syndrome : a comprehensive clinical
approach / edited by James A. Russell, Keith R. Walley.
    p. cm.
    1. Respiratory distress syndrome, Adult. –   I. Russell, James A.
II. Walley, Keith R. (Keith Robert)
    [DNLM: 1. Respiratory Distress Syndrome, Adult.   WF 140 A18346
1999]
RC776.R38A27984   1999
616.2 – dc21
DNLM/DLC   98-46408
                                                           CIP

ISBN   0 521 65410 6   paperback

Every effort has been made in preparing this book to provide accurate and up-to-date information that is in accord with accepted standards and practice at the time of publication.
Nevertheless, the authors, editors, and publisher can make no warranties that the information contained herein is totally free from error, not least because clinical standards are constantly changing through research and regulation. The authors, editors, and publisher therefore disclaim all liability for direct or consequential damages resulting from the use of material contained in this book. Readers are strongly advised to pay careful attention to information provided by the manufacturer of any drugs or equipment that they plan to use.

*With thanks to Sharon Stuart for her excellent secretarial assistance
and to Jo-Ann Strangis for her guidance throughout the editing process.*

*For Betty and Russ for their love, support, and vision for me;
For my daughters Francey and Allie for their fun and love,
And for Frances, the woman of my dreams, for her love, laughter,
and zest for life.*

– JAMES RUSSELL

*To Pat and our children for their love and for keeping the really important
things in focus.*

– KEITH WALLEY

Contributors

Richard K. Albert, M.D.
Chief, Department of Medicine
Denver Health Medical Center
Denver, Colorado

Ahmed Bahammam, M.D.
Clinical Fellow
Respiratory and Critical Care Medicine
Department of Internal Medicine
University of Manitoba
Winnipeg, Manitoba
CANADA

Gordon R. Bernard, M.D.
Professor of Medicine
Division of Pulmonary and Critical Care
　Medicine
Vanderbilt University School of Medicine
Nashville, Tennessee

Russell Bowler, M.D.
Division of Pulmonary and Critical Care
　Medicine
School of Medicine
University of California, San Francisco
San Francisco, California

Cary Caldwell, M.D.
Department of Gastroenterology
The University of Michigan Medical
　School
Ann Arbor, Michigan

Rajiv Dhand, M.D.
Associate Professor
Division of Pulmonary and Critical Care
　Medicine
Loyola University of Chicago
Stritch School of Medicine
Chicago, Illinois

Vinay Dhingra, M.D.
Program of Critical Care Medicine
University of British Columbia
Vancouver, British Columbia
CANADA

Chrystelle Garat, M.S.
Division of Pulmonary and Critical Care
　Medicine
School of Medicine
University of California, San Francisco
San Francisco, California

Bryan G. Garber, M.D.
Assistant Professor of Surgery
University of Ottawa
Ottawa, Ontario
CANADA

Paul C. Hébert, M.D.
Department of Medicine
Ottawa General Hospital
Ottawa, Ontario
CANADA

Steven L. Kunkel, Ph.D.
Professor, Department of Pathology
The University of Michigan Medical
  School
Ann Arbor, Michigan

R. Bruce Light, M.D.
Professor of Medicine and Medical
  Microbiology
Departments of Internal Medicine and
  Medical Microbiology
University of Manitoba
Winnipeg, Manitoba
CANADA

Nicholas Lukacs, Ph.D.
Department of Pathology
The University of Michigan Medical
  School
Ann Arbor, Michigan

Michael A. Matthay, M.D
Professor, Medicine and Anesthesia
Senior Associate, Cardiovascular Research
  Institute
Associate Director, Intensive Care Unit
School of Medicine/Cardiovascular
  Research Institute
University of California, San Francisco
San Francisco, California

James A. Russell, M.D.
Professor and Chairman, Department
  of Medicine
St. Paul's Hospital
University of British Columbia
Vancouver, British Columbia
CANADA

Gregory A. Schmidt, M.D.
Professor of Medicine
Section of Pulmonary and Critical Care
  Medicine
The University of Chicago
Chicago, Illinois

Theodore Standiford, M.D.
Pulmonary and Critical Care Medicine
The University of Michigan Medical
  School
Ann Arbor, Michigan

Robert M. Strieter, M.D.
Professor of Medicine
Pulmonary and Critical Care Medicine
The University of Michigan Medical
  School
Ann Arbor, Michigan

Martin J. Tobin, M.D.
Professor of Medicine and Director
Division of Pulmonary and Critical Care
  Medicine
Loyola University of Chicago
Stritch School of Medicine
Chicago, Illinois

Ari Uusaro, M.D.
Department of Anesthesiology and Inten-
  sive Care
Division of Critical Care
Critical Care Research Program
Kuopio University Hospital
Kuopio
FINLAND

Keith R. Walley, M.D.
Professor of Medicine
St. Paul's Hospital
University of British Columbia
Vancouver, British Columbia
CANADA

J. L. Wright, M.D.
Professor of Pathology
Vancouver Hospital
University of British Columbia Site
Vancouver, British Columbia
CANADA

Contents

Preface   xi

Introduction   1
James A. Russell and Keith R. Walley

1. *Overview, Clinical Evaluation, and Chest Radiology
   of ARDS*   6
   Vinay Dhingra, James A. Russell, and Keith R. Walley

2. *The Epidemiology of ARDS*   28
   Bryan G. Garber and Paul C. Hébert

3. *The Pathology of ARDS*   48
   J. L. Wright

4. *Cytokine-Induced Mechanisms of Acute Lung Injury Leading
   to ARDS*   63
   Steven L. Kunkel, Theodore Standiford, Cary Caldwell, Nicholas Lukacs,
   and Robert M. Strieter

5. *Pulmonary Pathophysiology in ARDS*   80
   Keith R. Walley and James A. Russell

6. *Cardiovascular Management of ARDS*   107
   Keith R. Walley and James A. Russell

7. *Mechanical Ventilation*   *139*
   Gregory A. Schmidt

8. *Respiratory Muscles and Liberation from Mechanical Ventilation*   *163*
   Rajiv Dhand and Martin J. Tobin

9. *Clinical Assessment and Total Patient Care*   *183*
   James A. Russell, Vinay Dhingra, and Keith R. Walley

10. *ARDS: Innovative Therapy*   *233*
    Gordon R. Bernard

11. *Nosocomial Pneumonia in ARDS*   *251*
    Ahmed Bahammam and R. Bruce Light

12. *Resolution and Repair of Acute Lung Injury*   *275*
    Russell Bowler, Chrystelle Garat, and Michael A. Matthay

13. *Multiple System Organ Failure*   *304*
    Ari Uusaro and James A. Russell

14. *Outcome and Long-Term Care of ARDS*   *334*
    Richard K. Albert

    Index   *345*

Preface

Acute respiratory distress syndrome (ARDS) is an important problem in critical care medicine because ARDS care is expensive, ARDS commonly affects young, previously healthy individuals, management is complex, and mortality is high. Indeed, management of the unstable, profoundly hypoxemic patient who has ARDS is one of the most challenging and potentially rewarding clinical scenarios we face in critical care medicine.

There are suggestions that the mortality of ARDS may be decreasing, yet large trials of innovative therapies continue to seek further improvements in outcome. It is not clear why mortality of ARDS may be decreasing, but some have proposed that comprehensive, organized intensive care is the reason.

We identified a great need for a comprehensive, clinically oriented handbook on ARDS to assist clinicians who manage patients with ARDS. We recognized that sound understanding of the pathophysiology and epidemiology of ARDS leads to improved clinical management. Furthermore, we have been stimulated by the challenge of balancing multiple competing aspects of our patients' physiology when managing our own patients who have ARDS. So we decided to write and edit this textbook on ARDS for a clinical audience of students, residents, and attending physicians in critical care, respiratory medicine, anesthesiology, internal medicine, and surgery.

Why do we think this book will be a useful addition to your textbook collection? First, we are extremely proud of the outstanding group of internationally recognized authors who have written lucid chapters covering topics in their areas of expertise. Second, we have emphasized a sound understanding of epidemiology, molecular mechanisms, and whole organ pathophysiology as the basis for clinical care. To provide continuity, we edited the text so it provides a clinical perspective that will make it valuable and useful at the bedside in the ICU as well as in the office and library. Lastly, we both love the challenges and rewards of successfully resuscitating the profoundly unstable, hypoxemic patient who has ARDS, and we hope this book helps you enjoy this clinical challenge as well.

Introduction

James A. Russell and Keith R. Walley

Acute respiratory distress syndrome (ARDS) is a very important problem in critical care medicine. First, ARDS occurs commonly in young, previously well individuals who have major insults such as multiple trauma, sepsis, and aspiration of gastric contents. Second, the mortality of ARDS remains relatively high at 40% to 60% despite improvements in drug therapy, mechanical ventilation, hemodynamic management, more potent antibiotics, better prevention of complications (e.g., stress ulceration), better supportive care (e.g., nutrition), and more effective methods of weaning from ventilation. Encouragingly, there are some indications that the mortality of ARDS may be decreasing. Third, the health care costs of ARDS are considerable because patients are almost exclusively managed in an expensive ICU setting. There is considerable pressure to contain costs and to improve the cost effectiveness of ARDS. Finally, ARDS is important because the quality of life for survivors of ARDS is good with generally very good to excellent return of pulmonary function, good return to quality of life in many, and even preliminary reports of excellent return of quality of life in most.

ARDS has been defined more precisely by an American-European Consensus Conference. Acute lung injury preceding ARDS is defined by presence of bilateral infiltrates on chest roentgenogram, no evidence of congestive heart failure (or pulmonary artery occlusion pressure less than 19 mmHg if a pulmonary artery catheter is in place), need for mechanical ventilation, and PaO_2/FiO_2 less than 200. Severe ARDS is similarly defined, except the PaO_2/FiO_2 ratio must be less than 100.

This textbook provides a comprehensive approach to the clinical management of patients who have ARDS. Our approach focuses heavily on underlying pathophysiology and provides recommendations for cost-effective investigation and management of ARDS, information regarding controversial areas in ARDS, and updates regarding the results of clinical trials of new therapy in ARDS. We have recruited an outstanding group of contributors who are internationally acknowledged experts in fundamental and clinical issues in ARDS.

Chapter 1 offers an overview of ARDS, an approach to clinical evaluation, and a review of radiologic assessment of ARDS. The overview component provides a stand-alone summary of some of the topics discussed in much greater detail later in the text in order to provide a general context for subsequent discussions. We also present an approach to the initial clinical evaluation of the patient with ARDS. Then radiologic examination, which is fundamental to the evaluation and management of patients with ARDS, is reviewed.

The clinical causes and epidemiology of ARDS are reviewed in Chapter 2 by Drs. Garber and Hébert. These authors present an approach to reviewing the literature that can be used to critically evaluate clinical studies in any field. Here they apply this approach to studies regarding the epidemiology of ARDS. Important risk factors for ARDS are identified using an evidence-based medicine approach. Finally, Drs. Garber and Hébert review studies regarding the morbidity and mortality of ARDS that suggest the mortality of ARDS may be decreasing for reasons that are as yet unclear.

In Chapter 3, Dr. Wright presents a concise review of the pathology of ARDS. The particular pathologic findings from early to late-phase ARDS are illustrated in detail. Dr. Wright identifies clinically important changes that have an impact on measures of pulmonary physiology.

In Chapter 4, Dr. Kunkel and colleagues review the molecular mechanisms of acute lung injury and ARDS. The key roles of early pro-inflammatory cytokines in initiating a pattern of recognition, recruitment, resolution, and repair are described. These authors point out the importance of the balance of pro- and anti-inflammatory mediators in determining the outcome of the inflammatory response characteristic of ARDS. Futhermore, Dr. Kunkel and colleagues discuss the concept of complex networks of signaling molecules and inflammatory effector cells that make up the pulmonary inflammatory response of ARDS. Finally, they present the changes over time in the inflammatory response in the lung in ARDS.

In Chapter 5, Drs. Walley and Russell discuss pulmonary physiology and approaches to monitoring clinically relevant aspects of the respiratory system of patients who have ARDS. Abnormal gas exchange is fundamental to the pathophysiology of ARDS, and appropriate monitoring using arterial blood gas analysis, transmission and reflectance oximetry, and metabolic cart measures of oxygen consumption and carbon dioxide production are discussed. Lung and airway mechanics are significantly impaired in ARDS. Dynamic and static pressure-volume relationships of ARDS, auto-PEEP, the importance of respiratory muscles, and control of respiratory drive are explained together with clinical approaches to evaluating and therapeutically altering these parameters.

Drs. Walley and Russell then discuss cardiovascular physiology and management in Chapter 6. Using basic concepts from cardiovascular physiology, the authors discuss the sepsis-like circulation of ARDS. Derangements in microvascular control and how these relate to the impaired peripheral oxygen extraction that occurs in sepsis, and may occur in ARDS, are discussed. Drs. Walley and Russell describe the oxygen delivery/consumption controversy as it relates to patients who have ARDS. They review the role of supranormal oxygen delivery in management of ARDS, the role of the pulmonary artery catheter, and the usefulness of gastric tonometery.

Mechanical ventilation of patients who have ARDS is probably the most complex form of ventilation in critical care. The fundamental issues in mechanical ventilation of patients who have ARDS are discussed by Dr. Schmidt in Chapter 7. These include the mechanics of mechanical ventilation, the effects of mechanical ventilation on normal and abnormal pulmonary and cardiovascular physiology, and the effects of mechanical ventilation on the peripheral vascular system. This review of physiology is used as a basis for understanding conventional and newer modes of ventilation. After discussing conventional modes of ventilation, Dr. Schmidt discusses new methods of mechanical ventilation in severe ARDS with very impaired gas exchange and decreased respiratory compliance including the use of pressure control ventilation, inverse ratio ventilation, and permissive hypercapnia ventilation. One major issue in mechanical ventilation of patients who have ARDS is the controversy surrounding ventilator-induced lung injury.

There have been many changes in techniques for weaning a patient from mechanical ventilation and those that are relevant to management of ARDS are reviewed by Drs. Dhand and Tobin in Chapter 8. They first examine the pathophysiologic determinants of weaning outcome including pulmonary gas exchange, respiratory muscle pump failure, decreased neuromuscular capacity, respiratory muscle dysfunction, increased respiratory muscle pump load, increased work of breathing, and psychological problems. Next, they consider how to predict which patients will be weaned successfully. Drs. Dhand and Tobin then discuss clinical approaches to weaning from mechanical ventilation. The discussion includes simple trials of spontaneous breathing through a T-tube system that were employed at the onset of mechanical ventilation; intermittent mandatory ventilation (IMV), which is the most popular weaning technique in North America; and pressure support ventilation (PSV). A once-daily trial of spontaneous breathing may be the most expeditious approach.

The cornerstones of therapy of patients who have ARDS are (1) reversal of the underlying cause(s) of ARDS (e.g., sepsis) and (2) excellent total patient care to keep the patient alive and free of complication while the patient's inflammatory response runs its course to resolution and repair. Aspects of total patient care are reviewed in Chapter 9 by Drs. Russell, Dhingra, and Walley. Complications occurring during the course of ARDS are reviewed. Prevention or rapid correction of these complications is fundamental in avoiding "second hits" that too frequently lead to multiple organ failure and death.

At present no proven therapy exists that either resolves or shortens the duration of established ARDS. In Chapter 10, Dr. Bernard discusses innovative therapies that are potentially useful and are under investigation in basic science and clinical studies of ARDS. Based on the molecular mechanisms of ARDS (Chapter 4), Dr. Bernard discusses a rationale for use of therapies designed to interrupt pro-inflammatory mediators. Futhermore, Dr. Bernard discusses therapies specific for management of ARDS such as surfactant replacement, inhaled nitric oxide, use of steroids in early ARDS, use of steroids in the late stage of ARDS, and other novel therapies currently being tested in trials of sepsis and ARDS.

Nosocomial pneumonia, discussed in Chapter 11 by Drs. Bahammaman and Light, is a major complication of patients who have ARDS. The microbiology of nosocomial pneumonia is important to understand from both a pathophysiologic and therapeutic perspective. They discuss the pathogenesis of nosocomial pneumonia including the role of microbial colonization such as oropharyngeal colonization, gastric colonization, and contamination of respiratory therapy equipment. Drs. Bahammaman and Light examine the host factors predisposing to respiratory infection including the roles of endotracheal intubation and aspiration, pulmonary changes that predispose to infection in ARDS, and systemic alterations in the patient who has ARDS that led to infection. The diagnosis of nosocomial infection in ARDS can be problematic, and they discuss issues such as the roles of chest roentgenogram, clinical evaluation, microbiological evaluation, and more sophisticated techniques such as bronchial alveolar lavage. In particularly, they review nonbronchoscopic techniques. The role of fibroptic bronchoscopy combined with protected specimen brushing or bronchial alveolar lavage is discussed. Then they review the pharmacologic considerations as a background to antimicrobial therapy for ARDS. Pending culture results report, empiric therapy is most often necessary when the diagnosis of pneumonia is suspected, and they make suggestions for initial empiric therapy. Prevention of pneumonia is preferable to treatment of established pneumonia because of the very high mortality, approaching 60%, of nosocomial pneumonia in general and of the even higher mortality, 60% to 80%, of nosocomial pneumonia in patients who have ARDS. Preventive measurements include body position, airway care, nutrition, and infection control and resistance.

In Chapter 12, Drs. Bowler, Garat, and Matthay review resolution and repair of acute lung injury. They discuss how excess alveolar fluid and protein are normally removed and how changes in alveolar removal may have prognostic implications. They then discuss fibrosing alveolitis in acute lung injury including the role of fibrin and fibrinogen, fibronectin, collagens, and cellular changes in the pathophysiology of fibrosis. They discuss growth factors relevant to acute lung injury such as platelet-derived growth factor, epidermal growth factor, transforming growth factor-alpha, transforming growth factor-beta, hepatocyte growth factor, and keratinocyte growth factor. They then discuss cytokines important in resolution of lung injury including tumor necrosis factor, IL-1, and IL-10.

Most patients who die of ARDS do not die of hypoxia but rather die of progressive multiple system organ failure (MSOF). In Chapter 13, Drs. Uusaro and Russell review aspects of multiple system organ failure that are relevant to patients who have ARDS. After defining and reviewing the epidemiology of MSOF, they review the evidence that multiple system organ failure is caused by overt or covert tissue hypoxia in patients who have ARDS. The oxygen delivery/consumption relationship as it relates to evidence for occult tissue hypoxia as a cause of MSOF is discussed. They suggest that the pathologic dependence of oxygen consumption on oxygen delivery has not been established in ARDS and very little evidence supports this as a cause of multiple system organ failure. They then review other mechanisms for multiple system organ failure such as ischemia-reperfusion injury and the role of reactive oxygen metabolites, leukocyte-mediated injury and leukocyte adherence and injury to endothelial cells, cytokine injury mechanisms, and other potential pathways.

Finally, in Chapter 14, Dr. Albert reviews the outcome and long-term care of patients who have ARDS. Dr. Albert again reviews the evidence that mortality of ARDs may be decreasing and discusses potential explanations. He then discusses the symptoms and limitations in survivors of ARDS, the roentgenographic changes in survivors of ARDS, and then reviews pulmonary function test abnormalities in survivors of ARDS. In general, there are mild to moderate reductions in spirometry, increased airway reactivity, modestly reduced lung volumes, somewhat increased dead space and, most commonly, decreased diffusing capacity in survivors of ARDS. Furthermore, survivors of ARDS have abnormal gas exchange that becomes more evident during exercise. Dr. Albert concludes that in the first year after ARDS most physiologic abnormalities will improve, with most of the improvement occurring in the first three months. Deficits persisting beyond one year are unlikely to improve any further. He also discusses the quality of life of survivors of ARDS and studies with somewhat divergent results. One study suggested moderately impaired quality of life, whereas another more recent study suggested relatively good quality of life in survivors or ARDS.

1

Overview, Clinical Evaluation, and Chest Radiology of ARDS

Vinay Dhingra, James A. Russell, and Keith R. Walley

Introduction

The acute respiratory distress syndrome is a relatively new disease that emerged as intensive care units developed. Before mechanical ventilation and ICUs existed, most patients with moderate or severe ARDS would have died. In this chapter we present an overview of ARDS and introduce other concepts dealt with in detail in subsequent chapters. For example, epidemiology is touched on here but is presented in much greater detail in Chapter 2. This overview chapter is also intended to be a stand-alone review of ARDS from a clinically oriented perspective. That is, we have tried to include the most important clinical concepts, present an approach to evaluating and managing the patient, and focus on chest radiology as an integral component of this process.

Definition

Acute lung injury associated with increased capillary–alveolar permeability has been termed the acute respiratory distress syndrome (ARDS). ARDS has many causes. The onset of ARDS is acute, and the duration is usually days to weeks.[1,2] The clinical hallmarks of ARDS are hypoxemia, reduced lung compliance, diffuse bilateral pulmonary infiltrates on chest radiograph, and need for mechanical ventilation.[3–6] Since its initial description in 1967, the criteria for defining ARDS have changed. Normal left ventricular (LV) filling pressures (i.e., PCWP < 18 mmHg)[7–12] and the presence of a risk factor were added as inclusion criteria after introduction of pulmonary artery catheters and after better understanding of the epidemiology of ARDS, respectively.[3–5]

Table 1.1. Lung injury score

Component	Score
1. Chest roentgenogram	
Alveolar consolidation	0
Alveolar consolidation confined to 1 quadrant	1
Alveolar consolidation confined to 2 quadrants	2
Alveolar consolidation confined to 3 quadrants	3
Alveolar consolidation confined to 4 quadrants	4
2. PaO_2/FiO_2	
≥ 300	0
225–299	1
175–224	2
100–174	3
<100	4
3. PEEP (cm H_2O) (when ventilated)	
≤ 5	0
6–8	1
9–11	2
12–14	3
≥ 15	4
4. Respiratory compliance (mL/cm H_2O) (when available)	
≥ 80	0
60–79	1
40–59	2
20–39	3
≤ 19	4

The final lung injury score is the average score of the components that were used.

	Lung injury score
No lung injury	0
Mild-to-moderate lung injury	0.1–2.5
Severe lung injury (ARDS)	> 2.5

Source: Adapted from Murray JF, Matthay MA, Luce JM, Flick MR. An expanded definition of the adult respiratory distress syndrome. Am Rev Respir Dis 1988; 138:720–723.

The criteria for the diagnosis of ARDS have evolved further since the original description.[1] In 1988 Murray and colleagues published the "acute lung injury score" in patients who have a risk factor for ARDS.[3] The score consists of two to four components, and each component is a score from 0 to 4 (Table 1.1). The components are added to yield the total score. This lung injury score has been used in a number of clinical trials to define ARDS. A meeting in 1992 of the American Thoracic Society and the European Society of Intensive Care Medicine produced a consensus statement for the diagnosis of acute lung injury (ALI) and of ARDS. Both ALI and ARDS require the onset to be acute with bilateral infiltrates on chest radiograph and a pulmonary capillary wedge pressure less than 19 mmHg or no clinical evidence of left atrial hypertension. The ratio of the partial pressure of arterial oxygen to the fraction of inspired oxygen (PaO_2/FiO_2) needs to be less than or equal to 300 mmHg for ALI and less than 200 mmHg for ARDS.[5] The ATS/ESICM definition of ARDS was recommended for clinical research such as epidemiology and clinical trials of new therapy for ARDS. There is still controversy regarding the current diagnostic criteria.[6,13]

History

Although clinical and pathologic descriptions of ARDS date back to the time of Osler and World War I,[14–19] Ashbaugh and colleagues are credited with the first descriptive study of ARDS in 1967. They described 12 patients who had acute onset of tachypnea, hypoxemia, decreased respiratory compliance, and diffuse infiltrates on chest radiograph.[1] Four years later this constellation of features was termed the adult respiratory distress syndrome. In 1992 the term *acute respiratory distress syndrome* replaced adult respiratory distress syndrome because the syndrome can occur in children, although it is much less common in children than adults.

Epidemiology and Risk Factors

In 1972 the National Institutes of Health estimated the incidence of ARDS at 60 cases per 100,000 population per year.[20] Since then, several methodologically sound studies of the incidence of ARDS have yielded a surprisingly wide range of incidence rates of 1.5 to 8.3 cases per 100,000 per year.[11,21,22] The range in incidence of ARDS in these studies is explained in part by variability in definition of ARDS used in the studies, by the methods used to identify cases, and by the reference sample population.

ARDS can be caused by a variety of risk factors that may be direct or indirect pulmonary insults. Garber and colleagues did an evidence-based literature review of the risk factors of ARDS. The epidemiologic literature indicates that the major risk factors of ARDS are sepsis, aspiration of gastric contents, multiple trauma, multiple transfusions, pulmonary contusion, pneumonia, and near-drowning.[1,2,7–12,22–24] DIC, fat embolism, and cardiopulmonary bypass had the lowest causation scores, indicating weak evidence as risk factors of ARDS. The presence of more than one risk factor further increases the risk of developing ARDS.

The mortality rate of ARDS is reported as 36% to 70%.[22,25–27] Several recent reports[28–30] suggest the mortality rate of ARDS may be decreasing.[28] In a study from the University of Washington,[28] the decreased mortality rate was accounted for by a decreased mortality rate of ARDS secondary to trauma. In contrast, there was no change over 10 years (1983–1993) in the mortality rate of ARDS associated with sepsis. The mortality rate of sepsis-induced ARDS is higher (40%) than for other causes of multitrauma. Using the American-European Consensus Conference definition,

Doyle and colleagues[31] found a mortality rate of ARDS of 59% in San Francisco. The mortality rate of severe ARDS may also be decreasing. The first North American multicenter trial of extracorporeal membrane oxygenation (ECMO) found a mortality rate of approximately 90% in both ECMO and conventionally treated patients who had severe acute hypoxemic respiratory failure. A later randomized controlled trial in North America of extracorporeal CO_2 removal (ECCOR) used very similar entry criteria to define patients who had severe acute hypoxemic respiratory failure.[29] There was no difference in mortality rate between patients treated with ECCOR and patients treated by a clinical algorithm of usual ventilatory care. More importantly, the mortality rate of the control group was only 65% – much lower than the expected 90% mortality rate of the original ECMO trial. The authors concluded that either mortality rate of severe acute hypoxemic resporatory failure has decreased over 30 years or the rigorous algorithms used to make clinical decisions decreased variance of care and also decreased mortality.

The major causes of death of patients who have ARDS are multiple system organ failure and refractory (irreversible) respiratory failure followed by cardiac, neurologic, hematologic, and other causes of death related to the underlying cause(s) of ARDS. Montgomery and colleagues[32] found that in the first three days after onset of ARDS most deaths were caused by the underlying condition that led to ARDS. Deaths more than three days after onset of ARDS were most often caused by multiple system organ failure (84%). Irreversible respiratory failure accounted for only 16% of deaths.

Pathology

The pathology of ARDS is diffuse alveolar damage (DAD). DAD is a nonspecific pattern of lung injury that can occur from many primary insults. Hemorrhage and protein-rich edema fluid accumulate in the alveoli. The pathologic changes can be divided into three phases. The acute or exudative phase (up to 6 days) is characterized by lung tissue edema and eosinophilic hyaline membranes along the walls of the alveolar ducts.[33,34] The proliferative phase (4 to 10 days) has less edema and a decrease in hyaline membranes but the start of interstitial fibrosis seen as proliferation of fibroblasts.[34,35] The final fibrotic phase (from 8 days onward) displays prominent fibrosis, which may obliterate the alveolar and bronchiolar spaces. Emphysematous changes as well as changes in the pulmonary circulation may also be seen in the fibrotic phase.[33–36]

Pathophysiology

The injury sustained by the lung produces progressive damage to the alveolar-capillary membrane and leads to increased vascular permeability, lung inflammation, and pulmonary edema.[37,38] In ARDS there is an increase in hydraulic conductivity for water and a decrease in the reflection coefficient for protein of the alveolar-capillary membrane, both of which lead to an increase in vascular permeability.[13,37,38] When vascular permeability increases, unopposed hydrostatic pressure effects dominate. As a result, small increases in hydrostatic pressure produce large increases in extravascular lung water, as shown in Figure 1.1. Thus excessive fluid resuscitation in patients

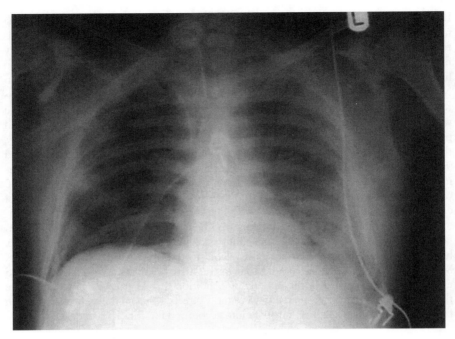

Figure 1.1. Typical chest radiograph of a patient with ARDS.

at risk of ARDS and patients who have ARDS will increase lung water more than normal patients because lung water increases even at normal left atrial pressures.[13] These effects culminate in alveolar flooding and pulmonary edema that is often rapid, progressive, and rich in protein.[37–39]

The pulmonary physiologic consequence of these changes is a decrease in lung compliance.[40] The decrease of lung compliance is a result of loss of aeratable lung volume and not due to changes in the intrinsic elastic properties of the lung.[41,42] Therefore, in early ARDS, the loss of pulmonary compliance reflects the degree of pulmonary edema and atelectasis – not lung injury per se.

The hypoxemia of ARDS is secondary to increased right to left intrapulmonary shunting of blood associated with alveolar flooding and loss of hypoxemic pulmonary vasoconstriction. Ventilation perfusion mismatching plays a much smaller role as a cause of hypoxemia.[13,43] Because of intrapulmonary shunting, hypoxemia is relatively resistant to increased FiO_2. The clinical consequences of high intrapulmonary shunt are that high FiO_2, mask BiPAP, or mechanical ventilation with positive airway pressure are required to correct hypoxemia.

Cardiovascular physiology and cardiopulmonary interaction are important in ARDS because of the effects of ARDS, the underlying cause(s) of ARDS (e.g., sepsis), and positive pressure ventilation.[44] The lung injury of ARDS produces pulmonary hypertension secondary to both a loss of pulmonary artery cross-sectional area as well as increased pulmonary vascular reactivity.[44,45] Pulmonary hypertension increases right ventricular (RV) afterload, which increases RV pressure, dimension, and stroke work.[46] Increased RV dimension shifts the intraventricular septum from right to left, decreases left ventricular compliance, and, if severe, impairs LV diastolic filling. Positive airway pressure and positive end-expiratory pressure (PEEP) decrease RV preload, increase RV afterload, and therefore decrease RV output.[44] RV diastolic compliance may also be reduced because of lung expansion compressing the heart.[47] These effects also subsequently decrease LV filling and LV output. RV volume is increased and RV ejection fraction is decreased in patients who have ARDS.[48–50] Survival has been inversely related to RV dimension. High PEEP can further accentuate these problems.[51] Survivors of ARDS have higher ventricular preload, higher cardiac output, and higher oxygen delivery than do nonsurvivors of ARDS.[49]

Mediators of Injury

The mediators of acute lung injury are discussed in Chapter 4. Several different pathways of mediators induce lung injury. These multiple cascades interact with one another to both amplify and suppress one another. TNF and IL-1 are two important pro-inflammatory cytokines released early after pulmonary or extrapulmonary injury or infection. Pro-inflammatory cytokines activate the complement system and cause release of additional mediators of inflammation, which in turn cause activation and aggregation of neutrophils in the pulmonary vasculature.[52,53] Neutrophil activation and adherence are important in acute lung injury and in other organ dysfunction.[54–56] The activated neutrophils can release additional inflammatory cytokines.[56] Subsequent events include increased platelet activating factor, prostaglandin and leukotriene release, platelet aggregation, induction of nitric oxide synthase, and enhanced cellular oxidant production.[56–60] Activation of leukocytes and adherence to pulmonary vascular endothelium is followed by release of products that directly injure endothelium and increase vascular permeability.[58] Activation of these various pathways causes ongoing endothelial injury and may also set up the conditions for secondary sepsis. ARDS and secondary sepsis may then lead to multiple system organ failure.[56,60,61]

Clinical Evaluation of Patients with ARDS

Primary Survey and Resuscitation

The initial assessment of a patient with acute respiratory failure is of paramount importance. We organize the assessment as simultaneous primary survey and resuscitation similar to the principles of advanced trauma life support (ATLS). Most patients with ARDS are extremely anxious, agitated, and in acute respiratory distress. Tachypnea, tachycardia, diaphoresis, and increased work of breathing demonstrated by intercostal indrawing and use of accessory muscles are characteristic.[1,2,13] Auscultation of the chest is often surprisingly clear but may reveal crackles and expiratory wheezes. Impending respiratory arrest is indicated by rapid shallow breathing, abdominal paradoxical movements, respiratory alternans, and declining level of consciousness. Tachypnea is not an indication for intubation; however, a respiratory rate >35 breaths per minute, use of accessory muscles, and intercostal indrawing suggest nonsustainable increased respiratory workload. Patients in extreme respiratory distress concentrate on breathing and no longer respond appropriately to external stimuli. Severe hypoxemia and respiratory fatigue lead to decreased level of consciousness, obtundation, and coma. In this situation urgent intubation is necessary because severe hypoxemia may cause permanent neurologic sequelae and may herald the onset of cardiorespiratory arrest.

A nonintubated patient must be assessed rapidly to determine whether additional respiratory support is necessary. The spontaneously breathing individual with respiratory distress should have high-flow oxygen with maximal FiO_2, ECG monitoring, frequent blood pressure assessment, and establishment of intravenous access. Pulse oximetry should be considered the "fifth vital sign" and should always be used to give continuous arterial oxygen saturation.

Airway protection and anatomy must be evaluated quickly for urgent intubation and to assess whether intubation is potentially difficult. Micrognathia, short neck, large tongue, temporomandibular joint disease, or cervical spine immobility may make direct laryngoscopy difficult. An easy and clinically useful screen of ease of intubation is to determine whether the uvula can be easily seen above the base of the tongue, an indication of less difficult intubation.

Cardiovascular assessment includes pulse, blood pressure, central filling pressures (jugular venous pulse), adequacy of skin perfusion, mentation, and assessment of cyanosis. Cyanosis is a late insensitive and unreliable sign of hypoxemia. Abnormal hemodynamics are frequently found at the onset of ARDS and are accentuated by sepsis and blood loss from trauma. Tachycardia, vasoconstriction, and hypotension may be present in some patients.[9,13]

The initial assessment includes a brief so-called AMPLE history that includes medication *a*llergies ("A"), current list of *m*edications ("M"), significantly *p*ast or recent illnesses ("P"), aspiration risk (time of *l*ast oral intake or gastric feed) ("L"), and *e*vents surrounding presentation ("E"). Significant illnesses and events that are relevant in ARDS include previous intubation problems, cardiovascular history (e.g., angina, ischemia, myocardial infarction, dysrhythmias, and valvular heart disease), neurologic status (e.g., increased intracranial pressure, intracranial hemorrhage, ischemia, and cervical spine pathology), musculoskeletal status (cord denervation injuries, crush injuries), burns, and coagulation status (e.g., coagulopathy).

The entire assessment should take less than a few minutes and, based upon it, a decision regarding intubation and mechanical ventilation is made. The indications for intubation with ARDS are to correct intractable hypoxemia, to decrease excessive work of breathing, to correct respiratory muscle fatigue, to provide airway protection, to improve tracheobronchial toilet, and to correct hypercapnia and acute respiratory acidosis, and, when ARDS is accompanied by evidence of shock, to divert blood flow from respiratory muscles to vital organ perfusion.[19] The importance of having proper equipment, personnel, and adequate clinical skills during the dynamic period of securing of the airway cannot be overstated and are discussed in detail in Chapters 7 and 9.

At the end of the primary survey and resuscitation, most patients should have respiratory and hemodynamic stability. The goals of intubation and mechanical ventilation are to achieve arterial oxygen saturation greater than 90% in the absence of severe respiratory acidemia, to decrease work of breathing, and to clear airway secretions or hemorrhage. We recommend assist-control ventilation, tidal volume of 6 to 8 mL/kg, respiratory rate of 20 to 25 breaths per minute, PEEP of 5 cm of H_2O, and FiO_2 of 0.95 as initial ventilator settings in most patients. Cardiovascular stability should be achieved as indicated by the absence of excessive tachycardia (heart rate > 140), extreme hypotension (systolic blood pressure < 80 mmHg or mean arterial blood pressure < 60 mmHg), the presence of good capillary refill, and adequate urine output (> 30 mL/hour) with or without inotropic support.

Secondary Survey – The Detailed Assessment

Once the patient is stabilized from a respiratory and cardiovascular standpoint and out of danger of immediate demise, a more detailed history, physical, radiologic, and laboratory examination may take place. The purposes of secondary assessment are to consider the etiology of acute respiratory failure, to plan ongoing therapy, and to assess complications.

Medical History

Three features of the history are important to elicit from patients who have ARDS: data relevant to diagnosis of ARDS, data necessary to identify the underlying cause of ARDS, and data relevant to complications of ARDS and complications of the underlying cause.

ARDS is heralded by the onset of tachypnea, followed by dyspnea and progressive hypoxemia.[1,2,62] There is a delay of several hours to days between the inciting event and the onset of respiratory distress.[13] This delay is less than 24 hours in the majority of patients with a range of 1 to 72 hours in 90% of patients.[1,2,9,10,62] Rare reports of delays as long as 1 week are most often associated with a second risk factor.[9] The delay time is also risk factor dependent, with aspiration of gastric contents being the shortest.[12]

It is important when obtaining the history to consider the differential diagnosis of ARDS. Cardiogenic pulmonary edema must be differentiated from ARDS. Cardiogenic pulmonary edema is caused by increased left atrial pressure or PCWP. Thus patients with cardiogenic pulmonary edema may have a history of angina, myocardial infarction, congestive heart failure, or acute renal failure. Acute cardiogenic pulmonary edema may be triggered by further myocardial dysfunction, by uncontrolled hypertension, by acute infection, and by noncompliance with medications.[63]

Other causes of acute hypoxemic respiratory failure and pulmonary infiltrates include extensive pneumonia, extensive atelectasis, chronic interstitial lung disease with acute exacerbation, and diffuse pulmonary hemorrhage. Usually these diagnoses can be differentiated from ARDS.

A detailed history of events leading up to acute respiratory failure is necessary to identify the underlying cause of ARDS. The astute clinician obtains the history using knowledge of the common risk factors for ARDS and evaluates evidence for each. Review of medical records, discussion with previous caregivers, and history from family members and witnesses may be helpful. For example, it is important to assess whether features of systemic inflammatory response syndrome (fever, tachycardia, tachypnea, and organ dysfunction) are present and to recognize that many of these features overlap with features of ARDS. Therefore, more detailed assessment of potential sources of sepsis, prior results of cultures, prior antibiotics, and prior surgery or drainage procedures are important in assessing whether sepsis is present.

Shock in patients with ARDS is caused by the underlying etiology of ARDS (e.g., sepsis, multiple trauma), severe ARDS itself and/or complications of ARDS (e.g., pulmonary hypertension), RV failure, or pneumothorax. Hypotension is present in up to 90% of patients at onset of ARDS.[9] Furthermore, shock increases the risk of ARDS in patients who have sepsis. Fein and colleagues found in a retrospective review of 116 patients with septicemia that all 21 patients who developed ARDS had shock compared with only 15% in those who did not.[8]

Sepsis is a very common risk factor of ARDS. Systemic inflammatory response syndrome is diagnosed by presence of fever, tachycardia, tachypnea (or mechanical ventilation), and one new organ dysfunction that could be caused by sepsis. Organ dysfunction that could be caused by sepsis includes hypotension (cardiovascular dysfunction), impaired oxygenation (pulmonary dysfunction), oliguria (renal dysfunction), thrombocytopenia and features of DIC (coagulation dysfunction), and decreased Glasgow Coma Score (GCS) (neurologic dysfunction). Finally, the diagnosis of severe sepsis also requires a proven or suspected source of sepsis.

Aspiration of gastric contents is often preceded by a decreased level of consciousness. Direct observation of aspiration may occur at the time of endotracheal intubation.

Physical Examination

A careful, systematic physical examination of the critically ill is fundamental. The initial physical exam of critically ill patients focuses on airway, breathing, and circulation (ABCs) by using general inspection, vital signs, and rapid cardiopulmonary assessment. In the nonintubated patient, assessment of the airway takes priority followed by evaluation of breathing as described in Chapters 7 and 9. The rapid ABC assessment may necessitate a rapid decision to intubate the patient who has inadequate airway protection, severe respiratory distress (with hypoxemia and increased work of breathing), or refractory shock.

Important features of general inspection to note are level of consciousness, evidence of acute distress, increased work of breathing (e.g., accessory muscle use), presence of diaphoresis, cyanosis (central or peripheral), anemia, and evidence of external uncontrolled hemorrhage (in trauma).

The respiratory exam begins with the airway and in the intubated patient includes inspecting the endotracheal tube for position and complications such as kinking, obstruction, and injury to the upper airway. Respiratory examination includes indrawing, use of accessory muscles, examination of tracheal position, chest expansion, breath sounds, and palpation for subcutaneous emphysema. The respiratory examination should be supplemented by inspection of secretions suctioned from the endotracheal tube. The experienced clinician will often assess simple respiratory mechanics of ventilated patients by noting tidal volume, peak airway pressure, PEEP, and plateau pressure at this time.

The cardiovascular exam includes assessment of heart rate and rhythm by bedside ECG monitoring, jugular venous pressure, skin perfusion, and a precordial examination. During the precordial exam the patient should be manually bagged to control for respiratory sounds in order to assess extra heart sounds, murmurs, and rubs. ARDS must be distinguished from congestive heart failure. The initial findings may mimic ARDS with respiratory distress, peripheral vasoconstriction, and hypotension. Features on examination that suggest cardiac failure include an elevated JVP, a diffuse and displaced apex impulse, and a third heart sound. The intensive care clinician supplements the cardiovascular examination by measuring CVP, PCWP, and cardiac output if the patient has a pulmonary artery catheter. Hemodynamic characteristics of cardiac failure include a low cardiac output and an elevated PCWP,[13] in contrast to those of ARDS, which often include an elevated cardiac output with a normal or low PCWP. However, we emphasize that a careful physical examination is a critical step to accurate interpretation of hemodynamics.

Severe abdominal crises (such as peritonitis, pancreatitis, and intra-abdominal abscess) and postoperative complications such as abdominal sepsis can cause ARDS. Abdominal examination focuses on evaluation of findings of peritonitis, assessment of incisions and drains in surgical patients, presence of ileus, and specific examination for right upper quadrant tenderness. Finally, examination of NG returns for the presence of blood should also be performed.

Examination of the extremities focuses on potential causes of ARDS and assessment of perfusion. Severe soft tissue infection and high-risk fractures are potential causes of ARDS. Long bone fractures and unstable pelvic fractures have an incidence of ARDS of 5% to 11%.[9,12] Complications of ARDS include deep venous thrombosis, tissue ischemia secondary to shock, and the skin rash of systemic air emboli from ventilation.[64]

The neurologic examination is often limited by sedating medications and paralysis. Clinical neurologic examination should again focus on causes and complications of ARDS, level of consciousness (GCS), assessment of brainstem reflexes, and evidence of focal neurologic deficits. Neurogenic pulmonary edema can complicate severe head injuries, status epilepticus, and intracranial hemorrhage. ARDS can also complicate aspiration of gastric contents as a result of depressed level of consciousness. Neurologic complications of ARDS include hypoxic encephalopathy, septic encephalopathy, systemic air emboli, and obtundation/coma as a component of multiple organ failure. ARDS with central nervous system dysfunction is associated with a high mortality.[65]

Chest Radiology

The plain portable AP chest radiograph is an important extension of the physical examination of patients who have acute hypoxemic respiratory failure. The chest radiograph is used to establish the diagnosis of ARDS, to exclude other diagnoses, to assess tube and line placement, to search for complications, and to grade severity of ARDS. The chest radiograph is often scored based on the number of quadrants involved.[3,66]

Establishing the Diagnosis of ARDS

The pathology of ARDS has three phases.[34] Similarly, the chest radiograph of patients who have ARDS mirrors the pathologic changes. The chest radiograph appearance of ARDS also depends on the stage, severity, and occasionally the etiology of ARDS.[67]

The first stage or radiologically latent stage is the most transient and occurs in the first few hours following presence of a risk factor for ARDS.[67,68] The patient may be clinically in respiratory distress; however, the chest radiograph may be surprisingly normal. The few abnormalities present at this stage may include a small increase in extravascular lung water reflected in the radiograph with subtle peribronchovascular cuffing (indicating interstitial edema) or ground glass opacification.[69] The radiograph often progresses to diffuse bilateral alveolar infiltrates over the ensuing 24 hours (Figure 1.1).[67] This delay in radiologic evidence of ARDS may reflect increasing edema over this time. The correlation between extravascular lung water and chest radiographs is not uniform.[13]

The etiology of ARDS may be suspected on chest radiograph. Direct pulmonary insults, such as near-drowning, aspiration, or pneumonia, may be diagnosed by finding typical focal parenchymal consolidation. Blunt chest trauma may show rib fractures, pneumothorax, patchy pulmonary contusion, and full-blown ARDS. Most other causes of ARDS are indistinguishable on plain chest films.

As ARDS advances over the next 24 to 72 hours there is progressive airspace consolidation. Air bronchograms are often bilateral, may be asymmetrical, and are usually in the peripheral lung regions associated with progressive decrease in lung volume. Infiltrates are often patchy, nonconfluent, nonsegmental, and slightly asymmetric at this stage. The patient will most often require mechanical ventilation with positive pressure at this time. The effects of positive airway pressure and PEEP are to increase lung volume and decrease the degree of parenchymal opacification.[67] Small pleural effusions are common but may not be apparent on plain portable AP chest radiograph. Moderate pleural effusions are reported on CT scan in clinical and studies of ARDS[70,71] and occur in experimental models of ARDS.

Over the next 4 to 10 days as the acute phase settles there is less pulmonary edema and increasing pulmonary fibrosis. The chest radiograph changes with a decrease in confluent consolidation and progressive increase of interstitial and ground glass patterns as a result of pulmonary fibrosis. The peripheral areas that were consolidated often become more lucent.[67]

Exclusion of Other Diagnoses

There are two steps in differential diagnosis of ARDS: first, consider other causes of airspace consolidation, and second, consider cardiogenic versus noncardiogenic pulmonary edema.

The radiographic features of other causes of acute hypoxemic respiratory failure are usually quite distinct from ARDS. Pulmonary embolus will frequently have no chest radiograph abnormalities or may show pleural-based infiltrates, patchy atelectasis, underperfusion of lung tissue, dilated main pulmonary artery, and small pleural effusions. Pulmonary infarction causes peripheral-based densities or rounded densities near the costophrenic sinus (Hampton's hump).[72] Signs of atelectasis include loss of lung volume, air bronchograms, shifts of the mediastinum and/or diaphragm, with little or no airspace consolidation, and enhanced definition of major or minor fissures in lobar atelectasis. The chest radiograph of pneumonia may include focal, unilateral, or bilateral consolidation. Atypical pneumonia usually causes a diffuse interstitial pattern that may be indistinguishable from ARDS.[72]

Several radiographic features may allow differentiation of cardiogenic pulmonary edema from ARDS. The three most helpful differentiating features on chest radiograph of cardiogenic pulmonary edema are the width of vascular pedicle, the distribution of pulmonary blood flow ,and the distribution of pulmonary edema.[73] In cardiogenic pulmonary edema, the vascular pedicle is engorged and thus widened on chest radiograph, there is redistribution of pulmonary blood flow such that the normal increase in pulmonary vasculature from apex to base is lost, and pulmonary edema is perihilar, a so-called bat wing appearance. However, these findings are more clearly evident on upright PA chest radiographs done in the radiology department than they are on a portable, supine AP chest radiograph in the ICU. In particular, the redistribution of pulmonary vasculature is helpful only in upright films because pulmonary vasculature is uniform from apex to base in a supine radiograph.

Other features of the chest radiograph distinguish ARDS from cardiogenic pulmonary edema. ARDS exhibits predominately patchy airspace consolidation and is often peripheral. Cardiogenic failure more often shows interstitial edema patterns such as septal lines, vascular redistribution, congestion, pleural effusions, and cardiomegaly.[67,69,73] Several studies suggest these features can be used to differentiate ARDS from cardiac failure in 70% to 85% of cases.[67] When severe pulmonary edema occurs, distinction of cardiogenic versus noncardiogenic edema may be impossible.

Finally, some patients have both cardiogenic and noncardiogenic pulmonary edema, making radiographic distinction even more difficult.[67,69,73]

Assessment of Tube and Line Placement

A major purpose of plain portable AP chest films in patients who have ARDS is to assess line and tube placement. Lines and tubes include central venous and pulmonary artery catheters, transvenous pacemakers, chest tubes, NG suction tubes, enteral feeding tubes, endotracheal tubes, and tracheostomy tubes.

Clinical assessment of endotracheal tube position may be difficult and therefore should always be assessed by chest radiograph. Optimal endotracheal tube position should be between 2 and 5 cm above the carina – or midway between the thoracic inlet and the carina – limiting the likelihood of inadvertent extubation or right mainstem intubation with changes in head position. Intubation of the right mainstem bronchus is the most frequent complication of endotracheal intubation and estimated to occur in 10% to 15% of intubations.[74,75] Esophageal intubation should be detected clinically. On frontal chest radiographs the diagnosis of esophageal intubation may be difficult but should be suspected if any of the following are present: unexplained gastric distension, distension of the distal esophagus with air, or the endotracheal tube tip is lateral to the tracheal air column.[67]

Endotracheal intubation can also be complicated by injury to the airways and barotrauma from positive pressure ventilation. Tracheal injury may be secondary to the endotracheal tube itself or the balloon cuff. Endotracheal intubation has been associated with pharyngeal, tracheal, and esophageal perforation. Plain chest radiographs may thus show air in soft tissue, esophageal distension, or mediastinal air. Balloon cuff overdistension may cause ischemia of the tracheal mucosa and will manifest on chest radiograph as focal distension of the tracheal air column.[67,75]

NG tubes are often used to prevent gastric distension and to deliver enteral nutrition. The tip of the NG tube or feeding tube should be more than 10 cm below the diaphragm, and the proximal openings of the NG tube should be below the diaphragm on plain chest radiograph.[76] Feeding tubes have a 1% incidence of malposition, most often into the tracheobronchial tree.[76,77] Pneumothorax may complicate inadvertent tracheobronchial placement of enteral feeding tubes, and the risk of this complication is higher in sedated and paralyzed patients.

Plain chest radiograph is necessary to assess central venous and pulmonary artery catheter placement and to detect complications. The tip of a venous catheter should be just above the level of the right atrium. Pulmonary artery catheter position is determined by the pressure wave form, the volume required for balloon inflation and radiographic documentation of catheter tip position in a central pulmonary artery.[67] Complications of central venous cannulation that may be apparent on plain chest radiograph include pneumothorax, hemothorax, pleural effusion secondary to fluid infusion, pericardial effusion, pulmonary hemorrhage secondary to pulmonary artery rupture, and triangular densities opposite the tip of the PA catheter secondary to pulmonary infarction.[78]

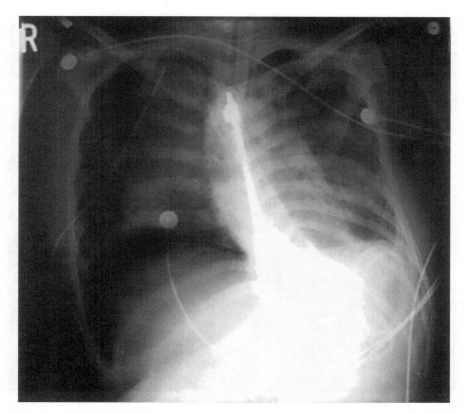

Figure 1.2. Pneumothorax in a patient with ARDS. Extension of the pneumothorax to the subpulmonic space results in lucency extending below the distinct upper border of the right hemidiaphragm.

Complications Evident on Chest Radiograph

The noncompliant lungs of ARDS render them extremely susceptible to barotrauma. Pulmonary interstitial emphysema frequently precedes pneumothorax, pneumomediastinum, and subcutaneous emphysema.[67,69] Pneumothorax results from the direct dissection of pulmonary air into the pleural space or from extension of pneumomediastinum into the pleural space.

Pneumothorax may present as a classic peripheral collection of air with clear delineation of a thin pleural line separated by air lucency from the inner chest wall (Figure 1.2). No lung markings in the area of pleural air and the air lucency may be visible in the pleural space from apex of lung to diaphragm. Occasionally, a skin fold on chest radiograph needs to be differentiated from pneumothorax. Findings that

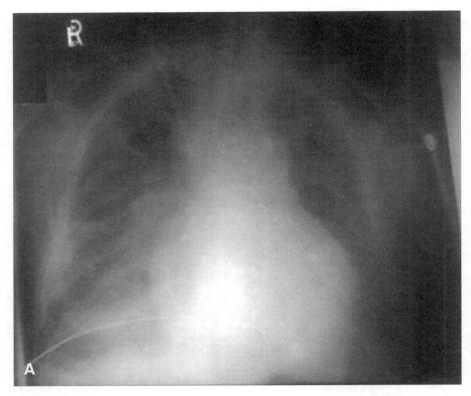

Figure 1.3 (A) A pneumothorax is difficult to appreciate on this AP portable supine chest film.

distinguish a skin fold from a pneumothorax include vertical lines that extend beyond the diaphragm or chest wall, sudden discontinuation of the line in the chest cavity, and gradual increase in water density from medial to the lateral margin of the skin fold line.

Pneumothorax may also have less common appearances on plain portable supine chest radiographs of mechanically ventilated critically ill patients. Pneumothoraces in the supine film may present as air collections in the least dependent areas such as the subpulmonic and anteromedial recesses (Figure 1.3). Anteromedial pneumothoraces cause hyperlucency of the anterior cardiophrenic sulcus or sharp delineation of the heart border, pericardial fat pad, or medial diaphragm. If a pneumothorax becomes large enough it will extend into the subpulmonic space producing a relative lucency of the upper abdomen or a deep diaphragmatic sulcus, the so-called deep sulcus sign (Figure 1.2).[67] The appearance of air in the pleural space may also be influenced by pleural adhesions. Pneumothoraces may also be loculated. The use of decubitus chest

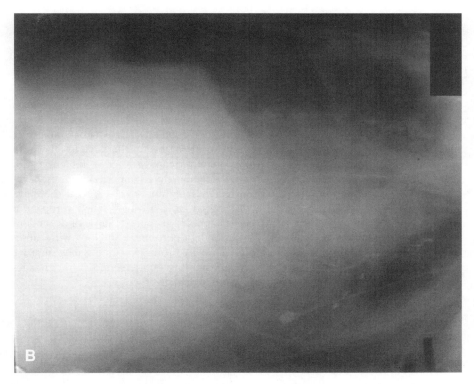

Figure 1.3 (B) A left-side-down decubitus chest radiograph now clearly identifies a right-sided pneumothorax.

radiographs (Figure 1.3) or CT scans can be helpful because up to 30% of pneumothoraces are missed on supine and semirecumbent chest radiographs.[79]

The radiographic appearance of pneumomediastinum is a sharp radiolucent line along the cardiomediastinal shadow, which results from the dissection of air along the peribronchovascular sheaths into the mediastinum.[67] Differentiation of pneumomediastinum from medial pneumothorax may be difficult on a supine chest radiograph. On decubitus chest radiography pleural air moves to the nondependent side; the air of a pneumomediastinum does not change appearance and certainly does not shift to the nondependent pleural space. Other radiographic features of pneumomediastinum are greater definition of the thymus and great vessels, discrete lines along the left paratracheal and mainstem bronchial walls, and a continuous diaphragm sign.[67] Dissection of mediastinal air along fascial planes causes subcutaneous emphysema of the neck or, less commonly, peritoneal or retroperitoneal air.[80] Pneumopericardium is a rare complication of pneumomediastinum that, except in small children, rarely results in hemodynamically significant cardiac tamponade.[67]

CT Scanning of the Thorax in ARDS

CT scans add considerable detail to the anatomic information available from the chest radiograph. As discussed this can aid in detecting pneumothoraces, particularly loculated pneumothoraces or those in unusual locations. Occasionally chest CT scans aid in assessing the likelihood of a loculated pneumothorax contributing to hemodynamically significant tamponade. In selected cases this can be inferred from location of the pneumothorax adjacent to the heart and shift or compression of surrounding structures. CT scans may also aid in detection and subsequent drainage of pleural effusions. This is particularly important in the febrile patient in whom empyema or lung abscess may be an inadequately treated source of infection. CT scans in large numbers of ARDS patients have demonstrated important lung involvement in the inflammatory response even in relatively normal regions on the chest radiograph.[81] Early in ARDS edema is distributed fairly homogeneously throughout the lung. Increased lung weight due to edema appears to cause collapse of dependent lung units. Distribution of edema fluid in dependent portions of the lung with subsequent ventilation-perfusion mismatch illustrate why prone positioning may improve arterial oxygenation. In later phases of ARDS the lungs undergo structural changes with the development of emphasematous parenchymal destruction.[81]

Laboratory Assessment

Laboratory assessment is useful to establish the diagnosis and severity of ARDS, to investigate the cause(s) of ARDS, to measure severity of illness, and to evaluate complications of ARDS. The severity of ARDS is most often evaluated using measures of gas exchange such as the PaO_2/FiO_2 ratio. As shown in Table 1.2, the ATS/European Consensus Conference definition uses $PaO_2/FiO_2 < 300$, < 200, and < 100 to define acute lung injury, ARDS, and severe ARDS, respectively.[5] The other usual measures of severity of ARDS are static compliance and radiographic appearance.

Laboratory evaluation is important to investigate the potential causes of ARDS. In particular, gram stain and culture of blood, sputum, urine, and fluid drainage (e.g., pleural, abdominal) is routine in evaluation of ARDS at onset and during the course of ARDS to assist in the diagnosis of sepsis. In addition, certain patients, such as the immunocompromised, often require fiberoptic bronchoscopy with brushings, washings, and occasionally bronchoalveolar lavage for the assessment of common bacterial pathogens, fungi (e.g., Candida), protozoa (e.g., Pneumocystis carinii), and for bacterial causes of atypical pneumonia (e.g., Legionnaires' disease, mycoplasma). The approach to investigation and diagnosis of pneumonia in ARDS is discussed in Chapter 11. Other causes of ARDS (e.g., pancreatitis, diabetic ketoacidosis) require laboratory evaluation based on clinical presentation.

Laboratory assessment is used to evaluate complications of ARDS such as multiple organ failure (Chapter 13). Organ function is assessed by baseline hematology panel (complete blood count with differential platelet count and coagulation), liver function (bilirubin, albumin, protein, enzymes), and renal function (serum urea and

Table 1.2. Recommended criteria for acute lung injury (ALI) and acute respiratory disease syndrome (ARDS)

	Timing	Oxygenation	Chest radiograph	Pulmonary artery wedge pressure
ALI criteria	Acute onset	$PaO_2/FiO_2 \leq 300$ mmHg (regardless of PEEP level)	Bilateral infiltrates seen on frontal chest radiograph	≤ 18 mmHg when measured or no clinical evidence of left atrial hypertension
ARDS criteria	Acute onset	$PaO_2/FiO_2 \leq 200$ mmHg (regardless of PEEPlevel)	Bilateral infiltrates seen on frontal chest radiograph	≤ 18 mmHg when measured or no clinical evidence of left atrial hypertension

Adapted from Bernard GR, Artigas A, Brigham K, et al. The American-European Consensus Conference on ARDS. Definitions, mechanisms, relevant outcomes, and clinical trial coordination. Am J Respir Crit Care Med 149:818–824, 1994.

creatinine). Multiple organ failure scoring is described in more detail in Chapter 13. MOF scoring (e.g., APACHE II, III, SAPS II, MPMII) can be used to assess severity of illness,[82] to estimate prognosis, and to evaluate the clinical course.

Summary

In summary, clinical evaluation of ARDS patients begins with a stepwise approach starting with the primary assessment ABCs. The detailed secondary survey looks for causes of ARDS, seeks for evidence of associated problems and organ system dysfunction, and considers carefully the laboratory abnormalities – including the chest radiograph. A clear epidemiologic understanding of ARDS in the individual patient and a clear understanding of the physiologic issues in the individual patient lead to rational therapy aimed at reversing pathologic processes that can be reversed, preventing further injury, and allowing the resolution and repair to proceed without adverse sequelae.

References

1. Ashbaugh DG, Bigelow DB, Petty TL, Levine BE. Acute respiratory distress in adults. Lancet 1967; 2:319–323.

2. Petty TL, Ashbaugh DG. The adult respiratory distress syndrome clinical features, factors influencing prognosis and principles of management. Chest 1971; 60(3):233–239.
3. Murray JF, Matthay MA, Luce JM, Flick MR. An expanded definition of the adult respiratory distress syndrome. Am Rev Respir Dis 1988; 138:720–723.
4. Matthay MA. The adult respiratory distress syndrome: definition and prognosis. Clin Chest Med 1990; 11(4):575–580.
5. Bernard GR, Artigas A, Brigham KL, et al. The American-European Consensus Conference on ARDS. Am J Respir Crit Care Med 1994; 149:818–824.
6. Schuster DP. What is acute lung injury? What is ARDS? Chest 1995; 107(6):1721–1726.
7. Pepe PE, Potkin RT, Holtman Reus D, et al. Clinical predictors of the adult respiratory distress syndrome. Am J Surg 1982; 144:124–130.
8. Fein AM, Lippmann M, Holtzman H, et al. The risk factors, incidence, and prognosis of ARDS following septicemia. Chest 1983; 83 (1):40–42.
9. Fowler AA, Hamman RF, Good JT, et al. Adult respiratory distress syndrome: risk with common predispositions. Ann Intern Med 1983; 98:593–597.
10. Mancebo J, Artigas A. A clinical study of the adult respiratory distress syndrome. Crit Care Med 1987; 15(3):243–246.
11. Villar J, Slutsky AS. The incidence of the adult respiratory distress syndrome. Am Rev Respir Dis 1989; 140:814–816.
12. Hudson LD, Milberg JA, Anardi D, Maunder RJ. Clinical risks for development of the acute respiratory distress syndrome. Am J Respir Crit Care Med 1995; 151:293–301.
13. Schuster DP, Kollef MH. Acute respiratory distress syndrome. Disease a Month 1996; 42(5):270–326.
14. Petty TL. The acute respiratory distress syndrome: historic perspective. Chest 1994; 105(3): Suppl:44S-47S.
15. Jenkins MT, Jones RF, Wilson B, Moyer GA. Congestive atelectasis: a complication of the intravenous infusion of fluids. Ann Surg 1950; 132(3):327–347.
16. Montgomery AB. Early description of ARDS. Chest 1991; 99(1):261–262.
17. Simeone FA. Pulmonary complications of nonthoracic wounds: a historical perspective. J Trauma 1968; 8(5):625–648.
18. Sibbald WJ, Anderson RR, Holliday RL. Pathogenesis of pulmonary edema associated with the adult respiratory distress syndrome. CMAJ 1979; 120:445–450.
19. Russell JA. Pathophysiology of acute respiratory failure. Chest Surg Clin NA 1991; 1(2):209–237.
20. National Heart and Lung Institute, National Institutes of Health. Respiratory distress syndromes: task force report on problems, research approaches, needs. U.S. Government Printing Office, Washington DC. 1972 DHEW Publication No. (NIH) 73–432:165–180.
21. Thomsen GE, Morris AH. Incidence of the adult respiratory distress syndrome in the state of Utah. Am J Respir Crit Care Med 1995; 152:965–971.
22. Garber BG, Hebert PC, Yelle J-D, Hodder RV, McGowan J. Adult respiratory distress syndrome: a systematic overview of incidence and risk factors. Crit Care Med 1996; 24 (4):687–695.
23. Sloane PJ, Gee MH, Gottlieb JE, et al. A multicenter registry of patients with acute respiratory distress syndrome: physiology and outcome. Am Rev Respir Dis 1992; 146:419–426.

24. Fowler AA, Hamman RF, Zerbe GO, Benson KN, Hyers TM. Adult respiratory distress syndrome prognosis after onset. Am Rev Respir Dis 1985; 132:472–479.
25. Suchyta MR, Clemmer TP, Elliott CG, et al. The adult respiratory distress syndrome: a report of survival and modifying factors. Chest 1992; 101(4):1074–1079.
26. Rinaldo JE. The prognosis of the adult respiratory distress syndrome: inappropriate pessimism? Chest 1986; 90:470–471.
27. Suchyta MR, Clemmer TP, Elliott CG, et al. Increased mortality of older patients with acute respiratory distress syndrome. Chest 1997; 111:1334–1339.
28. Milberg JA, Davis DR, Steinberg KP, Hudson LD. Improved survival of patients with acute respiratory distress syndrome (ARDS): 1983–1993. JAMA 1995; 273(4): 306–309.
29. Morris AH, Wallace CJ, Menlove RL, et al. Randomized clinical trial of pressure-controlled inverse ratio ventilation and extracorporeal CO_2 removal for adult respiratory distress syndrome. Am J Respir Crit Care Med 1994; 149:295–305.
30. Steinberg KP, McHugh LG, Hudson LD. Causes of mortality in patients with the adult respiratory distress syndrome (ARDS): an update. Am Rev Respir Dis 1993; 147: Suppl:A347, abstract.
31. Doyle RL, Szaflarski N, Gunnard WM, Wiener-Kronish JP, Matthay MA. Identification of patients with acute lung injury: predictors of mortality. Am J Respir Crit Care Med 1995; 152:1818–1824.
32. Montgomery AB, Stager MA, Carrico CJ, Hudson LD. Causes of mortality in patients with the adult respiratory distress syndrome. Am Rev Respir Dis 1985; 132:485–489.
33. Orell SR. Lung pathology in respiratory distress following shock in the adult. Acta Path Microbiol Scand Section A 1971; 79:65–76.
34. Tomashefski JF. Pulmonary pathology of the adult respiratory distress syndrome. Clin Chest Med 1990; 11(4):593–619.
35. Meyrick B. Pathology of adult respiratory distress syndrome. Crit Care Clin 1986; 2(3):403–428.
36. Tomashefski JF, Davies P, Boggis C, et al. The pulmonary vascular lesions of the adult respiratory distress syndrome. Am J Pathol 1983; 112:112–126.
37. Rinaldo JE, Rogers RM. Adult respiratory distress syndrome: changing concepts of lung injury and repair. NEJM 1982; 306(15):900–909.
38. Fulkerson WJ, MacIntyre N, Stamlet J, Crapo JD. Pathogenesis and treatment of the adult respiratory distress syndrome. Arch Intern Med 1996; 156:29–38.
39. Matthay MA. The acute respiratory distress syndrome. NEJM 1996; 334(22):1469–1470.
40. Marini JJ. Lung mechanics in the adult respiratory distress syndrome: recent conceptual advances and implications for management. Clin Chest Med 1990; 11(4):673–690.
41. Gattinoni L, Pesenti A, Avalli L, Rossi F, Bombino M. Pressure-volume curve of total respiratory system in acute respiratory failure computed tomographic scan study. Am Rev Respir Dis 1987; 136:730–738.
42. Slutsky AS, Scharf SM, Brown R, Ingram RH Jr. The effect of oleic acid induced pulmonary edema on pulmonary and chest wall mechanics in dogs. Am Rev Respir Dis 1980; 121:91–96.
43. Dantzker DR, Brook CJ, Dehart P, Lynch JP, Weg JG. Ventilation-perfusion distributions in the adult respiratory distress syndrome. Am Rev Respir Dis 1979; 120:1039–1052.

44. Biondi JW, Schulman DS, Wiedemann HP, Matthay RA. Mechanical heart-lung interactions in the adult respiratory distress syndrome. Clin Chest Med 1990; 11(4):691–714.
45. Zapol WM, Snider MT. Pulmonary hypertension in severe acute respiratory failure. NEJM 1977; 296(9):476–480.
46. Stool EW, Mullins CB, Leshin SJ, Mitchell JH. Dimensional changes of the left ventricle during acute pulmonary arterial hypertension in dogs. Am J Cardiol 1974; 33:868–875.
47. Marini JJ, Culver BH, Butler J. Mechanical effect of lung distention with positive pressure on cardiac function. Am Rev Respir Dis 1981; 124:382–386.
48. Brunet F, Dhainaut JF, Devaus JY, et al. Right ventricular performance in patients with acute respiratory failure. Int Care Med 1988; 14:474–477.
49. Russell JA, Ronco JJ, Lockhat D, Belzberg A, Kiess M, Dodek PM. Oxygen delivery and consumption and ventricular preload are greater in survivors than in nonsurvivors of the adult respiratory distress syndrome. Am Rev Respir Dis. 1990; 141:659–665.
50. Sibbald WJ, Driedger AA, Myers ML, Short AIK, Wells GA. Biventricular function in adult respiratory distress syndrome. Hemodynamic and radionuclide assessment with special emphasis on right ventricular function. Chest 1983; 84:126–134.
51. Biondi JW, Schulman DS, Soufer R, et al. The effect of incremental positive end-expiratory pressure on right ventricular hemodynamics and ejection fraction. Anesthesiol Analg 1988; 67:144–151.
52. Repine JE. Scientific perspectives on adult respiratory distress syndrome. Lancet 1992; 339:466–472.
53. Tate RM, Repine JE. Neutrophils and the adult respiratory distress syndrome. Am Rev Respir Dis 1983; 128:552–559.
54. Hammond B, Kontos HA, Hess ML. Oxygen radicals in the adult respiratory distress syndrome, in myocardial ischemia and reperfusion injury, and in cerebral vascular damage. Can J Physiol Pharmacol 1985; 63:173–187.
55. Ward PA, Johnson KJ, Till GO. Oxygen radicals and microvascular injury of lungs and kidney. Acta Physiologica Scandinavia. Suppl. 1986; 548:79–85.
56. Rinaldo JE, Christman JW. Mechanisms and mediators of the adult respiratory distress syndrome. Clin Chest Med 1990; 11(4):621–632.
57. Rinaldo JE, Rogers RM. Adult respiratory distress syndrome. NEJM 1986; 315(9): 578–580.
58. Rocker GM, Wiseman MS, Pearson D, Shale DJ. Diagnostic criteria for adult respiratory distress syndrome: time for reappraisal. Lancet 1989; 1:120–123.
59. Pittet JF, Mackersie RC, Martin TR, Matthay MA. Biological markers of acute lung injury: prognostic and pathogenetic significance. Am J Respir Crit Care Med 1997; 155:1187–1205.
60. Headley AS, Tolley E, Meduri U. Infections and the inflammatory response in acute respiratory distress syndrome. Chest 1997; 111(5):1306–1321.
61. Dorinsky PM, Gadek JE. Mechanisms of multiple nonpulmonary organ failure in ARDS. Chest 1989; 96(4):885–892.
62. Petty TL. Acute respiratory distress syndrome. Disease a Month 1990; 36(1):1–58.
63. Young JB. Contemporary management of patients with heart failure. Med Clin NA 1995; 79(5):1171–1190.
64. Marini JJ, Culver BH. Systemic gas embolism complicating mechanical ventilation in the adult respiratory distress syndrome. Ann Intern Med 1989; 110:699–703.

65. Bell RC, Coalson JJ, Smith JD, Johanson WG. Multiple organ system failure and infection in adult respiratory distress syndrome. Ann Intern Med 1983; 99(3):293–298.
66. Bombino M, Gattinoni L, Pesenti A, Pistolesi M, Miniati M. The value of portable chest roentgenography in adult respiratory distress syndrome: comparison with computed tomography. Chest 1991; 100(3):762–769.
67. Aberle DR, Brown K. Radiologic considerations in the adult respiratory distress syndrome. Clin Chest Med 1990; 11(4):737–754.
68. Greene R. Adult respiratory distress syndrome: acute alveolar damage. Radiology 1987; 163:57–66.
69. Morgan PW, Goodman LR. Pulmonary edema and adult respiratory distress syndrome. Radiol Clin NA 1991; 29(5):943–963.
70. Wiener-Kronish JP, Broaddus VC, Albertine KH, et al. Relationship of pleural effusions to increased permeability pulmonary edema in anesthetized sheep. J Clin Invest 1988; 82:1422–1429.
71. Wiener-Kronish JP, Matthay MA. Pleural effusions associated with hydrostatic and increased permeability pulmonary edema. Chest 1988; 93 (4):852–858.
72. Klein JS, Fischbein NJ. The lung. In Fundamentals of diagnostic radiology, eds WE Brant, CA Helms, Williams & Wilkins, Baltimore, 1994, pp. 412–494.
73. Milne EN, Pistolesi M, Miniati M, Giuntini C. The radiologic distinction of cardiogenic and noncardiogenic edema. AJR 1985; 144:879–894.
74. Ovenfors CO. Iatrogenic trauma to the thorax. J Thorac Imag 1987; 2:18–31.
75. Pingleton SK. Complications of acute respiratory failure. Med Clin NA 1983; 67(3):725–746.
76. McWey RE, Curry NS, Schabel SI, et al. Complications of nasoenteric feeding tubes. Am J Surg 1988; 155:253–257.
77. Harris MR, Huseby JS. Pulmonary complications from nasoenteral feeding tube insertion in the intensive care unit: incidence and prevention. Crit Care Med 1989; 17(9):917–919.
78. Boyd KD, Thomas SJ, Gold J, Boyd AD. A prospective study of complications of pulmonary artery catheterizations in 500 consecutive patients. Chest 1983; 84(3):245–249.
79. Tocino IM, Miller MH, Fairfax WR. Distribution of pneumothorax in the supine and semirecumbent critically ill adult. AJR 1985; 144:901–905.
80. Goodman LR, Putman CE. Diagnostic imaging in acute cardiopulmonary disease. Clin Chest Med 1984; 5(2):247–264.
81. Pelosi P, Crotti S, Brazzi L, Gattinoni L. Computed tomography in adult respiratory distress syndrome: what has it taught us? Eur Respir J. 1996; 9:1055–1062.
82. Gregoire G, Russell JA. Assessment of severity of illness. In Principles of critical care, eds JB Hall, GA Schmidt, LDH Wood, McGraw-Hill, New York, 1998, pp. 57–69.

2

The Epidemiology of ARDS

Bryan G. Garber and Paul C. Hébert

Introduction

More than 25 years ago, Ashbaugh and colleagues described a series of patients whose striking but uniform clinical, physiologic, roentgenographic, and pathologic abnormalities distinguished them from other patients who developed respiratory failure.[1,2] This syndrome has since become known as *adult* or *acute respiratory distress syndrome (ARDS)*. Despite extensive research and literature devoted to ARDS,[3–5] overall mortality rates have remained in excess of 40%.[6–10] The inability to find new therapeutic modalities that decrease mortality rates from this syndrome has been a source of disappointment in this field.[5] Consequently, prevention or early intervention appears to be an important and necessary approach in the management of ARDS. The high mortality rate and lack of success of new interventions have also led to a reevaluation of our basic understanding of ARDS. Thus, revisiting the epidemiology of this syndrome is of paramount importance. By determining the incidence and establishing risk factors for ARDS, invaluable information required to develop preventative strategies or targeted early therapy may surface, offering the hope for improved outcomes in patients afflicted with this syndrome.

In this chapter, we begin by describing possible study designs used in determining epidemiologic features of any disease, including ARDS, in order to better appreciate the strengths and weaknesses of the existing literature. We then describe the major studies estimating the incidence, risk factors, and case-fatality rate of ARDS. We also briefly discuss the long-term outcomes of this illness. In order to provide the reader with the most reliable epidemiologic inferences from the literature, we have primarily based our comments on a systematic search, selection, and appraisal of the published literature.

Defining ARDS in Epidemiologic Studies

Most definitions of ARDS primarily rely on a prespecified degree of hypoxia, diffuse bilateral x-ray opacities, and decreased pulmonary compliance as principal features. Other criteria used in various definitions include the absence of clinical evidence of congestive heart failure (CHF) often not explicitly outlined, a pulmonary capillary wedge pressure less than 18 mmHg, and the presence of a predisposing illness. Murray et al.[11] incorporated the operational characteristics of hypoxia, chest x-ray findings, compliance, and PEEP values into a standardized scoring system termed the *acute lung injury score*. This scoring system may also identify less severe lung injury, which may then go on to become ARDS. The American-European Consensus Conference definition[12] encompasses most of these elements and has been proposed as the standard for future research.

Even though there is a substantial variation in the use of definitions for ARDS, a review of the literature noted that 49% of epidemiologic studies did not provide any definition of ARDS whatsoever[13] (Table 2.1). When a definition was provided, the lack of a gold standard diagnostic test for ARDS may ultimately lead to the inappropriate identification of ARDS or controls in a study. This is termed *misclassification* and means that some patients are falsely labeled with a diagnosis of ARDS or inappropriately categorized as not having this condition when it is truly present. Consequently, an incidence study may either over- or underestimate the true incidence rate of this syndrome. Misclassification in a study examining risk factors may occur for both the outcome (ARDS) and the exposure (risk factors). The ultimate effect will depend on whether the misclassification was random or differential. In random misclassification, the diagnosis of disease is incorrect in the same proportion of subjects in the groups with and without the risk factor. The net effect is a diminished strength of association between the disease and the risk factor. In contrast, differential misclassification, where the proportion of subjects misclassified in the exposed and unexposed groups are unequal, could either result in an exaggeration or underestimation of the true effect. Differential misclassification usually results from a selection or measurement bias where a disproportionate number of outcomes or exposures are attributed to one group. Because of either a lack of definition or the variability in definitions of ARDS employed in the literature, the potential effects of misclassification may be significant in many clinical studies. Misclassification may be minimized by adopting reproducible operational definitions for both ARDS and risk factors as well as by blinding the ascertainment of these to prevent differential misclassification.

Types and Quality of Studies Documenting the Epidemiology of ARDS

In studies describing incidence, case-fatality rates, and risk (or prognostic) factors, a group of patients with a specific disease or syndrome must be assembled to compare their characteristics and outcomes. Often, studies will also attempt to demonstrate

Table 2.1. Operational characteristics of all major definitions of ARDS

Source	Hypoxemia	PEEP (cm H_2O)	Bilat CXR infiltrates	Compliance (mL/cm H_2O)	PCWP (mmHg)	Other
American–European Conference[12]	$PaO_2/FiO_2 \leq 200$	No	Yes	No	≤ 18[a]	No
Hudson et al.[25]	$PaO_2/FiO_2 < 150$ or < 200	No + PEEP	Yes	No	≤ 18[a]	Yes[b]
Bone et al.[30]	$PaO_2/FiO_2 < 150$ or < 200	No + PEEP	Yes	No	No	No
Fowler et al.[6]	A-a gradient < 0.2	No	Yes	< 50	< 12	No
Pepe et al.[26]	$PaO_2 < 75$ torr $FiO_2 > 0.5$	No	Yes	No	≤ 18	Yes[b]
Sloane et al.[32]	$PaO_2/FiO_2 \leq 250$	No	Yes	No	No	Yes[c]
Murray et al.[11]	$PaO_2/FiO_2 < 100$	≥ 15	All four quadrants	≤ 19	No	Yes[d]

[a]Or no evidence of left atrial hypertension.
[b]No other causes to explain findings.
[c]In appropriate clinical setting (trauma, sepsis, shock, posttransfusion, pancreatitis, inhalation/aspiration, pregnancy).
[d]Used scoring system classifying levels of acute lung injury.

that certain attributes might predispose a patient to develop a disease. These attributes are referred to as *risk factors*. If the attributes modify the patient's outcome once a disease has been diagnosed, they are by definition called *prognostic factors*. For example, massive red cell transfusions might predispose trauma victims to develop ARDS (a risk factor) but have little impact on prognosis. However, patients who develop ARDS because of septic shock (a risk factor) may also have a significantly greater mortality rate as compared to other patients with ARDS (also a prognostic factor).

Different types of studies provide information regarding the epidemiology of ARDS. A *case series* is a description of a selected group of patients. Despite being diagnosed with the same disease, the patients may be quite dissimilar in terms of severity and staging of disease as well as therapeutic interventions. The information derived from a case series may be very useful in rare diseases or as an initial description of a disease or new treatment. Inference regarding incidence, risk, and case-fatality rates is quite limited using this type of study. A *case-control* study is somewhat better in that "cases" of patients with a certain disease are compared retrospectively to other patients without the disease. However, this design relies on the selection of appropriate controls as a comparator. Thus, a case series describes a disease, whereas a case-control study is better able to compare risks. Neither study type reliably estimates incidences or case-fatality rates, and both are prone to all sorts of biases even when estimating risk or prognostic factors. In summary, case-control designs are most useful in very rare diseases or as preliminary studies. In a *cohort study*, patients with the same disease are followed over time and outcomes are documented. If no interventions are performed on the patients, the natural history of a disease without treatment may be determined. If standard therapies are administered then a cohort may still describe the prognosis of patients once treated. Finally, the control arm of a *randomized controlled trial* may also describe the natural history or the prognosis of a disease because patients are given either a placebo or standard accepted therapy. Each study design has advantages and disadvantages, as described in Table 2.2.

When reading a study, first verify that the authors have provided valid and reproducible definitions of ARDS, the risk factors, and the outcomes of interest, as previously outlined. Once the presence or absence of adequate definitions has been established, ascertain the strength of the study design. A well-executed prospective cohort study is the preferred and most powerful design option in ascertaining incidence and case-fatality rates as well as in establishing risk and prognostic factors.[14] The association between some putative risk factors, such as certain therapeutic modalities (multiple transfusions and early facture stabilization), and the development of ARDS might best be determined through randomized controlled clinical trial designs. Retrospective case reports and case series were considered the weakest designs if the factor is modifiable or an aspect of therapy. In a prospective cohort design (or the placebo arm of a clinical trial), determine next if the authors established an inception cohort, reproducibly described all baseline characteristics of the population at risk, reported a complete follow-up, and had enough patients to document a statistically valid association.[15,16] The term *inception cohort* means that all patients in the study should be either "disease free" or at an easily identified point early in the illness and be at a comparable stage in the natural history of

Table 2.2. Types of primary studies used to assess risk factors, incidence, and prognosis

Study design	Description	Advantage	Disadvantage
Case report/series	Observations of patient or a group with disease	Initial description Very useful in rare disease Inexpensive and quick	Very selective Prone to bias
Case-control	Patients compared to controls	Useful in defining risk or prognosis factors Very useful in rare disease Inexpensive and quick	Prone to selection bias Limited generalizability
Retrospective cohort study	Patients with same disease identified in the past and followed forward in time	Describes natural history and incidences of outcomes Efficient and inexpensive	Prone to losses to follow-up Prone to biases Very difficult in rare diseases
Prospective cohort study	Patients with same disease followed forward in time	Describes natural history and incidences of outcomes	Time consuming and expensive Very difficult in rare diseases
Randomized controlled study	Patients in the control group of a randomized controlled study	Similar to cohort	Similar to cohort

the disease under study. The inability to assemble a proper inception cohort may significantly influence the description of prognosis and risk. Ideally, risk factor studies should also describe the strength of association by reporting an odds ratio or relative risk measurement. To report such measures of association, a study must clearly describe the exposure to the risk factor as well as the lack of exposure or risk.

In order to infer causality, it is not sufficient to simply document a statistical association. Indeed, if a statistical association between a risk factor and ARDS is observed, causation should be considered if the clinical evidence also demonstrated biologic credibility, there is consistency from study to study, a correct temporal sequence of exposure followed by the outcome is observed, and there is the absence of an analogous cause-and-effect relationship that might confound the association.[17] The term *confounding* refers to a condition, a therapy, or something else about the patient or the disease that is related to both the risk factor and the development of ARDS. By virtue of this relationship, the "confounder" can influence the outcome more than the risk factor under study. An example of confounding might be the observation of a statistical association between blood transfusion and ARDS. Blood transfusion may be a marker of the extent of tissue injury in trauma rather than be truly a causative agent of ARDS. To detect confounding in clinical studies, authors should report on more advanced statistical methods such as a stratified or multivariate analysis.

Incidence of ARDS

The term *incidence* is an epidemiologic concept that quantifies the number of new cases of a disease in all persons at risk of developing the disease. The unit for this rate is measured in the number of cases per 100,000 population per year or the number of cases per person-years (number of persons at risk multiplied by the period of time at risk is actually referred to as an *incidence density*). Incidence rates may also be reported for specific groups such as hospitalized patients, or all patients admitted to the ICU as the number of cases per 1,000 admissions. Prevalence refers to all new and old cases of a disease at a specific point in time and is reported simply as the number of cases per 100,000 population (or per 1,000 admissions) without reference to a time period. Incidence rates are most accurately ascertained in a well-conducted cohort study; prevalence rates may be most easily determined in a survey or any other cross-sectional study. Prevalence and incidence rates are most useful for individuals interested in the health of populations. For clinicians, a rough appreciation of whether a disease is common or rare will often suffice.

ARDS, by all accounts, would be considered a rare disease despite the large variation in published estimates ranging from 1.5 to 71 cases per 10^5 general population (Table 2.3). In 1972 the National Institute's Heart and Lung Task Force on Respiratory Diseases estimated that 150,000 persons developed ARDS each year in the United States, which results in an incidence of 71 cases per 10^5 population per year based on cross-sectional survey data.[18] This estimate was derived using a consensus panel of experts and did not include a reproducible operational definition. Even though the NIH estimate is based on the weakest evidence, it remains the most widely quoted.

Table 2.3. Study design, population, and reported incidence of ARDS from the five reported studies

Study/Year of publication	Design	Population	Definition of ARDS	Incidence (cases/10⁵ population)
NIH[18] (1972)	Consensus conference	Population	No operational definition	71
Baumann et al.[19] (1986)	Prospective cohort	Hospital	1. New infiltrate on CXR 2. Hypoxemia 3. Compliance < 50 mL/cm H_2O 4. PCWP < 15 mmHg	1.8%
Webster et al.[23] (1988)	Survey	Population	1. "Characteristic CXR" 2. Hypoxemia (PaO_2 < 8 torr on FiO_2 0.5)	4.5
Villar and Slutsky[21] (1989)	Prospective cohort	Population	1. Condition associated with ARDS 2. Hypoxemia (PaO_2 < 55 FiO_2 0.5 + % cm PEEP)	1.5
Thomsen and Morris[20] (1995)	Prospective cohort	Population	1. P(a/A) O_2 ≤ 0.2 2. Bilat CXR infiltrates 3. PCWP < 15 mmHg 4. Compliance ≤ 50 mL/cm H_2O	4.8–8.3
Lewandowski et al.[22] (1995)	Prospective cohort	Population	Murray criteria[25]	3.0

Four subsequent studies were designed to determine specifically the incidence of ARDS[19-22] using a prospective cohort design. Thomsen et al.,[20] using well-documented operational definitions, prospectively followed all admissions to 6 out of 8 Utah hospitals that regularly managed patients with ARDS and reported an incidence ranging from 4.8 to 8.3 cases/10^5 for the population of Utah. Mathematical adjustments were employed to correct for the occurrence of ARDS in non-Utah residents, the occurrence of ARDS in Utah residents outside of the state, and the approximate number of ARDS cases occurring in nonscreened Utah hospitals. Given that 2 out of 8 major referral hospitals as well as 32 smaller hospitals in the state were not actively screened, the accuracy of their estimate is entirely placed on the robustness of their mathematical corrections. Villar and Slutsky[21] performed a population-based prospective cohort study in which they examined the incidence of ARDS on an isolated island with a single large hospital. The authors examined all ICU admissions occurring over a 3-year period and reported an ARDS incidence of 1.5 cases/10^5 population. When more liberal criteria were employed the incidence increased to 3.5 cases/10^5 population. Although an inception cohort was identified, the results of this study may not be generalizable to large metropolitan centers given that the incidence of blunt trauma as well as other ARDS risk factors are presumably not comparable. In addition, the determination of ARDS may not have been free of bias given the lack of blinded outcome assessment. A multicenter prospective study from Berlin, Germany,[22] prospectively followed all adult admissions to 72 of 74 ICUs in that city over a 2-month period to document the incidence rate, severity, and mortality of acute respiratory failure in that city with a population of 3.44 million. Using the Murray criteria of an Acute Lung Injury Score > 2.5, these researchers[22] documented an incidence of ARDS of 3.0 cases/10^5 population/year. The fourth study, by Baumann and colleagues,[19] prospectively identified 11,112 emergency admissions. Of 11,112 emergency admissions, 4,920 patients had at least 1 of 9 predetermined risk factors for ARDS. The high-risk cohort was followed over a period of 7 days for the onset of the syndrome. The reported incidence of ARDS was 1.8% (90/4,920) in the high-risk group but would be reported as 8.1 cases per 1,000 admissions if all emergency admissions were considered in the denominator.

Other investigators used inferior types of study design to determine incidence rates. A British study using a retrospective survey design[23] reported a population incidence of 4.5 cases/10^5 population. The use of broad definitions of the syndrome and the retrospective nature of the design made this study particularly prone to selection and recall bias as well as misclassification of cases. Difficulties with incomplete records may have also been a serious concern. Two further incidence estimates have been provided in the literature. Villar and Slutsky[21] quote the 88 incident cases identified in the 1-year prospective risk factor study on ARDS reported by Fowler et al. and derived an incidence estimate of 5.2 cases/10^5 population/year.[6] Because this study only followed patients with one or more of eight risk factors for ARDS, it is possible that there were other cases which may have been missed because they did not qualify as a high-risk group. Finally, Evans et al.[24] reported an incidence of ARDS in San Francisco of 25 cases/10^5 population/year. This study was abandoned before completion and was published only in abstract form. In this study, 20% of patients had pneumocystis carinii owing to the high incidence of human immunodeficiency virus (HIV) in San Francisco. The investigators were unable to determine the number of nonresident cases referred from other parts of California and obtain complete information from all participating hospitals.

Therefore, the published evidence suggests that the true population incidence ranges from 1.5 to 8.3 cases/10^5 population/year. It is also safe to conclude that the widely quoted NIH estimate derived from expert opinion is likely an overestimate of the true population incidence rate. Factors such as changing definitions of the syndrome, varying prevalence of risk factors within populations, and differences in the study designs likely account for the large range in incidences among the more reliable estimates.

Risk Factors for ARDS

The concept of establishing risk in clinical studies requires further explanation prior to describing the literature. In epidemiology, we determine risk by comparing patients who are exposed (have the risk factor) to a group who is not exposed (absence of the specific risk factor in the control group). A case-control study or, better yet, a well-conducted cohort study are the most appropriate design approaches to be considered by an investigator attempting to define risk factors for a specific condition. Despite convincing laboratory data, the clinical evidence supporting a causal relationship between most proposed risk factors and ARDS is quite limited. The evidence reported in this section suggests that the association is strongest for sepsis, trauma, multiple transfusions, aspiration of gastric contents, pulmonary contusion, pneumonia, and near-drowning. It is weakest for DIC, fat embolism, and cardiopulmonary bypass (Table 2.4).

Studies by Hudson,[25] Pepe,[26] and Fowler[6] reported on multiple risk factors including sepsis, sepsis syndrome or bacteremia, aspiration, multiple transfusions, cardiopulmonary bypass, disseminated intravascular coagulation (DIC), fractures, near-drowning, pancreatitis, pneumonia, pulmonary contusion, shock, and trauma. All studies assembled a prospective cohort and followed them for the onset of ARDS using slightly different operational definitions (Table 2.1). In 695 patients at risk, Hudson et al.[25] reported the highest incidence of ARDS with sepsis syndrome (75 of 176; 43%), trauma (69 of 271; 25%), emergency transfusions of more than 15 units (46 of 115; 40%), and aspiration (13 of 59; 22%). In this study, the risk of ARDS increased by 10% to 20% for each individual risk factor if more than one factor was present. Age and severity of illness measured using APACHE II scores were both directly related to the risk of developing ARDS. Thus, it appears that classically reported risk factors are not alone in increasing the risk of ARDS. An earlier study of 88 patients from the same institution[26] identified similar clinical risk factors with the highest event rate in patients with sepsis syndrome (38%) and aspiration of gastric

Table 2.4. Summary of the clinical evidence for risk factors and incidence rates for ARDS

Risk factor	References	Number of articles	NUMBER OF ARTICLES WITH DEFINITION OF		Incidence of ARDS (%)
			ARDS	Exposure	
Aspiration of gastric contents	1, 2, 6, 25, 26, 32, 45–49	11	9/11	7/11	12–36
Pulmonary contusion	1, 2, 25, 26, 47, 49–55	12	5/12	6/12	5–21.8
Pneumonia	1, 2, 6, 32, 56–59	8	6/8	4/9	12–31
Near-drowning	25, 26, 47, 60	4	3/4	4/4	33
Smoke inhalation	6, 61–66	7	2/7	7/7	1.8–17
Sepsis	6, 25, 26, 32, 33, 46–49, 67–77	20	12/20	12/20	11–80
DIC	6, 30, 78	3	2/3	3/3	23
Shock	2, 26–28, 49, 54, 68, 69, 79, 80	10	6/10	5/10	25–32
Multiple transfusions	3, 6, 25, 26, 32, 47, 49, 81–88	15	8/15	13/15	5–36.4
Fat embolism	1, 89–92	5	2/3	3/3	–
Fractures	6, 25, 26, 47, 93–97	9	9/9	9/9	2–21
Pancreatitis	1, 5, 26, 32, 46, 98–100	8	5/8	8/8	6–18
Cardiopulmonary bypass	6, 101, 102	3	2/3	3/3	1.3–1.7
Trauma	1, 2, 28, 32, 33, 46, 49–51, 54, 58, 69, 77, 79, 81, 87, 102–111	25	11/25	25/25	1.2–39

contents (30%). Among 993 patients in a large prospective cohort, Fowler et al.[6] noted the highest rates of ARDS with pneumonia (10 of 84;12%), DIC (2 of 9; 22%), and pulmonary aspiration(16 of 45; 36%). In this study, the risk of ARDS was uniformly increased with the presence of multiple risk factors. Table 2.4 describes all publications that identify specific risk factors.

As a risk factor for ARDS, trauma is somewhat unique, given that injury patterns may be quite heterogeneous and that other risk factors discussed in Table 2.4 may also be present. Trauma may therefore be a confounder and be associated with ARDS only by virtue of its relationship to other risk factors. Yet laboratory evidence indicates that trauma independently activates the inflammatory response and thereby may independently act as a risk factor for ARDS.[27] Hoyt and colleagues[28] attempted to address this question in a large single center prospective cohort study examining post-traumatic pulmonary complications. The 3,289 trauma admissions to a level I trauma center who either died, were admitted for more than 3 days, or admitted to the ICU had a reported rate of pulmonary complications of 11.2% (368/3,289). The reported incidence of post-traumatic ARDS based on an acceptable operational definition was 1.2%. The authors then made use of a case-control design within the cohort in which cases of ARDS were compared to trauma victims in the cohort who did not develop ARDS. These groups were compared and analyzed to identify potential risk factors using logistic regression analysis. These statistical procedures control for the interaction and potential confounding between the different risk factors. They identified blunt trauma, an injury severity score (ISS) > 16, trauma score < 13, and surgery to the head as significant risk factors in trauma patients for the development of ARDS. Unfortunately, they did not attempt to examine whether any of the other risk factors described in Table 2.4 were also associated with the development of ARDS. In this study as well as in the study published by Hudson,[25] severity of illness seems to be associated with the development of ARDS.

All of the studies discussed in this section adopted similar designs and therefore have similar strengths and weaknesses. Each of the studies primarily identifies the proportion of patients with a specific risk factor that eventually go on to develop ARDS. For the clinician, this type of data is useful in potentially targeting specialized care as well as diagnostic and preventative therapeutic strategies. However, given that all patients have either the specific risk factor under study or another risk factor, we are unable to conclude if the risk factor per se has a causal role in the development of the disease. Because none of these studies employed a control group, they were considered as large prospective case series and are incapable of providing a common measure of risk such as an odds ratio or relative risk estimate. The ability to ascertain a relative risk or an odds ratio for an individual risk factor provides a powerful means of identifying patient and disease characteristics as well as other clinical features that may be related to the development of the disease. Doing so may provide a better understanding of the pathophysiology of ARDS or at worst possibly point to potential avenues for further research. Patients who develop ARDS are often complex such that the development of ARDS cannot be easily attributed to a single risk factor. While searching for potential risk factors, one would usually control for the potential effects of confounding factors. Confounding may occur when another variable is associated with both the specific risk factor and with the outcome (ARDS) of interest. Multivariate analysis or stratified analysis should be used to identify confounding. Only the study by Hoyt et al.[28] employed techniques to control for the potential effects of confounding in this way.

In a previous study attempting to define the level of clinical evidence supporting a causal relationship between risk factors and ARDS, sepsis as well as all of the direct injury mechanism risk factors such as aspiration, pulmonary contusion, and pneumonia ranked high on biologic plausibility because of strong laboratory evidence suggesting their association with ARDS.[29] Almost all of the risk factors with the exception of shock and multiple transfusion demonstrated consistency in their association with ARDS across studies. Similarly, virtually all of the risk factors showed the appropriate temporal sequence of exposure followed by outcome. DIC was the one exception[30] where a temporal sequence was not demonstrated, suggesting it was a manifestation of organ failure and not causally associated with ARDS.

In summary, evidence from the literature strongly suggests that direct mechanisms of lung injury such as the aspiration of gastric contents, pneumonia, and possibly trauma to the lungs have a significant role to play in the development of ARDS. Further, indirect or systemic mechanisms of lung injury such as sepsis syndrome, fat embolism syndrome, and multiple emergency transfusions are also related to the development of ARDS. However, we are unable to quantify the magnitude and importance attributed to specific risk factors, given the limitations in the literature.

Case-Fatality Rates from ARDS

Mortality rates following the development of ARDS have been reported between 40% and 60%.[1,2,6-10] However, one study from Harborview Medical Center in Seattle[7] suggested that overall case fatality rates were possibly decreasing.[7] In 918 patients gathered between 1983 and 1993, Milberg and colleagues observed a mortality ranging from 53% to 68% between 1983 and 1987, then decreasing below 50% in 1991 to as low as 36% in 1993.[7] These crude rates were reported as essentially unchanged following adjustments for age and disease severity. Despite a higher APACHE II score, patients whose admitting diagnosis was sepsis demonstrated case-fatality rates that declined from 67% to 41% during the period between 1990 and 1992. Similar crude and adjusted decreases in mortality rates were observed in trauma victims. The lowest case-fatality rate was 17% overall in 1993. Although this was a well-conducted study that adopted standard definitions for ARDS as well as reproducible and consistent eligibility criteria over the 10-year period, the reasons for the decline in case-fatality rates remain unclear and possibly center specific. Indeed, one prospective study using the American-European Consensus Conference definition for ARDS documented a mortality rate of 59%, consistent with observations from earlier studies.[31]

Other studies have ascertained the case-fatality rate in patients with specific etiologies or risk factors causing ARDS.[9,10,25,32,33] In terms of a diagnosis as a risk factor, ARDS resulting from sepsis has a higher mortality rate than other causes,[7,31,32] whereas post-traumatic ARDS appears to have a lower mortality rate (40% vs. 17% in 1993).[7] Similarly, there is evidence from a number of studies[7,10,22,32,34] that increasing age is directly related to increased mortality from ARDS. Quite clearly, severity of illness and significant co-morbid illnesses will influence all outcomes from ARDS. Other clinical characteristics related to increased mortality include nonpulmonary organ dysfunction occurring after admission (odds ratio of 8.1, suggesting that a patient is 8 times more likely to die if nonpulmonary organ dysfunction is present) and chronic liver disease (OR = 5.2).[31]

Respiratory failure is rarely the cause of death following the development of ARDS.

Several studies examining mortality from ARDS identified sepsis syndrome and multiple system organ failure as the primary causes of death.[8–10,34] Even though several therapeutic interventions have been developed and evaluated in randomized clinical trials,[5] none have demonstrated a decrease in mortality rates from this syndrome.

Morbidity from ARDS

In the literature, a large number of laboratory studies have examined the early pulmonary complications associated with the treatment of ARDS. Investigators have focused on the deleterious consequences associated with oxygen toxicity,[35–37] ventilator-induced lung injury,[38] and barotrauma.[39]

The majority of literature on the long-term consequences of ARDS focused primarily on changes in pulmonary function.[40,41] Although most patients had abnormal pulmonary function measurements initially, the majority of patients improved substantially within the first 6 to 12 months. Pulmonary function impairment was also correlated with age, ARDS severity, and duration of mechanical ventilation.[42] Findings from these studies are limited by the length of follow-up over time.

A more complete picture of recovery was provided by a prospective cohort study performed at Harborview Medical Center.[43] The authors adopted a standard operational definition of ARDS and identified all patients who survived and were successfully extubated. Fifty-two of 82 eligible patients consented, 42% of survivors had at least two examinations, and 24% had complete follow-up that was performed at 3, 6, and 12 months. The 24% who had complete follow-up were similar in characteristics to those who refused participation. Subjects underwent pulmonary function studies and also completed the Sickness Impact Profile (SIP), a self-administered questionnaire designed to determine illness-related dysfunction. The authors noted that abnormal pulmonary function tests improved substantially between extubation and 3 months, with additional improvement at 6 months. No further improvement was detected at 1 year. By the sixth month FVC remained abnormal in 55%, TLC in 45%, and DLco in 26% of patients followed. When the standard for low DLco was changed to those of previous studies, abnormalities were present in 80%. A modified lung injury score was created to adjust for the severity of ARDS. Using this score, only 10% of patients with low scores had residual impairment at 6 months compared to 60% with high lung injury scores.

The physiologic findings of pulmonary function abnormalities are of questionable clinical significance when we review quality of life assessments in ARDS survivors. Even though the total health SIP scores generally paralleled changes in pulmonary function, few patients reported that their functional impairment was related to their lungs in the study by McHugh et al.[43] This is probably because ARDS survivors, in addition to suffering acute lung injury, also experience a variety of injuries to other organ systems that have long-term effects on daily living. A subsequent study examined both a focus group of 6 acute lung injury survivors and performed a survey of 24 survivors from 6 to 41 months after their acute illness to examine their health-related quality of life.[44] Acute lung injury was defined using the American European Consensus conference definition.[12] Significant decrements in health-related quality of life were found even at median of 15 months with profiles similar to outpatients with serious medical illnesses. Respiratory and psychological symptoms were reported in a quarter to a third of patients. However, a significant number of these ARDS survivors had other premorbid medical illnesses prior to their episode of ARDS, suggesting they may have had serious functional limitations prior to their illness. Secondly, the use of a retrospective cross-sectional survey may not have been representative of all ARDS survivors. These concerns raise some doubts about the generalizability of the latter study's findings.

In conclusion, the literature shows that most ARDS survivors have significant improvement in pulmonary function that usually levels out at 6 months. Up to one-half of patients show persistent abnormalities of pulmonary function manifested as either a mild restrictive or diffusing capacity impairment. However, the significance of these physiologic changes may well be overshadowed by other associated organ dysfunction.

Summary

Acute respiratory distress syndrome results in severe aberrations in pulmonary mechanics. Numerous attempts have been made to develop clinically sensible definitions for this syndrome.[1,11,12] Until recently, many studies did not adopt standardized definitions for the syndrome or potential risk factors, limiting inferences from the published literature. Despite these many limitations, studies have consistently documented that ARDS is a rare disease occurring between 1.5 to 8.3 cases per 10^5 population per year. A number of risk factors, often classified as direct mechanisms such as inhalational injury or indirect mechanisms such as sepsis, have been identified. Unfortunately, the magnitude of the risk cannot be quantified because few studies have included proper controls. Studies using stronger designs such as properly conceived and conducted cohort designs might further elucidate the mechanisms of injury for complex etiologies such as trauma and sepsis.

The case-fatality rate from this syndrome depends on the etiology. Mortality approximates 20% for post-traumatic ARDS to more than 60% for sepsis-induced ARDS. Most importantly, a recent study suggests that overall crude and adjusted mortality rates have decreased in the past seven years. Although we remain somewhat skeptical that there has been a 20% improvement in the survival rates from ARDS in the past few years, we remain hopeful that new therapeutic strategies will be developed and result in significant advances in the care of patients with this devastating illness. Future studies are necessary to better quantify long-term outcomes from this syndrome.

References

1. Ashbaugh DG, Bigelow DB, Petty TL, Levine BE. Acute respiratory distress in adults. Lancet 1967; 2:319–323.
2. Ashbaugh DG, Petty TL, Bigelow DB, Harris TM. Continuous positive-pressure breathing (CPPB) in adult respiratory distress syndrome. J Thorac Cardiovasc Surg 1969; 57:31–41.
3. Blaisdell FW. Pathophysiology of the respiratory distress syndrome. Arch Surg 1974; 108:44–49.
4. Petty TL. Adult respiratory distress syndrome: historical perspective and definition. Respir Med 1981; 2:99.
5. Kollef MH, Schuster DP. The acute respiratory distress syndrome. N Engl J Med 1995; 332:27–37.
6. Fowler AA, Hamman RF, Good JT, Benson KN, Baird M, Eberle DJ, et al. Adult respiratory distress syndrome: risk with common predispositions. Ann Intern Med 1983; 98:593–597.
7. Milberg JA, Davis DR, Steinberg KP, Hudson LD. Improved survival of patients with acute respiratory distress syndrome (ARDS): 1983–1993. JAMA 1995; 273:306–309.
8. Bell RC, Coalson JJ, Smith JD, Johanson WGJ. Multiple organ system failure and infection in adult respiratory distress syndrome. Ann Intern Med 1983; 99:293–298.
9. Montgomery AB, Stager MA, Carrico CJ, Hudson LD. Causes of mortality in patients with the adult respiratory distress syndrome. Am Rev Respir Dis 1985; 132:485–489.
10. Suchyta MR, Clemmer PT, Elliot CG, Orme JFJ, Weaver LK. The adult respiratory distress syndrome. A report of survival and modifying factors. Chest 1992; 101:1074–1079.
11. Murray JF, Matthay MA, Luce JM, Flick MR. An expanded definition of the adult respiratory distress syndrome. Am Rev Respir Dis 1988; 138:720–723.
12. Bernard GR, Artigas A, Brigham KL, Carlet J, Falke K, Hudson L, et al. Report of the American-European consensus conference on acute respiratory distress syndrome: definitions, mechanisms, relevant outcomes, and clinical trial coordination. J Crit Care 1994; 9:72–81.
13. Garber BG, Hebert PC, Yelle JD, Hodder RV, McGowan J. Adult respiratory distress syndrome: a systematic overview of incidence and risk factors. Crit Care Med 1996; 24:687–695.
14. Laupacis A, Wells G, Richardson S, Tugwell P. Users' guide to the medical literature: V. How to use an article about prognosis. JAMA 1994; 272:234–237.
15. Evidence-Based Medicine Working Group. How to read clinical journals: III.To learn the clinical course and prognosis of disease. Can Med Assoc J 1981; 124:869–872.
16. van Walraven C, Hebert PC. A reader's guide to the evaluation of prognostic studies. Postgrad Med J 1996; 72:6–11.
17. Henneken CH, Buring JE. Epidemiology in medicine. Little, Brown, Boston, 1987.
18. National Heart and Lung Institute, National Institutes of Health. Respiratory distress syndromes: task force report on problems, research approaches, needs. U.S. Government Printing Office, Washington, DC. 1972 DHEW Publication No. (NIH) 73; 432:165–180.
19. Baumann WR, Jung RC, Koss M, Boylen T, Navarro L, Sharma OP. Incidence and mor-

tality of adult respiratory distress syndrome: a prospective analysis from a large metropolitan hospital. Crit Care Med 1986; 14:1–4.

20. Thomsen GE, Morris AH. Incidence of the adult respiratory distress syndrome in the state of Utah. Am J Crit Care 1995; 152:965–971.

21. Villar J, Slutsky AS. The incidence of the adult respiratory distress syndrome. Am Rev Respir Dis 1989; 140:814–816.

22. Lewandowski K, Metz J, Deutschmann C, Preib H, Kuhlen R, Artigas A, et al. Incidence, severity, and mortality of acute respiratory failure in Berlin, Germany. Am J Respir Crit Care Med 1995; 151:1121–1125.

23. Webster NR, Cohen AT, Nunn JF. Adult respiratory distress syndrome – how many cases in the UK? Anaesthesia 1988; 43:923–926.

24. Evans B, Wachter R, Wiener-Kronish J, Luce J. Incidence of adult respiratory distress syndrome in an urban population. Am Rev Respir Dis 1988; 137:A469 Abstract.

25. Hudson LD, Milberg JA, Anardi D, Maunder RJ. Clinical risks for development of the acute respiratory distress syndrome. Am J Respir Crit Care Med 1995; 151:293–301.

26. Pepe PE, Potkin RT, Reus DH, Hudson LD, Carrico CJ. Clinical predictors of the adult respiratory distress syndrome. Am J Surg 1982; 144:124–130.

27. Moore FA, Moore EE, Read RA. Postinjury multiple organ failure: role of extrathoracic injury and sepsis in adult respiratory distress syndrome. New Horizons 1993; 1:538–549.

28. Hoyt DB, Simons RK, Winchell RJ, Cushman J, Hollingsworth-Fridlung P, Holbrook T, et al. A risk analysis of pulmonary complications following major trauma. J Trauma 1993; 35:524–531.

29. Hudson LD. Causes of the adult respiratory distress syndrome – clinical recognition. Clin Chest Med 1982; 3:195–212.

30. Bone RC, Francis PB, Pierce AK. Intravascular coagulation associated with the adult respiratory distress syndrome. Am J Med 1976; 61:585–589.

31. Doyle RL, Szaflarski N, Gunnard WM, Wiener-Kronish JP, Matthay MA. Identification of patients with acute lung injury: predictors of mortality. Am J Respir Crit Care Med 1995; 152:1818–1824.

32. Sloane PJ, Gee MH, Gottlieb JE, Albertine KH, Peters SP, Burns JR, et al. A multicenter registry of patients with acute respiratory distress syndrome. Physiology and outcome. Am Rev Respir Dis 1992; 146:419–426.

33. Fein AM, Lippmann M, Holtzman H, Eliraz A, Goldberg SK. The risk factors, incidence, and prognosis of ARDS following septicemia. Chest 1983; 83:40–42.

34. Suchyta MR, Clemmer PT, Elliott CG, Orme JFJ, Morris AH, Jacobson J, et al. Increased mortality of older patients with acute respiratory distress syndrome. Chest 1997; 111:1334–1339.

35. Jenkinson SG. Oxygen toxicity. New Horizons 1993; 1:504–511.

36. Fisher AB. Oxygen therapy: side effects and toxicity. Am Rev Respir Dis 1980; 122:61.

37. Moran JF, Robinson LA, Lowe JE, et al. Effects of oxygen toxicity on regional ventilation and perfusion in the primate lung. Surgery 1981; 89:575.

38. Marini JJ. New options for the ventilatory management of acute lung injury. New Horizons 1993; 1:489–503.

39. Meade MO, Cook DJ, Kernerman P, Bernard G. How to use articles about harm: the relationship between high tidal volumes, ventilating pressures, and ventilator-induced lung injury. Crit Care Med 1997; 25:1915–1922.

40. Elliott CG, Morris AH, Cengiz M. Pulmonary function and exercise gas exchange in survivors of adult respiratory distress syndrome. Am Rev Respir Dis 1981; 123:492–495.
41. Elliott CG, Rasmusson BY, Crapo RO, Morris AH, Jensen RL. Prediction of pulmonary function abnormalities after adult respiratory distress syndrome (ARDS). Am Rev Respir Dis 1987; 135:634–638.
42. Ghio AJ, Elliott CG, Crapo RO, et al. Impairment after adult respiratory distress syndrome. Am Rev Respir Dis 1989; 139:1158.
43. McHugh LG, Milberg JA, Whitcomb ME, Schoene RB, Maunder RJ, Hudson LD. Recovery of function in survivors of the acute respiratory distress syndrome. Am J Respir Crit Care Med 1994; 50:90–94.
44. Weinert CR, Gross CR, Kangas JR, Bury CL, Marinelli WA. Health related quality of life after acute lung injury. Am J Respir Crit Care Med 1997; 156:1120–1128.
45. Mendelson CL. The aspiration of stomach content into the lungs during obstetric anesthesia. Am J Obstet Gynecol 1946; 52:191–205.
46. Weigelt JA, Snyder WH, Mitchell RA. Early identification of patients prone to develop adult respiratory distress syndrome. Am J Surg 1981; 142:687–691.
47. Maunder RJ. Clinical prediction of the adult respiratory distress syndrome. Clin Chest Med 1985; 6:413–426.
48. Pepe PE. Early prediction of the adult respiratory distress syndrome by a simple scoring method. Ann Emerg Med 1983; 12:749–755.
49. Fulton RL, Jones CE. The cause of post-traumatic pulmonary insufficiency in man. Surg Gynecol Obstet 1975; 140:179–186.
50. Moseley RV, Doty DB, Pruitt BAJ. Physiologic changes following chest injury in combat casualties. Surg Gynecol Obstet 1969; 129:233–242.
51. Eiseman LWB. The changing pattern of post-traumatic respiratory distress syndrome. Ann Surg 1997; 181:693–697.
52. Roscher R, Bittner R, Stockmann U. Pulmonary contusion. Clinical experience. Arch Surg 1974; 109:508–510.
53. Wanebo H, van Dyke J. The high-velocity pulmonary injury. Relation to traumatic wet lung syndrome. J Thorac Cardiovasc Surg 1972; 64:537–550.
54. Simmons RL, Heisterkamp CA, Collins JA, Genslar S, Martin AMJ. Respiratory insufficiency in combat casualties: III. Arterial hypoxemia after wounding. Ann Surg 1969; 170:45–52.
55. Robertson HT, Lakshminarayan S, Hudson LD. Lung injury following a 50-meter fall into water. Thorax 1978; 33:175–180.
56. Ferstenfeld JE, Schlueter DP, Rytel MW, Molloy P. Recognition and treatment of adult respiratory distress syndrome secondary to viral interstitial pneumonia. Am J Med 1975; 58:709–718.
57. Torres A, Serra-Battles J, Ferrer A, Jimenez P, Celis R, Cobo E, et al. Severe community-acquired pneumonia. Epidemiology and prognostic factors. Am Rev Respir Dis 1991; 144:312–318.
58. Antonelli M, Moro ML, Capelli O, De Blasi RA, D'Errico RR, Conti G, et al. Risk factors for early onset pneumonia in trauma patients. Chest 1994; 105:224–228.
59. O'Brien PG, Sweeney DF. Interstitial viral pneumonitis complicated by severe respiratory failure. Successful management using intensive dehydration and steroids. Chest 1973; 63:314–322.

60. Modell JH, Graves SA, Ketover A. Clinical course of 91 consecutive near-drowning victims. Chest 1976; 70:231–238.
61. Nash G, Foley FD, Langlinais PC. Pulmonary interstitial edema and hyaline membranes in adult burn patients: electron microscopic observations. Human Pathol 1974; 5:149–160.
62. Pruitt BAJ, Flemma RJ, DiVincenti FC, Foley FD, Mason ADJ. Pulmonary complications in burn patients – a comparative study of 697 patients. J Thorac Cardiovasc Surg 1970; 59:7–18.
63. Hollingsed TC, Saffle JR, Barton RG, Craft WB, Morris SE. Etiology and consequences of respiratory failure in thermally injured patients. Am J Surg 1993; 166:592–597.
64. Aharoni A, Moscona R, Kremerman S, Paltieli Y, Hirshowitz B. Pulmonary complications in burn patients resuscitated with a low-volume colloid solution. Burns 1989; 15:281–284.
65. Getzen LG, Pollak EW. Fatal respiratory distress in burned patients. Surg Gynecol Obstet 1981; 152:741–744.
66. Pruit BAJ, Di Vincenti FC, Mason ADJ, Foley FD, Flemma RJ. The occurrence and significance of pneumonia and other pulmonary complications in burned patients: comparison of conventional and topical treatments. J Trauma 1970; 10:519–531.
67. Ziegler EJ, Fisher CJJ, Sprung CL, Straube RC, Sadoff JC, Foulke GE, et al. Treatment of gram-negative bacteremia and septic shock with HA-1A human monoclonal antibody against endotoxin. A randomized, double-blind, placebo-controlled trial. N Engl J Med 1991; 324:429–436.
68. Clowes GHAJ, Hirsch E, Williams L, Kwasnik E, O'Donnell TF, Cuevas P, et al. Septic lung and shock lung in man. Ann Surg 1975; 181:681–692.
69. Horovitz JH, Carrico CJ, Shires GT. Pulmonary response to major injury. Arch Surg 1974; 108:349–355.
70. Kaplan RL, Sahn SA, Petty TL. Incidence and outcome of the respiratory distress syndrome in gram-negative sepsis. Arch Intern Med 1979; 139:867–869.
71. Browdie DA, Deane R, Shinozaki T, Morgan J, DeMeules JE, Coffin LH, et al. Adult respiratory distress syndrome (ARDS) sepsis, and extracorporeal membrane oxygenation (ECMO). J Trauma 1977; 17:579–586.
72. Markham JD, Vitseck JR, O'Donohue WJJ. Acute adult respiratory distress syndrome associated with gonococcal septicemia. Chest 1976; 70:667–672.
73. Vito L, Dennis RC, Weisel RD, Hechtman HB. Sepsis presenting as acute respiratory insufficiency. Surg Gynecol Obstet 1974; B8:896–900.
74. Ashbaugh DG, Petty TL. Sepsis complicating the acute respiratory distress syndrome. Surg Gynecol Obstet 1972; 135:865–869.
75. McLean APH, Duff JH, MacLean D. Lung lesions associated with septic shock. J Trauma 1968; 8:891–898.
76. Greenman RL, Schein RMH, Martin MA, Wenzel RP, Macintyre NR, Emmanuel G, et al. A controlled clinical trial of E5 murine monoclonal IgM antibody to endotoxin in the treatment of gram-negative sepsis. JAMA 1991; 266:1097–1102.
77. Safar P, Grenvik A, Smith J. Progressive pulmonary consolidation: review of cases and pathogenesis. J Trauma 1972; 12:955–967.
78. Horwitz CA, Ward PCJ. Disseminated intravascular coagulation, nonbacterial thrombotic endocarditis and adult pulmonary hyaline membranes – an interrelated triad? Report of a case following small bowel resection for a strangulated inguinal hernia. Am J Med 1971; 51:272–280.

79. Shoemaker WC, Appel P, Czer LSC, Bland R, Schwartz S, Hopkins JA. Pathogenesis of respiratory failure (ARDS) after hemorrhage and trauma: I.Cardiorespiratory patterns preceding the development of ARDS. Crit Care Med 1980; 8:504–512.

80. Petty TL, Ashbaugh DG. The adult respiratory distress syndrome. Clinical features, factors influencing prognosis and principles of management. Chest 1971; 60:233–239.

81. Collins JA, James PM, Bredenberg CE, Anderson RW, Heisterkamp CA, Simmons RL. The relationship between transfusion and hypoxemia in combat casualties. Ann Surg 1978; 188:513–519.

82. Durtschi MB, Haisch CE, Reynolds L, Pavlin E, Kohler TR, Heimbach DM, et al. Effect of micropore filtration on pulmonary function after massive transfusion. Am J Surg 1979; 138:8–13.

83. Barrett J, Tahir AS, Litwin S. Increased pulmonary anteriovenous shunting in humans following blood transfusion. Relation to screen filtration pressure of transfused blood and prevention by Darcon Wool (Swank) filtration. Arch Surg 1978; 113:947–950.

84. Gridlinger GA, Vegas AM, Churchill WHJ, Valeri CR, Hechtman HB. Is respiratory failure a consequence of blood transfusion? J Trauma 1980; 20:627–631.

85. McNamara JJ, Molot MD, Stremple JF. Screen filtration pressure in combat casualties. Ann Surg 1970; 172:334–341.

86. Mosely RV, Doty DB. Death associated with multiple pulmonary emboli soon after battle injury. Ann Surg 1970; 171:336–346.

87. Reul GJJ, Beall ACJ, Greenberg SD. Protection of the pulmonary microvasculature by fine screen blood filtration. Chest 1974; 66:4–9.

88. Reul GJJ, Greenberg SD, Lefrak EA, McCollum WB, Beall ACJ, Jordan GLJ. Prevention of post-traumatic pulmonary insufficiency. Fine screen filtration of blood. Arch Surg 1973; 106:386–393.

89. Ashbaugh DG, Petty TL. The use of corticosteroids in the treatment of respiratory failure associated with massive fat embolism. Surg Gynecol Obstet 1966; 123:493–500.

90. Fischer JE, Turner RH, Herndon JH, Riseborough EJ. Massive steroid therapy in severe fat embolism. Surg Gynecol Obstet 1971; 132:667–672.

91. Pazell JA, Peltier LF. Experience with sixty-three patients with fat embolism. Surg Gynecol Obstet 1972; 135:77–80.

92. Burgher LW, Dines DE, Linscheid RL, Didier EP. Fat embolism and the adult respiratory distress syndrome. Mayo Clin Proc 1974; 49:107–109.

93. Johnson KD, Cadambi A, Seibert B. Incidence of adult respiratory distress syndrome in patients with multiple musculoskeletal injuries: effect of early operative stabilization of fractures. J Trauma 1985; 25:375–384.

94. Bone LB, Johnson KD, Weigelt J, Scheinberg R. Early versus delayed stabilization of femoral fractures. A prospective randomized study. J Bone Joint Surg 1989; 71-A:336–340.

95. Behrman SW, Fabian TC, Kudsk KA, Taylor JC. Improved outcome with femur fractures: early vs. delayed fixation. J Trauma 1990; 80:792–798.

96. Pape H-C, Auf'm'Kolk M, Paffrath T, Regel G, Sturm JA, Tscherne H. Primary intramedullary femur fixation in multiple trauma patients with associated lung contusion – a cause of posttraumatic ARDS. J Trauma 1993; 34:540–548.

97. Goris RJA, Gimbrere JSF, van Niekerk JLM, Schoots FJ, Booy LHD. Early osteosynthesis

and prophylactic mechanical ventilation in the multitrauma patient. J Trauma 1982; 22:895–903.

98. Hayes MFJ, Rosenbaum RW, Zibelman M, Matsumoto T. Acute respiratory distress syndrome in association with acute pancreatitis. Evaluation of positive end expiratory pressure ventilation and pharmacologic doses of steroids. Am J Surg 1974; 127:314–319.

99. Interiano B, Stuard ID, Hyde RW. Acute respiratory distress syndrome in pancreatitis. Ann Intern Med 1972; 77:923–926.

100. Warshaw AL, Lesser PB, Rie M, Cullen DJ. The pathogenesis of pulmonary edema in acute pancreatitis. Ann Surg 1975; 182:505–510.

101. Culliford AT, Thomas S, Spencer FC. Fulminating noncardiogenic pulmonary edema. A newly recognized hazard during cardiac operations. J Thorac Cardiovasc Surg 1980; 80:868–875.

102. Messent M, Sullivan K, Keogh BF, Morgan CJ, Evans TW. Adult respiratory distress syndrome following cardiopulmonary bypass: incidence and prediction. Anaesthesia 1992; 47:267–268.

103. Martin AMJ, Simmons RL, Heisterkamp CA. Respiratory insufficiency in combat casualties: I. Pathologic changes in the lungs of patients dying of wounds. Ann Surg 1969; 170:30–38.

104. Simmons RL, Heisterkamp CA, Collins JA, Bredenberg CE, Mills DE, Martin AMJ. Respiratory insufficiency in combat casualties: IV. Hypoxemia during convalescence. Ann Surg 1969; 170:53–62.

105. Simmons RL, Martin AMJ, Heisterkamp CA, Ducker TB. Respiratory insufficiency in combat casualties: II. Pulmonary edema following head injury. Ann Surg 1969; 170:39–44.

106. Lewis FRJ, Blaisdell FW, Schlobohm RM. Incidence and outcome of posttraumatic respiratory failure. Arch Surg 1977; 112:436–443.

107. Roumen RMH, Redl H, Schlag G, Sandtner W, Koller W, Goris RJA. Scoring systems and blood lactate concentrations in relation to the development of adult respiratory distress syndrome and multiple organ failure in severely traumatized patients. J Trauma 1993; 35:349–355.

108. Cole WG. Respiratory sequels to non-thoracic injury. Lancet 1972; 1:555–556.

109. Powers SRJ, Burdge R, Leather R, Monaco V, Newell J, Sardar S, et al. Studies of pulmonary insufficiency in non-thoracic trauma. J Trauma 1972; 12:1–14.

110. Olcott C, Barber RE, Blaisdell FW. Diagnosis and treatment of respiratory failure after civilian trauma. Am J Surg 1971; 122:260–268.

111. Geiger JP, Gielchinsky I. Acute pulmonary insufficiency. Treatment in Vietnam casualties. Arch Surg 1971; 102:400–405.

3

The Pathology of ARDS

J. L. Wright

Introduction

This chapter discusses the pathologic features of the clinical syndrome of adult respiratory distress. Mechanisms and common and uncommon etiologies are addressed in other chapters. This chapter first describes pathologic features in general and then focuses on the very few conditions in which the pathology is distinctive. A brief pathologic differential diagnosis is given in conclusion.

Classic Pathologic Features

The pathologic term for ARDS (diffuse alveolar damage, or DAD) is utilized because it reflects a morphologic process that can evolve from acute to chronic stages. It is usually separated into three histologic phases,[1-3] although there is extensive overlap between them. The initial phase, designated as acute and exudative, is generally seen in histologic sections up to 6 days after the initial event. The second phase, seen between 4 and 10 days, is characterized by a proliferative response; the chronic fibrotic phase is seen after a period of 8 to 10 days. Although DAD usually involves the lungs bilaterally and diffusely, certain etiologies such as aspiration or radiation can cause lesions localized to a lobe, a lobe segment, or a certain field (Figure 3.1). The sequence of the reaction in DAD appears to be stereotypic, and often no specific etiology can be suggested from the histology even after detailed pathologic examination.[4]

In the acute stage, the surgical or postmortem findings are striking, with the lungs

James A. Russell and Keith R. Walley, eds. *Acute Respiratory Distress Syndrome.* Printed in the United States of America. Copyright © 1999. Cambridge University Press. All rights reserved.

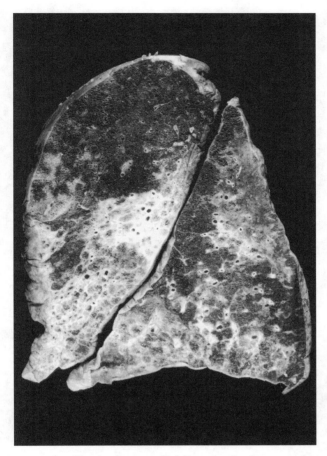

Figure 3.1. An example of localized organized diffuse alveolar damage in a patient who was irradiated. Note the sharp margins, indicative of the edge of the radiation field.

filling the pleural cavity and remaining in almost full inflation after the chest is opened. When the lungs are diffusely affected, they are characteristically heavy, each weighing 1,000 g or greater. The lung slices have a rubbery texture with a meaty gross appearance, which, after fixation, shows obliteration of the lung markings, and the lung appears homogeneous (Figure 3.2). Low-power microscopy is characteristic; the alveolar ducts and respiratory bronchioles are prominent, and adjacent alveoli are collapsed (Figure 3.3). Brightly eosinophilic hyaline membranes cover the surfaces of the respiratory bronchioles and alveolar ducts (Figure 3.4), and it is worth stressing that hyaline membranes are not commonly found in the alveoli. The membrane itself is composed of an admixture of fibrin and other plasma proteins. Although the alveolar

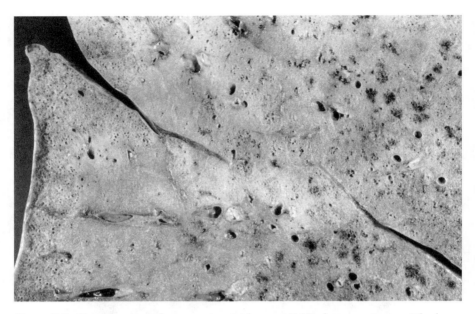

Figure 3.2. Gross specimen from a patient with acute DAD due to aspiration. The lungs were heavy and had a meaty texture. There is diffuse loss of the lung markings in the involved segments.

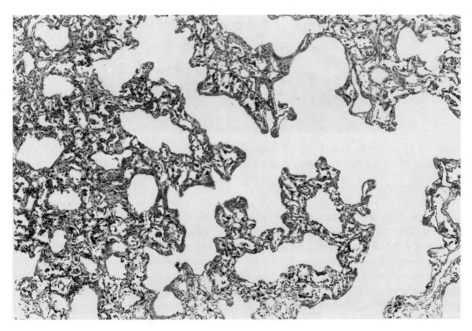

Figure 3.3. Photomicrograph of a lung with acute DAD. The alveolar ducts are prominent, and the adjacent alveoli are collapsed. H&E × 60

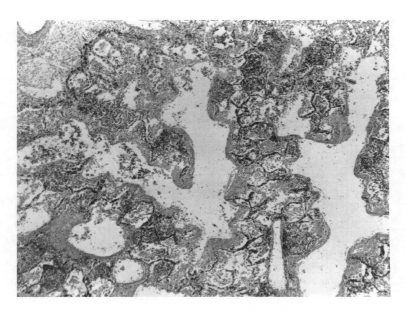

Figure 3.4. Photomicrograph from a patient with acute DAD illustrating the eosinophilic hyaline membranes lining the alveolar ducts. In the acute phase, they are generally acellular and brightly eosinophilic. H&E × 40

interstitium is widened, this is usually due primarily to edema, and there is only a minimal, and nonspecific, interstitial inflammatory infiltrate. Alveolar lining cells and capillary endothelial cells can completely slough, leaving their respective basement membranes denuded of cells. This degree of destruction can be confirmed by electron microscopy, which will show extensive pneumocyte damage and abundant surfactant debris. Microthrombi are common within the capillaries in acute DAD, and probably form around damaged or sloughed endothelial cells.

As DAD evolves into the second phase, the lungs are still enlarged grossly. However, the cut surface is altered with smooth firm areas of consolidated lung tissue and the formation of small cysts, which are usually in the peripheral portions of the lung (Figure 3.5). On microscopy, the interstitial infiltrate becomes more marked, but there is again a mixture of acute and chronic inflammatory cells and an increase in interstitial cells. The most marked cell proliferation, however, occurs in the airspaces, which show organization of the hyaline membranes by proliferating fibroblasts, along with cell debris and acute and chronic inflammatory cells (Figure 3.6). Alveolar collapse becomes more marked, and the alveolar ducts increasingly distorted. At this stage, the process may be reversible, and the lung parenchyma may return to normal. However, in cases of more severe damage, the repair reaction is marked, and tufts of granulation tissue can be seen in the alveoli as well as clusters of macrophages. The hyaline membranes become organized by fibroblastic tissue, epithelial cells proliferate over the surface, and ultimately the

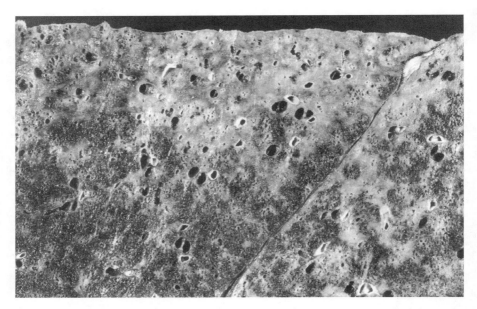

Figure 3.5. Gross specimen from a patient with organizing DAD. Note that the lung surface still has a homogeneous appearance. In addition, however, small cysts can be found in the periphery of the lung tissue, which represent early reorganization of the airspaces.

membranes become incorporated into the walls of revised and thickened airspaces (Figure 3.7). The pneumocytes are often prominent, with large nucleoli, which can be mistaken for viral inclusions, and show increased mitotic activity. Although once considered to be a hallmark of chemotherapeutic toxicity, these cells are entirely nonspecific and are seen in DAD from any etiology. Occasionally, the cytoskeleton is altered dramatically with the formation of Mallory's hyaline.[5] The newly formed type II cells tend to be closely spaced, forming a row along the alveolar septa (Figure 3.8). The airspaces can also show bronchiolar or squamous metaplasia (Figure 3.9), sometimes so atypical as to simulate malignancy.

In the final, fibrotic, stage, the lungs may be shrunken, but remain heavy, and show larger, irregular areas of dense consolidation with scattered areas of gray fibrous tissue. As fibrosis progresses, the pleural surface may show cobblestoning, characteristic of underlying fibrosis. In some cases, predominately those patients who required high-pressure ventilation with increased oxygen concentrations, adult DAD can be organized in the same fashion seen in infants,[6–11] producing radiographically hyperinflated lungs with cyst formation, a condition known in both as bronchopulmonary dysplasia (BPD). On gross inspection the lungs show extensive fibrosis with marked cyst formation secondary to reorganization of the airspaces (Figure 3.10). Once again, the cysts are typically most prominent in the lung periphery, but they can also

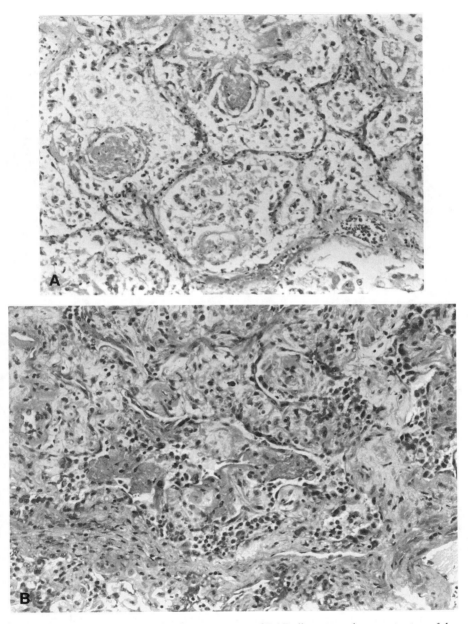

Figure 3.6. (A) An example of early organization of DAD illustrating the organization of the hyaline membranes. H&E × 120 (B) An example of a temporally later stage of organization. Note that the hyaline membrane and granulation tissue are being incorporated into the thickened wall of an airspace. H&E × 325

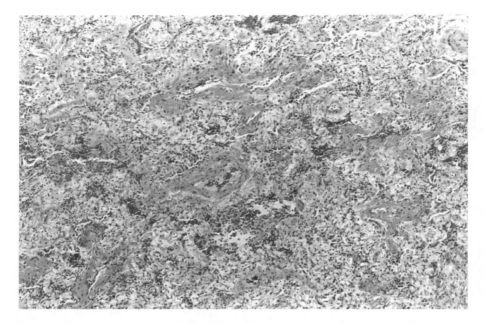

Figure 3.7. An example of organizing DAD illustrating extensive granulation tissue in the airspaces accompanied by fragments of hyaline membrane and inflammatory cells. The walls of the airspaces are thickened and distorted. Some tufts of granulation tissue are apparent in the airspace lumens; others have been incorporated into the airspace wall. H&E × 40

be found throughout the altered lung tissue. Characteristically, the cysts measure between 1 mm to several centimeters and can be distinguished from emphysematous bullae by their thick walls and fibrotic surrounding lung parenchyma. The cysts of BPD appear to be centered around alveolar ducts and consist of irregular, inflamed, and densely fibrotic walls with collapse of the adjacent alveoli (Figure 3.11). Within the scarred areas, the pulmonary vessels show thickened distorted walls with intimal fibrosis and narrowing or actual obliteration of their lumens.

Pathologic Features Suggesting Specific Etiologies

Infections

Obviously, infections require recognition of the infective agent, be it viral, protozoan, fungal, or bacterial. Pathologists must be very careful when ascribing DAD to a viral infection because, as noted earlier, the cells containing viral inclusions must be carefully differentiated from reactive cells.

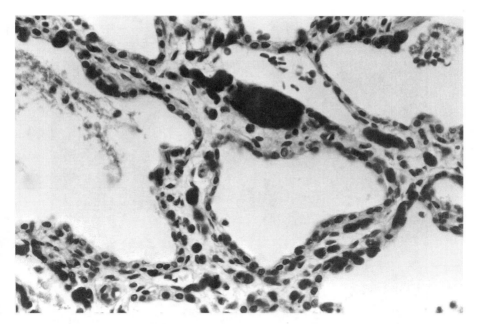

Figure 3.8. Early repair reaction in ARDS. Note the marked proliferation of peg-shaped type II cells over the alveolar surface. These cells have the capacity to differentiate into type I cells and thus restore the normal alveolar architecture. H&E × 325

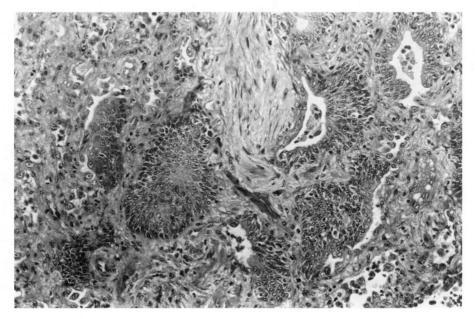

Figure 3.9. Squamous metaplasia is present in an area of organizing diffuse alveolar damage. H&E × 325

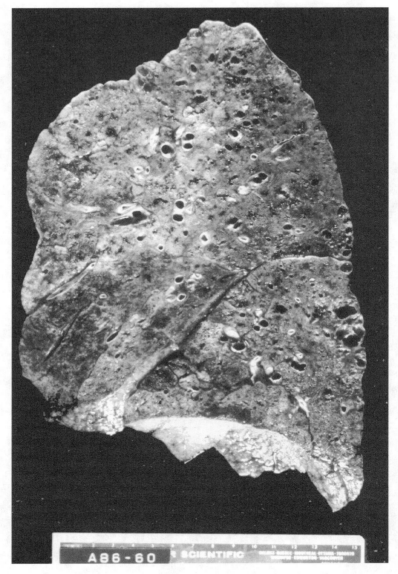

Figure 3.10. Gross photograph showing the adult form of bronchopulmonary dysplasia. Note the cystic rearrangement of the airspaces that can be distinguished from emphysema because of their thick walls.

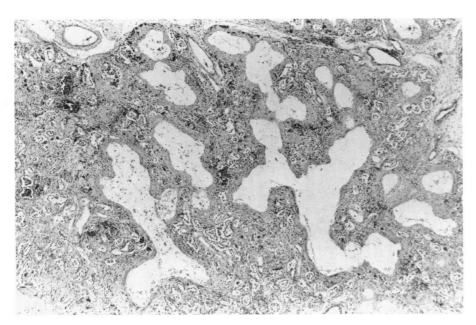

Figure 3.11. Low-power magnification of a section taken from a lung with adult bronchopulmonary dysplasia. Note that the architecture is completely rearranged, and the airspaces are irregular. The branching pattern of open spaces indicates residual alveolar ducts. H&E × 40

Liquid Aspiration

Aspiration of gastric contents in the unconscious patient is one of the most common insults resulting in ARDS (see Chapter 2). The severity of the injury depends on the pH of the liquid aspirated, and hydrochloric acid has been shown to cause a particularly florid form of DAD.[12] If only gastric acid is aspirated, pathologic findings are nonspecific, although aspiration may be suggested if abundant mouth flora is found in the airways or airspaces; only if vegetable or meat fibers are identified can the DAD be ascribed to aspiration.

Near-drowning[13] is associated with the filling of the lungs with either fresh or salt water. Although DAD is probably produced by osmotic damage to the alveolar capillary membrane,[13] there are no histologic markers that would definitely allow one to ascribe the changes solely to drowning rather than to infection by the large and varied numbers of organisms present in lake and sea water.

Inhalation of Noxious Gases and Fumes

Although inhalation of oxides of nitrogen and oxygen itself are associated with DAD, the pathologic features are entirely nonspecific. Patients who develop DAD

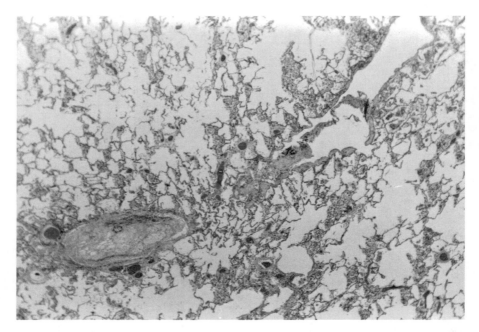

Figure 3.12. A photomicrograph demonstrating an airway in a patient who developed DAD after exposure to smoke and fumes in a house fire. Note the black pigment in the airway lumen, accompanied by an acute inflammatory infiltrate and epithelial necrosis. H&E × 20

after exposure to smoke and gases during a fire[14] may have an associated bronchiolitis, with black particulate embedded in the necrotic debris in the airway lumen (Figure 3.12).

Chemical and Drug Ingestion

Amiodarone[15–17] produces a phospholipidosis, with infiltrates of mural and intra-alveolar foamy macrophages (Figure 3.13).

Paraquat is a potent herbicide sold in various product forms, each containing different concentrations of the chemical. The histologic features of acute and organizing DAD are seen, but often the fibrosis has an unusual pattern with intra-alveolar fibrosis[18,19] (Figure 3.14), and when this is seen paraquat ingestion should be questioned.

Pathologic Differential Diagnosis

Histologic findings must always be interpreted in conjunction with the clinical findings, and failure to do so explains many of the misconceptions present in the older literature.

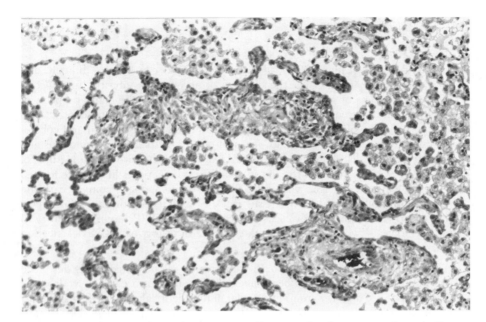

Figure 3.13. This case of amiodarone toxicity illustrates the characteristic foamy cells present in both the interstitium and alveolar airspaces. H&E × 325

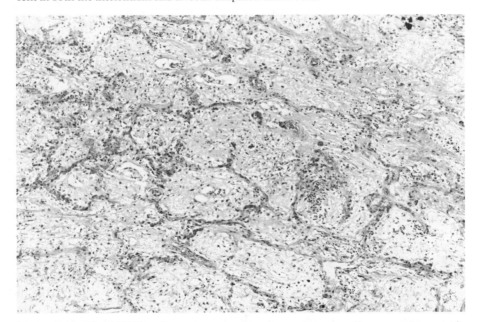

Figure 3.14. The ARDS in this patient was secondary to ingestion of paraquat in a suicide attempt. The alveoli are filled with loose granulation tissue. Their walls are apparent because of congested capillaries. This appearance is highly suggestive of diffuse alveolar damage due to paraquat. H&E × 120

1. *Idiopathic interstitial fibrosis (UIP, fibrosing alveolitis)*. It can be very difficult, and often impossible, to discover the etiology of an endstage fibrotic lung. When viewing CT scans or gross specimens, UIP tends to spare the central aspects of the lung and has greater severity of fibrosis in the lung periphery, whereas DAD affects the whole of the lung or lung lobe. Peripheral cyst formation and cobble-stoning of the pleura are hallmark features of UIP; cysts are less numerous and more irregularly distributed in organized DAD, even when it has the features of adult BPD. On microscopy, the fibrotic walls in the airspaces in UIP are formed of dense bands of collagen with little fibroblastic component compared to the more poorly collagenized fibrous tissue in DAD with its obvious fibroblastic pro-liferation. Clinically, the diseases are very distinct, UIP having a history of months to years, whereas DAD has the short-term history of ARDS described in Chapter 2.

2. *Acute interstitial pneumonia*. This entity constitutes what was generally described by Hamman-Rich,[20] and has been given this eponym as a clinical syndrome.[21] The time course and symptoms are similar, if not identical, to ARDS, also result-ing in the term *idiopathic ARDS*.[22] In fact, the distinction from ARDS is really rather semantic in that it is considered appropriate to use the term *acute intersti-tial pneumonia* if there is no known etiology, but to use *diffuse alveolar damage* if the condition can be ascribed to a known factor. Pathologically, acute interstitial pneumonia is identical to organizing DAD.

3. *Bronchiolitis obliterans and organizing pneumonia (BOOP)*. The clinical history of BOOP often dates weeks or months from an apparent initial respiratory tract infection or inhalational injury, rather than the acute illness of ARDS. Histologi-cally, DAD and BOOP can be difficult to separate if the latter is severe in inten-sity and diffuse in nature, but the granulation tissue plugs in BOOP are usually centered around respiratory bronchioles and alveolar ducts rather than within the alveoli as in severe organizing DAD. An extensive search for hyaline membranes will sometimes prove helpful in making the distinction because hyaline mem-branes are never seen in BOOP.

4. *Severe pneumonia*. In some types of pneumonia such as Legionnaires' disease, the inflammatory infiltrate consists primarily of macrophages, and there can be abun-dant intra-alveolar organization with granulation tissue tufts. Hyaline membranes are not, however, a feature of ordinary pneumonia. A common pathologic prob-lem can be differentiating severe pneumonia from DAD that has become superin-fected with bacterial or fungal organisms. When this occurs, the usual features of bacterial pneumonia with alveolar neutrophils and fluid exudate can be seen, and this will become organized in the usual fashion, with granulation tissue filling the affected alveoli. In severe cases, actual necrosis and abscess formation occurs. However, the background of DAD should also be apparent, and the organized granulation tissue should be at a temporally different stage than that associated with pneumonia.

Summary

Diffuse alveolar damage has a classical gross and histologic appearance that is temporally dependent. Although in the majority of cases the pathology is stereotypic and no etiology can be identified, the pathology can occasionally suggest a potential cause. In addition to pathologic examination, clinical history is important in distinguishing DAD from other inflammatory and fibrotic lung diseases.

References

1. Meyrick B. Pathology of the adult respiratory distress syndrome. Crit Care Clin 1986; 2:405–428.
2. Tomashefski JF. Pulmonary pathology of the adult respiratory distress syndrome. Clin Chest Med 1990; 11:593–619.
3. Moore FD, Lyons JH, Pierce EC. Characteristic clinical and chemical behavior; postmortem findings. In Post-traumatic pulmonary insufficiency, ed Anonymous, Saunders, Toronto, 1969, pp. 99–124.
4. Blennerhassett JB. Shock lung and diffuse alveolar damage: pathological and pathogenetic considerations. Pathology 1985; 17:239–247.
5. Warnock ML, Press M, Churg A. Further observations on cytoplasmic hyaline in the lung. Hum Pathol 1980; 11:59–65.
6. Churg A, Golden J, Fligiel S, Hogg JC. Bronchopulmonary dysplasia in the adult. Am Rev Respir Dis 1983; 127:117–120.
7. Taghizadeh A, Reynolds EOR. Pathogenesis of bronchopulmonary dysplasia following hyaline membrane disease. Am J Pathol 1976; 82:241–264.
8. Coalson JJ. Pathophysiologic features of respiratory distress in the infant and adult. In Textbook of critical care, eds Shoemaker WC, Thompson WL, Holbrook PR, Saunders, Philadelphia, 1984: pp. 344–354.
9. Bachofen M, Weibel ER. Structural alterations of lung parenchyma in the adult respiratory distress syndrome. Clin Chest Med 1982; 3:35–56.
10. Northway WH, Rosan RC, Porter DY. Pulmonary disease following respiratory therapy of hyaline membrane disease. N Engl J Med 1967; 276:357–368.
11. O'Brodovich HM, Mellins RB. Bronchopulmonary dysplasia. Unresolved neonatal acute lung injury. Am Rev Respir Dis 1985; 132:694–709.
12. Mornex J, Chytil-Weir A, Martinet Y, Courtney M, Lecocq J, Crystal RG. Expression of the alpha-1-antitrypsin gene in mononuclear phagocytes of normal and alpha-1-antitrypsin deficient individuals. J Clin Invest 1986; 77:1952–1961.
13. Modell JH, Graves SA, Ketover A. Clinical course of 91 consecutive near-drowning victims. Chest 1976; 70:231–238.
14. Fein A, Leff A, Hopewell PC. Pathophysiology and management of the complications resulting from fire and the inhaled products of combustion. Crit Care Med 1980; 8:94–98.

15. Costa-Jussa FR, Corrin B, Jacobs JM. Amiodarone lung toxicity: a human and experimental study. J Pathol 1984; 143:73–79.
16. Dean PJ, Groshart KD, Porterfield JG, Iansmith DH, Golden EB. Amiodarone-associated pulmonary toxicity. Am J Clin Pathol 1987; 87:7–13.
17. Myers JL, Kennedy JL, Plumb VJ. Amiodarone lung: pathologic findings in clinically toxic patients. Hum Pathol 1987; 18:349–354.
18. Rebello G, Mason JK. Pulmonary histological appearances in fatal paraquat poisoning. Histopathol 1978; 2:53–66.
19. Toner PG, Vetters JM, Spilg WG, Harland W. Fine structure of the lung lesion in a case of paraquat poisoning. J Pathol 1970; 102:182–185.
20. Hamman L, Rich AR. Acute diffuse interstitial fibrosis of the lungs. Int Clin Q 1995; 43:177–212.
21. Olson J, Colby TV, Elliott CG. Hamman-Rich syndrome revisited. Mayo Clin Proc 1990; 65:1538–1548.
22. Katzenstein AL. Katzenstein and Askin's surgical pathology of non-neoplastic lung disease. Saunders, Philadelphia, 1997.

4

Cytokine-Induced Mechanisms of Acute Lung Injury Leading to ARDS

Steven L. Kunkel, Theodore Standiford, Cary Caldwell, Nicholas Lukacs, and Robert M. Strieter

Introduction

As reported in Chapter 2, despite a number of important advances in mechanical ventilatory support, intensive care unit technology, and critical care training, the mortality due to complications of acute respiratory distress syndrome (ARDS) and/or multiorgan failure has not significantly changed during the past 20 years. The failure to fully advance new therapeutic schemes to treat patients with sepsis and ARDS likely reflects our limited knowledge regarding the basic mechanisms underlying these diseases.[1] Thus, the ability to further diminish morbidity and increase survival requires an in-depth understanding of the important mediators involved in the evolution of these syndromes. This information could in turn provide clues as to what exogenous (microorganisms and their products) and endogenous (host-derived) factors should be targeted for modification or elimination during the various phases of sepsis leading to ARDS.

The pathogenesis of ARDS and multiorgan failure–complicating sepsis remains to be fully elucidated. However, polymicrobial agents, products derived from these microorganisms, and the subsequent host response to these factors are key determinants for the initiation and later perpetuation of organ injury.[2] In fact, the host's own response to the initial challenge may be a more critical determinant to the outcome of sepsis and ARDS than the original inciting agent. This concept is supported by the findings that many of the multiple effects of bacterial-derived

James A. Russell and Keith R. Walley, eds. *Acute Respiratory Distress Syndrome.* Printed in the United States of America. Copyright © 1999. Cambridge University Press. All rights reserved.

products, such as endotoxin and muramyl dipeptide, are largely indirect. These compounds exert their biologic effects in vivo by initiating a variety of mediator-generating cascades, including coagulation and complement, vasoactive compounds, reactive oxygen and nitric oxide, arachidonic acid metabolites, and cytokines.[3] The establishment of cytokine networks involving pro- and anti-inflammatory mediators are of particular interest in that these multifunctional mediators have been shown to regulate the host's reactivity and influence subsequent tissue injury.[4,5]

Many of the historical studies assessing the therapy of ARDS have focused on improving both hemodynamics and the overall physiology of the host. These investigations have led to the development of therapeutic applications such as positive end-expiratory pressure (PEEP), which has been useful in decreasing intrapulmonary shunting and increasing lung volume.[6] Even though PEEP is efficacious in temporarily reducing both hypoxemia and early death due to low oxygenation, this intervention has not proven successful for increasing long-term survival. Additional strategies directed at using systems to optimize oxygen delivery and oxygen uptake, increase cardiac output, and improve hemodynamic parameters have been worthwhile goals. However, like PEEP, they have not significantly improved survival. These clinical attempts to alter the pathology of ARDS have focused mainly on modifying the symptoms of the disorder instead of suppressing the mechanisms responsible for the induction of the response. This information again reinforces our poor understanding of the fundamental basic mechanisms that initiate and maintain the responses leading to ARDS.

Interestingly, ARDS may be the common final pathway for a variety of maladies, including massive soft tissue injury, trauma, fat emboli, multiple transfusions, disseminated intravascular coagulation, abscess, and sepsis. All of these etiologies have pathologic processes that include altered physiology, microvascular injury, capillary permeability, leukocyte activation, and dysregulation of cytokine production. In many cases the salient feature that appears to be involved in the initiation of these disorders is the interactions of cellular and humoral immune/inflammatory mediators with the microvasculature. Unfortunately, systemic microvascular injury occurs throughout the host in acute septic shock, which often progresses to lung dysfunction. The outcome of this injury in the lung is diffuse alveolar-capillary membrane damage causing extravascular fluid accumulation, activation of coagulation pathways favoring a procoagulant state, intravascular accumulation of leukocytes in the pulmonary capillaries, and transendothelial leukocyte migration. The ability of the host to mount a vigorous inflammatory response is unquestionably important in the setting of normal defense mechanisms. However, when the sequence of inflammatory events results in dysregulation of mediator cascades, the host's inflammatory responses are no longer under normal control and dire clinical consequences result. These consequences translate into cases where treatment may not be efficacious and outcome is not predictable.

The Role of Cytokines in the Initiation and Maintenance of Systemic Inflammation Early Response Cytokines (IL-1 and TNF)

Defining the role of specific cytokines in disease and applying this information to develop therapeutic strategies to target sepsis has been a central theme in several scientific laboratories. A prototypic example of investigations that have led to an understanding of the interrelationship between cytokines, disease, and potential therapy is the accumulating information on the activity of interleukin-1 (IL-1) and tumor necrosis factor-alpha (TNF).[7,8] These two cytokines have been implicated in mediating the pathophysiology of various infectious diseases, septic shock, and sepsis syndrome. Interestingly, the biologic activity of IL-1 and TNF with regard to systemic inflammation are closely related, even though the two cytokines are structurally unrelated. Interleukin-1 was originally described as a polypeptide with lymphocyte activating properties and TNF was described as a soluble oncolytic factor found in the serum of bacillus Calmette-Guerin immunized mice treated with LPS. One of the striking features of IL-1 and TNF is the similar, multifunctional roles that these cytokines play during certain diseases, which is likely a manifestation of their ability to induce cytokine networks that initiate and maintain an inflammatory response. Evidence supports the notion that both of these mediators are early response cytokines generated during the initiation of an inflammatory response. The expression of IL-1 and/or TNF sets in motion a cascade of cellular events, resulting in the production of more distal cytokines necessary to promote and maintain the inflammatory response. Studies have shown that macrophage-derived IL-1 or TNF can activate either resident tissue cells or immune cells and induce the expression of a variety of cytokines, including interleukin-6 (IL-6), interleukin-8 (IL-8), monocyte chemoattractant protein-1 (MCP-1) and other chemotactic cytokines, growth factors and colony stimulating factors, as well as IL-1 and TNF themselves. TNF and IL-1 also induce endothelial cell, leukocyte, and pulmonary parenchymal cells to undergo cytoskeletal changes and increase expression of adhesion molecules leading to recruitment and retention of an active inflammatory cell infiltrate.

IL-1 and TNF-dependent cytokine networks are particularly important in the elicitation of specific leukocyte populations to an area of reactivity. The production of these early response cytokines can network with surrounding cells to generate potent neutrophil chemotactic cytokines. In this paradigm, early response cytokines can induce the surrounding normal resident cells to become important effector cells during inflammation via the generation of other cytokines needed to maintain the reaction.[4,9] The establishment of this cytokine network is especially important in infectious diseases because the rapid recruitment of leukocytes is critically important in clearing the infectious agent.

The activation of cytokine cascades is no doubt important to the normal elicitation of blood-borne leukocytes to an area of tissue injury or infection. However, when TNF and IL-1 are overexpressed and cytokine cascades are not appropriately regulated, the consequences may be life threatening. This is likely a contributing scenario to the pathology found in fulminant infections, sepsis, multiorgan failure, and acute respiratory distress syndrome. However, the use of biologics targeting IL-1 and/or TNF as efficacious therapeutics for the treatment of ARDS or sepsis have met with little clinical success.[10] For example, clinical protocols utilizing neutralizing monoclonal antibodies to human TNF have not proven beneficial for the treatment of sepsis in multicenter randomized clinical trials. In addition, clinical protocols developed to target IL-1 via the application of the interleukin-1 receptor antagonist have not been judged useful for the treatment of sepsis or ARDS. The outcome of many of these clinical trials may have been predicted knowing that the activity of IL-1 and TNF are so similar. With the present level of knowledge regarding cytokine biology, it is likely that the most efficacious approach would be a therapeutic cocktail targeting IL-1 and TNF and other cytokines.

Balance between Pro- and Anti-inflammatory Mediators

The early pro-inflammatory cytokines TNF and IL-1 initiate the pulmonary inflammatory response that mediates tissue injury but ultimately also leads to resolution and repair. Thus, the inflammatory response is necessarily a balance between (1) pro-inflammatory mediators that are important in clearing the initiating stimulus but also damage tissue, and (2) anti-inflammatory mediators that aid in regulation of tissue repair. For example, a number of cytokines whose expression is induced by TNF and IL-1 have significant anti-inflammatory properties. Soluble receptors for TNF bind circulating TNF and reduce its biologic activity, resulting in increased survival in some animal models of severe systemic inflammation. Similarly, IL-1 is modulated by an IL-1 receptor antagonist protein. IL-1 receptor antagonist is an endogenous molecule that acts as a competitive inhibitor, with no agonist activity, for binding to IL-1 receptors. When IL-1 receptor antagonist is administered in various animal models of inflammation, cell infiltration, edema, and tissue damage are reduced. IL-10 is an important cytokine that can downregulate the expression of TNF and other pro-inflammatory cytokines. Blocking endogenous IL-10 in an animal model of acute lung injury resulted in substantially increased pulmonary injury.[11]

One clinical study demonstrated that decreased concentrations of anti-inflammatory mediators in patients with ARDS was associated with increased mortality rates.[5] In this study of 28 ARDS patients, median IL-1 receptor antagonist concentrations were 1,600 pg/mL in survivors compared to 90 pg/mL in nonsurvivors. Similarly, the median IL-10 concentrations were 120 pg/mL in survivors compared to 40 pg/mL in nonsurvivors. These findings suggest that failure to mount an anti-inflammatory response early in ARDS contributes to more severe organ injury and mortality. Thus, the balance between the pro- and anti-inflammatory components in ARDS is important in mounting an appropriate, but not excessive, inflammatory response.

Chemokines

The identification of new chemotactic factors has provided an important impetus to assess leukocyte recruitment at the mechanistic level. Chemotactic cytokines, chemokines, appear to play fundamentally important roles in the early and late phases of ARDS.[12,13] One interesting aspect of the chemokine supergene family is the relative specificity that these polypeptide mediators display for the recruitment of certain peripheral blood leukocyte populations.[14-16] The importance of this biologic activity is exemplified by the redundancy of inflammatory mediators that display leukocyte chemotactic activity. As stated earlier, the recruitment response is a strict requirement for the normal operation of inflammation; thus, the host appears to possess a number of mechanisms that will target leukocytes to an area of immune/inflammatory reactivity. Previous investigations have identified a number of active participants in leukocyte locomotion. These factors represented a wide range of chemical entities, including biologically active lipids, split products of large polypeptides, small polypeptides, and peptides (24 amino acids). However, most of these early identified mediators of inflammation lacked specificity for the elicitation of a particular leukocyte population. During the mid-1980s, two supergene families of chemotactic peptides were identified that demonstrated relative specificity for movement and activation of leukocyte populations.[14] These chemokines belong to two main groups of related polypeptides, identified by the location of two of the four cysteine amino acids comprising their primary amino acid structure.

Accumulating evidence supports the concept that members of these supergene families have pro-inflammatory and reparative activities. In their monomeric form, most of these chemokines are less than 10,000 daltons, possess a basic isoelectric point, and are heparin-binding proteins. One of the chemokine families displays a conserved amino acid motif characterized by the location of two amino terminal cysteines separated by one nonconserved amino acid residue. This chemokine family is designated as the C-X-C chemokine supergene family and has a relatively high degree of specificity for the elicitation of neutrophils. The C-X-C chemokines are all clustered on human chromosome 4 and possess approximately 20% to 55% homology in their primary structure. Interest in this area is exemplified by investigations that have identified 12 different C-X-C chemokines, including platelet factor-4, platelet basic protein, connective tissue activating protein III, beta thromboglobulin, neutrophil activating factor-2, interleukin-8, growth-related oncogene alpha, beta, and gamma, gamma interferon-inducible protein (IP-10), epithelial neutrophil activating protein-78, monokine induced by gamma interferon (MIG), and granulocyte chemotactic protein-2 (GCP-2).[17] Connective tissue activating protein-III, beta thromboglobulin, and neutrophil activating protein-2 are all N-terminal truncations of platelet basic protein. These cleavage products are formed when platelet basic protein is released from platelet alpha granules and is proteolytically digested by leukocyte-derived proteases.

Recent investigations have demonstrated that an important feature in the primary structure of C-X-C chemokines may account for the neutrophil chemotactic and activating properties of these mediators (Table 4.1). These studies identified three critical amino acid residues immediately preceding the first N-terminal cysteine, which are important in binding to a neutrophil receptor and activating neutrophils. These amino acids are Glu-Leu-Arg or the ELR motif, which is absent in certain members of the C-X-C chemokine family. In particular, platelet factor-4, IP-10, and MIG all lack the ELR motif and do not possess potent neutrophil-activating properties. However, when the ELR motif was synthetically introduced into platelet factor-4, this polypeptide gained chemotactic activity. Therefore, certain members of the C-X-C supergene family may have different biologic activities. Interestingly, platelet factor-4 (a non-ELR containing C-X-C chemokine) was one of the first members of this family to be described. This factor was originally identified for its ability to bind heparin, leading to the inactivation of the anticoagulation function of heparin. Interleukin-8 has been the most studied C-X-C chemokine and is produced by an array of cells including primary cultures of monocytes, alveolar macrophages, neutrophils, keratinocytes, mesangial cells, epithelial cells, hepatocytes, fibroblasts, and endothelial cells. In addition, IL-8 is expressed by a number of neoplasms and transformed cell lines.

Recent investigations have identified IL-8 as an important cytokine in the pathogenesis of a number of human diseases, including diseases of the lung.[18,19] In one study, IL-8 has been found in the bronchoalveolar lavage (BAL) of patients at risk of developing ARDS, and this chemotactic mediator may be an important prognostic indicator for the clinical development of this syndrome.[12] It is generally believed that a significant contributing factor to the pathology of ARDS is the sequestration, emigration, and activation of neutrophils. Although ARDS has been described in patients with peripheral blood neutropenia, there is compelling evidence for the participation of neutrophils in most cases of ARDS. In these studies, high concentrations of IL-8 were found in the BAL from trauma patients, some within 1 hour of injury.[20] Patients who progressed to ARDS had significantly higher levels of IL-8 in the BAL than those patients who did not develop ARDS. One cellular source of IL-8 in these ARDS patients was the alveolar macrophage; however, it is likely other cells in the alveolar/capillary wall may also contribute to the elevated pulmonary levels of IL-8. An important aspect of these studies was identifying elevated IL-8 levels that preceded the presence of increased neutrophil numbers in the BAL. Although an earlier study also identified IL-8 in the BAL fluid of both ARDS patients and patients at risk of developing ARDS, a significant correlation with mortality was not found.[21] However, additional investigations identified elevated levels of IL-8 in the BAL of ARDS patients, as compared to controls, and the IL-8 levels significantly correlated with patient mortality.[22,23] These investigators also demonstrated a significant correlation between the percentage of neutrophils and the IL-8 concentration

Table 4.1 The C-X-C chemokine family
includes chemotactic cytokines, which may
contain or lack the amino terminal motif of
glutamic acid (E), leucine (L), and arginine (R).

C-X-C chemokines containing an ELR motif

Interleukin-8 (IL-8)
Epithelial neutrophil activating protein (ENA-78)
Neutrophil activating protein-2 (NAP-2)
Growth regulated oncogene alpha (GRO-alpha)
Growth regulated oncogene beta (GRO-beta)
Growth regulated oncogene gamma (GRO-gamma)
Granulocyte chemotactic protein-2 (GCP-2)

C-X-C chemokines lacking an ELR motif

Gamma-interferon inducible protein-10 (IP-10)
Monokine induced by gamma interferon (MIG)
Platelet factor-4 (PF4)

in the BAL fluid. Furthermore, the IL-8 levels in the lavage fluid was near the optimal concentration necessary to induce in vitro neutrophil chemotaxis. Thus, further investigations targeting the role of C-X-C chemokines, such as IL-8, may prove to be worthwhile in understanding the mechanisms leading to ARDS.

An additional family of polypeptide mediators related to the C-X-C chemokines is the C-C chemokine family.[24] This group is defined by the location of the first two N-terminal cysteines being found in juxtaposition to one another. In general terms, the C-C chemokine family has relative specificity for the elicitation of mononuclear cells. The C-C chemokine family includes macrophage inflammatory protein-1 alpha and beta, monocyte chemoattractant protein 1, 2, and 3, 1-309, and RANTES. Like the C-X-C family, certain members of the C-C family have been identified as products from a number of cellular sources, including a variety of noninflammatory cells and tumor cell lines.

Recent experiments have shown that RANTES, a member of the C-C supergene family, may play an important role during the evolution of endotoxemia.[25] These studies demonstrated that RANTES MRNA and protein could be compartmentalized within the lungs of endotoxin-challenged mice. In addition, the expression of RANTES protein could be temporally related to the influx of mononuclear phagocytic cells. This latter data was strengthened by the observation that passive immunization of animals with neutralizing antibodies to RANTES could significantly reduce monocyte, but not neutrophil infiltration in the lungs of endotoxin-challenged mice. The mechanism(s) whereby RANTES may interact with monocytes and influence their elicitation into the lungs could be via directly influencing monocyte chemotaxis, or RANTES may enhance monocyte transmigration by directly regulating the expression of monocyte beta 2 integrins. This latter phenomenon has also been shown for RANTES-treated eosinophils.

Further studies identified the cellular source of lung-derived RANTES in endotoxin-treated mice to be pulmonary epithelial cells. These data were generated using an immunohistochemical analysis of lung sections recovered from endotoxin-treated mice. Interestingly, primary cultures of rat type 11 pneumocytes challenged with TNF expressed detectable levels of RANTES protein, as shown by Western blot analysis. This information further supports the notion that the cellular source of RANTES in the lung, after an in vivo challenge with endotoxin, is the epithelium. The production of RANTES by pulmonary epithelium is via a cytokine network driven by early response cytokines such as IL-1 and TNF. This common theme of IL-1 and TNF–driven cytokine networks can be observed a number of times during the evolution of inflammation, leading to leukocyte recruitment. Interestingly, RANTES was not expressed by lung macrophages in vivo, as initially shown by immunohistochemistry. Further data from isolated normal alveolar macrophages challenged with LPS, IL-1, or TNF demonstrated that these stimulated cells did not express steady-state levels of RANTES MRNA or protein, suggesting that noninflammatory resident cells may be the most significant sources of RANTES during certain inflammatory responses.

Chemokine Expression by Noninflammatory Cells

The expression of various chemokines by noninflammatory cells raises an intriguing question regarding the specific role that resident tissue cells play during the initiation and maintenance of an inflammatory response. Historically, investigations have suggested that monokines and lymphokines were expressed only by monocytes and lymphocytes; however, this does not accurately reflect the cell-specific cytokine production pattern during inflammation. This is especially true regarding the production of chemokines because stromal cells, epithelial cells, endothelial cells, and hepatocytes can all express significant levels of these polypeptide mediators of inflammation.[6,26–28,29,30] These studies support the notion that normal resident tissue cells can support an inflammatory response via the induction of appropriate chemokines. The production of either C-C or C-X-C family members by local resident cells depends on a cytokine network. In this network or cascade, early response cytokines or master cytokines, such as IL-1 or TNF, can dictate the expression of subsequent chemokines.

This communication process is likely controlled at the tissue level by fixed, resident macrophages. These sentinel macrophages can respond rapidly to injury or a foreign challenge and release IL-1 and/or TNF, which can activate the surrounding resident tissue cells in a cytokine-specific manner (Table 4.2). During the evolution of sepsis the early insult of particular microorganisms or products derived from microorganisms may provide the signal to activate the resident tissue macrophage, which in turn releases IL-1 and/or TNF to activate the surrounding cells that nor-

Table 4.2. The expression of IL-8 is induced in a stimulus-specific network. In particular, early-response cytokines, such as IL-1 and TNF, are potent inducing cytokines for IL-8 expression by a variety of cells.

	STIMULUS			
Cellular source	LPS	TNF	IL-1	IL-6
Monocytes	+++	++	+++	–
Alveolar macrophages	+++	++	+++	–
Epithelial cells	–	++	+++	–
Fibroblasts	+/–	++	+++	–
Endothelial cells	++	++	+++	–

mally comprises the tissue. Resident nonimmune cells are usually not susceptible to a challenge with specific inflammatory activating agents like lipopolysaccharide or immune complexes. Therefore, the production of IL-1 or TNF by local resident macrophages can magnify the response needed to initiate and maintain the recruitment process. These networks have been assessed in the context of both the lung and liver, where early response cytokines released by alveolar macrophages or Kupffer cells can interact with surrounding type 11 alveolar epithelial cells or hepatocytes, respectively.

The Gut-Liver-Lung Connection during the Evolution of Sepsis

The multiorgan involvement that can be observed during the evolution of sepsis is an enigmatic clinical feature associated with increased mortality as the number of involved organs increase. Although ARDS is associated with pulmonary inflammation and loss of lung function, it is clearly not the only organ involved in the pathology of sepsis. The susceptibility of the lung to inflammation and injury during systemic inflammation appears to be due to its anatomic attribute of possessing a large capillary bed. This vascular component of the lung is indeed necessary for gas exchange, but it is also the location of the initial interactions between leukocytes and endothelium during the evolution of systemic inflammation. As one of a number of different etiologies initiates the systemic inflammatory response that can ultimately lead to sepsis, the lung is usually one of the first organs to exhibit signs of dysfunction. The cellular composition of the lung coupled with its anatomic location in relation to the liver and intestinal tract place this organ at significant risk during systemic inflammation. The gut-liver-lung triad is particularly interesting in that alterations in the integrity of the gut can provide the systemic signals which activate circulating blood leukocytes or resident inflammatory cells in the liver. This event can cause local hepatic inflammation and the systemic release of mediators that influence the next target organ, the lungs. Thus, the lung ultimately is the recipient of cytokines, microorganisms and their products, and activated leukocytes, which are derived from "downstream" organs and passed on via the blood to the lungs.

Experimentally, this phenomenon can be demonstrated using a model of endotoxemia.[7] Mice intraperitoneally challenged with lipopolysaccharide (LPS) demonstrate a rapid systemic cytokine response followed by pathologic alteration in the small intestine and recruitment of leukocytes to the liver and lungs. The pathology of the small intestines is characterized by a loss in the integrity of the gut microvilli, revealing a cytologic picture similar to an ischemic gut. Microorganisms and their products can easily enter the systemic circulation and impact the vascular bed found in the liver. The fixed tissue macrophages or Kupffer cells in the liver can respond to factors released in the gut and generate a new set of mediators that enter the circulation and travel to the lungs. As previously stated, the lung with its vast vascular bed of capillaries receives a mixed insult of endogenous host mediators and exogenous factors that precipitates a vigorous inflammatory response in the lungs. The organ-to-organ communication that occurs between the gut-liver-lung is one of the key components leading to the pathology of ARDS.

Cell-to-Cell Communication during Systemic Inflammation

There is little doubt that organ-to-organ communication is an important connection in the establishment of ARDS that may progress to multiorgan failure. However, superimposed on the organ communication pathway is cell-to-cell communication that is established within each afflicted organ. Thus, interorgan communication appears to provide the major signals to drive the local communication circuits at the tissue level. Although parameters such as fever, acute phase proteins, hematocrit PO_2, and liver function enzymes are useful to decipher global systemic and organ function, concomitant alterations are also occurring at the cellular and molecular levels. Recent studies have shown that a number of common inflammatory cascades depend on a balance of early response pro-inflammatory mediators and their subsequent systemic and local regulation by antagonists, inhibitors, and suppressive cytokines. It is likely that common, local cytokine pathways are established during systemic responses which are required for the generation of specific leukocyte-recruiting mediators in each organ.

One well-characterized cytokine cascade has been identified between resident macrophages and structural cells of the lung. Initially, this network was demonstrated in vitro using LPS-stimulated alveolar macrophage conditioned media as a stimulus for lung fibroblasts in a macrophage-fibroblast co-culture system.[31] In a series of experiments, normal human alveolar macrophages were either left unchallenged or challenged with LPS for 18 hours and the conditioned media collected and overlaid on normal lung fibroblasts. After 18 hours, the human fibroblasts were assessed for the expression of steady-state levels of IL-8 MRNA in response to the various conditioned media. The addition of the alveolar macrophage conditioned media to normal lung fibroblasts resulted in significant expression of steady-state IL-8 MRNA, as assessed by laser densitometry. To further explore the potential mechanism responsible for the increase in fibroblast IL-8 MRNA expression, the alveolar macrophage conditioned media was first incubated with neutralizing antibodies to either interleukin-1 (IL-1) or tumor necrosis factor (TNF) prior to fibroblast stimulation. In these studies the neutralizing antibodies significantly reduced the expression of fibroblast-derived IL-8 MRNA. Antibodies to human IL-1 reduced the expression of fibroblast-derived IL-8 by approximately 50%, whereas antibodies to human TNF reduced the expression by approximately 20%. However, the combination of neutralizing antibodies directed against both IL-1 and TNF resulted in an 80% reduction in steady-state levels of fibroblast-derived IL-8 MRNA. Only minimal IL-8 expression was observed by nonconditioned media treated fibroblasts, and normal lung fibroblasts treated with LPS were not responsive.

These studies demonstrated that LPS-stimulated macrophages can generate soluble mediators, such as IL-1 and TNF, which network with nonimmune tissue cells and induce their expression of IL-8. In an extension of the studies just described, an alveolar macrophage/pulmonary fibroblast co-culture system was utilized to further explore cytokine networking. At time 0, the co-culture system was challenged with LPS, and at specified time points the co-culture was assessed for the expression of antigenic IL-8 by immunolocalization. A very rapid expression of antigenic IL-8 was observed by the LPS-challenged alveolar macrophages, and the expression of pulmonary fibroblast IL-8 was markedly delayed. The maximum percentage of alveolar macrophage that were IL-8 positive occurred by 3 to 4 hours post LPS stimulation. However, the maximum percentage of IL-8 positive co-cultured fibroblasts was not observed until 24 hours. These data are interesting in light of the fact that lung fibroblasts do not respond to an LPS challenge. Thus, cells that are normal constituents of tissue can become important effector cells during both the initiation and maintenance of an inflammatory response via a process of cytokine networks. This process of cytokine networking is not limited to cells in the lung; a similar process has also been observed to occur between hepatocytes and Kupffer cells in the liver.[32] In these studies, isolated human Kupffer cells challenged with LPS were shown to produce mediators that could induce the expression of IL-8 by normal human hepatocytes. Again, LPS-conditioned media recovered from Kupffer cells was found to generate IL-1 and TNF that could network with hepatocytes and induce the expression of IL-8. These studies support the notion that cell-to-cell communication is likely superimposed on organ-to-organ communication during the evolution of systemic inflammation.

Animal Models of Systemic Inflammation That Leads to Lung Injury

The initiation and maintenance of acute pulmonary inflammation is known to involve a complex series of events that depend on the expression and regulation of various cytokines. Initial efforts centered around an assessment of TNF and IL-1 as prominent early response mediators of endotoxin-induced inflammation. Experimental animals challenged intraperitoneally with LPS demonstrated a rapid rise in the expression of TNF MRNA and biologic activity in both the ascites fluid and plasma, which was followed by pulmonary neutrophilia and systemic lymphopenia.[7] A kinetic analysis demonstrated that the expression of TNF in response to an in vivo LPS challenge was extremely rapid. Within the ascites, TNF activity was present by 30 minutes after LPS administration and peaked by 1 to 2 hours. Levels of plasma TNF were also rapidly induced: circulating TNF levels reached a zenith by 1 hour post LPS administration. A similar time course for cell-associated TNF was observed with peritoneal macrophages and peripheral blood mononuclear cells. IL-1-like activity was also identified in the ascites fluid as early as 1 hour post LPS challenge. In contrast to the rapid time course for the expression of TNF, the levels of ascites IL-1 persisted for 4 to 8 hours. These data indicate that the in vivo induction of TNF is a rapid event under tight endogenous control. Further studies demonstrated that the in vivo expression of steady-state levels of TNF MRNA by peritoneal cells was clearly detectable by 15 minutes post LPS challenge, peaked at 30 minutes, and declined by 60 minutes. The peak in macrophage TNF MRNA in these studies was assessed by both Northern blot and in situ hybridizational analyses.

Additional investigations, assessing the cellular source of cytokines post LPS challenge, demonstrated that the Kupffer cell was important in vivo for generating TNF.[33] Immunolocalization of TNF, IL-1 alpha, and IL-1 beta in the liver exhibited a distinct pattern for each of the cytokines, as the peak in cytokine antigen occurred at 1, 6, and 3 hours, respectively. Interestingly, antigenic staining for all of the cytokines was clearly restricted to sinusoidal lining cells and was not observed in hepatocytes, ductal cells, or endothelial cells. Cytokine antigen was localized to sessile macrophages (Kupffer cells), and the staining distribution was identical to that for a mouse macrophage marker. Staining was not observed in non-LPS-challenged mice. The immunolocalization pattern for TNF and IL-1, within the Kupffer cells, was quite different. Interleukin-1 staining was diffusely cytoplasmic, whereas TNF staining tended to be more localized within the cytoplasm. The kinetics of TNF immunolocalization in Kupffer cells demonstrated that this cytokine was consistently the first cytokine expressed after an in vivo challenge with LPS, reaching a maximal expression by 1 hour, then rapidly disappearing by 3 hours. Interleukin-1 beta also rapidly appeared and reached a high expression level by 2 to 3 hours. IL-1 alpha followed a more prolonged time course, reaching a maximum at 3 to 6 hours. Both forms of IL-1 were no longer detectable by 18 hours.

Pathophysiologic alterations have been correlated with the cytokine profile in the endotoxemia models.[7] In association with a profound circulating neutrophilia, which developed by 1 hour post LPS challenge, most of the major organs examined demonstrated neutrophil infiltrates. This was particularly true in the lungs. Morphometric analysis of the lungs demonstrated an 8-fold increase in neutrophil numbers in LPS-treated animals. Additional analysis using a myeloperoxidase (MPO) assay, as an indirect assessment of neutrophil accumulation, demonstrated a striking increase in lung MPO activity that histologically correlated with neutrophil infiltration. Subsequent studies were conducted to determine the ameliorating effect of TNF inhibition on the pathology induced by LPS. Passive immunization with neutralizing anti-TNF antibodies, prior to LPS administration, demonstrated a significant reduction in recoverable plasma TNF levels, which correlated with reduced neutrophil accumulation in the lungs. In addition, the profound neutrophilia was significantly reduced in the antibody-treated animals. In further studies directed at understanding the regulation of TNF, cyclosporin A was assessed for its modulating effects on LPS-induced pathology. This immunosuppressive agent was found to cause a dose-dependent reduction in circulating TNF levels and a decrease in a number of the pathologic parameters usually associated with endotoxemia. Interestingly, cyclosporin A altered the production of biologically active TNF, but did not alter the expression of steady-state levels of TNF MRNA.

One of the major drawbacks to using endotoxemia as a model to study the multiple alterations that are occurring during systemic inflammation is that endotoxemia does not exactly model an infectious process. Many of the investigations that have utilized endotoxin as a model are studying grossly altered physiology and not an infectious process. This is important because most septic patients are likely to have a polymicrobial etiology underlying their disorders. In order to understand the etiology and pathogenicity of polymicrobial-induced sepsis, investigators have turned to the cecal ligation/puncture model (CLP) as a system to study the cellular and molecular mechanisms involved in a more physiologic relevant model of systemic inflammation.

The use of CLP has generated renewed interest because it is relevant, possesses a polymicrobial etiology, and mortality and/or morbidity can be altered depending on the size of the puncture to the cecum.[34] A rapidly progressing systemic inflammatory response can be initiated with 80% mortality in 24 to 48 hours with a puncture wound using an 18 gauge needle, or a more prolonged systemic response can be induced with low mortality in 24 to 48 hours using a small (26 gauge needle) puncture wound. Histologically, the lungs appear to be a sensitive target organ in the CLP model. By 8 hours after establishing an 18 gauge puncture model, thickening of the pulmonary septa could be observed accompanied by leukocyte infiltration. Especially prominent are the significant numbers of neutrophils within the pulmonary interstitium. The histology of sham-operated animals exhibited no significant changes at the same time point.

Studies were next performed to quantitate changes in specific cytokine levels and correlate these data with the survival curve. Cytokine concentrations from samples recovered from 18 gauge CLP animals were compared to samples recovered from the 26 gauge model. The kinetics in MIP2, sTNFr (p75), and IL-10 levels from serum samples recovered from the 18 gauge CLP model were dramatically accelerated and peaked within the first 6 hours. Similar kinetics were observed for TNF. On the contrary, the kinetics and levels of MIP-2, sTNFr (p75), and IL-10 were quite different in the 26 gauge model.

The expression of plasma levels of antigenic MIP-2, sTNFr (p75), and IL-10 were reduced, as compared to the 18 gauge model. Moreover, the kinetics of pro- and anti-inflammatory mediator production in the 26 gauge model demonstrated a delay in peak expression with a pattern of high levels occurring between 6 to 12 hours for MIP-2 and 12 to 24 hours for sTNFr (p75) and IL-10. These polypeptides were not significantly elevated in the plasma of sham controls. A similar correlative pattern of mediator expression was also found in the peritoneal lavage of the CLP animals.

Additional studies demonstrated the presence of MIP-2 antigen in the aqueous extracts of lungs and liver for 48 to 72 hours after the initiation of the CLP response. Interestingly, significant levels of IL-10 were found in aqueous extracts of liver in naive mice (baseline) that subsequently declined during the evolution of systemic inflammation in both the 18 and 26 gauge models. The decrease in IL-10 levels was more precipitous in the 18 gauge than the 26 gauge CLP model and correlated with higher mortality at 48 hours. This latter observation suggested that IL-10 is constitutively produced in the liver and may be locally released during inflammation. The difference in the mediator profiles in the two CLP models may directly reflect the distinct pathologic profiles found in these two systems. In the 18 gauge CLP model, an overwhelming systemic inflammatory response occurs with elevated levels of pro-inflammatory cytokines such as TNF and MIP-2. In this model the expression of the regulatory mediators, IL-10 and sTNFr, were also significantly elevated during the first 6 hours, but these modulating polypeptides were not sustained in the 18 gauge CLP model. This altered balance in the production of pro-inflammatory and regulatory polypeptides is likely a key component to leukocyte activation, elicitation, and subsequent tissue injury found in acute systemic inflammation. The accelerated expression pattern supports the hypothesis that early and aggressive therapy is important in treating multiorgan injury syndromes. In the 26 gauge model of systemic inflammation, both IL-10 and sTNFr (p75) remain elevated, reaching their zenith in expression between 12 and 24 hours. This is a time point when the levels of MIP-2 decline. The sustained production of these regulatory mediators is likely an important aspect relating to the in vivo cytokine balance that dictates resolution of inflammation, and may be a positive prognostic indicator for recovery/survival.

Summary

The information in this chapter demonstrates that the pathophysiologic alterations that occur during the initiation and maintenance of ARDS are truly complex. Organ-to-organ communication networks are clearly important in providing the stimuli that lead to the initiation of multiorgan injury and ARDS. However, superimposed on this organ communication loop is the aspect of cell-to-cell communication. This interaction is key to the local perpetuation of the response and depends on cytokine networks, whereby early response cytokines (IL-1 and TNF) can induce the expression of more distal cytokines (IL-6 and IL-8). These cytokine networks involve both pro- and anti-inflammatory mediators. The cell-to-cell communication networks are likely initiated by the activation of resident fixed macrophages or tissue dendritic cells that can rapidly release a set repertoire of newly synthesized cytokines. IL-1 and TNF are classical examples of these early polypeptide mediators that in turn activate surrounding resident tissue cells in a cascadelike mechanism and promote the expression of additional cytokines needed to maintain the cellular inflammatory response. Cell-to-cell communication is an important means to continue the elicitation of leukocyte subpopulations to an area of tissue injury because the in vivo production of chemokines depends on this interaction. Investigations using both animal models and human samples have clearly demonstrated that various cytokines play a significant role in the initiation and maintenance of multiorgan injury, including ARDS. Unfortunately, many clinical trials based on the elimination of a particular cytokine or competing with a cytokine at the receptor level and blocking the activity of a particular cytokine have not been very successful. These observations point out the importance of the balance between pro- and anti-inflammatory mediators in the inflammatory response. These therapeutic approaches have targeted biologically potent early response cytokines, such as IL-1 and TNF, which may not be the most amenable cytokines for eliminating when patients present with ARDS. Thus, strategies based on targeting cytokines are turning to regulating more distal inflammatory cytokines or regulating cytokine networks that influence cell viability.

Acknowledgments

These studies were supported in part by National Institutes of Health grants HL50057, P50HL46487, HL319634, and HL35276.

References

1. Rinaldo JER, Rogers RM. Adult respiratory distress syndrome: changing concepts of lung injury and repair. N Engl J Med 1982; 306:900–909.
2. Brigham KL, Meyrick B. Endotoxin and lung injury. Am Rev Respir Dis 1986; 133:913–927.
3. McGuire WW, Spragg RG, Cohen AB. Studies on the pathogenesis of the adult respiratory distress syndrome. J Clin Invest 1982; 69:543–553.
4. Standiford TJ, Kunkel SL, Basha MA, Chensue SW, Lynch JP, Toews GB, Strieter RM. Interleukin-8 gene expression by a pulmonary epithelial cell line: a model for cytokine networks in the lung. J Clin Invest 1990; 86:1945–1953.

5. Donnelly SC, Strieter RM, Reid PT, Kunkel SL, Burdick MD, Armstrong I, Mackenzie A, Haslett, C. The association between mortality rates and decreased concentrations of interleukin-10 and interleukin-1 receptor antagonist in the lung fluids of patients with the adult respiratory distress syndrome. Ann Intern Med 1996; 125:191–196.

6. Strieter RM, Kasahara K, Allen R, Showell HJ, Standiford TJ, Kunkel SL. Human neutrophils exhibit disparate chemotactic factor gene expression. Biochem Biophys Res Comm 1990; 173:725–730.

7. Remick DG, Strieter RM, Eskandari DT, Nguyen D, Genord MA, Kunkel SL. Role of tumor necrosis factor in lipopolysaccharide-induced pathologic alterations. Am J Pathol 1990; 136:49–60.

8. Xing Z, Jordana M, Kirpalani H, Driscoll KE, Schall TJ, Gauldie J. Cytokine expression by neutrophils and macrophages in vivo: endotoxin induces TNF, MIP-2, IL-1, IL-6, but not RANTES or TGF MRNA expression in acute lung inflammation. Am J Respir Cell Mol Biol 1994; 10:148–153.

9. Luster AD. Chemokines – chemotactic cytokines that mediate inflammation. N Engl J Med 1998; 338:436–445.

10. Zeni F, Freeman B, Natanson C. Anti-inflammatory therapies to treat sepsis and septic shock: a reassessment. Crit Care Med 1997; 25:1095–1100.

11. Shanley TP, Warner RL, Ward PA. The role of cytokines and adhesion molecules in the development of inflammation and injury. Mol Med Today 1995; 1:40–45.

12. Goodman RB, Strieter RM, Martin DP, Steinberg KP, Milberg JA, Maunder RJ, Kunkel SL, Walz A, Hudson LD, Martin TR. Inflammatory cytokines in patients with persistence of the acute respiratory distress syndrome. Am J Respir Crit Care Med 1996; 154:602–611.

13. Smith RE, Strieter RM, Phan SH, Kunkel SL. C-C chemokines: novel mediators of the profibrotic inflammatory response to bleomycin challenge. Am J Respir Cell Mol Biol 1996; 15:693–702.

14. Matsushima K, Oppenheim JJ. Interleukin-8 and MCAF: novel inflammatory cytokines inducible by IL-1 and TNF. Cytokine 1989; 1:2–13

15. Baggiolini M, Walz A, Kunkel SL. Neutrophil-activating peptide-1/interleukin-8, a novel cytokine that activates neutrophils. J Clin Invest 1989; 84:1045–1049.

16. Oppenheim JJ, Zachariae OC, Mukaida N, Matsushima K. Properties of the novel proinflammatory supergene "intercrine" cytokine family. Ann Rev Immunol 1991; 9:617–648.

17. Miller MD, Krangel MS. Biology and biochemistry of the chemokines: a family of chemotactic and inflammatory cytokines. Crit Rev Immunol 1992; 12:17–46.

18. Antony VB, Godbey SW, Kunkel SL, Hott JW, Hartman B, Burdick MD, Strieter RM. Recruitment of inflammatory cells to the pleural space. J Immunol 1993; 151:7216–7223.

19. Broaddus VC, Boylan AM, Hoeffel JM, Kim KJ, Sadick M, Chuntharapai A, Hebert CA. Neutralization of IL-8 inhibits neutrophil influx in a rabbit model of endotoxin-induced pleurisy. J Immunol 1994; 152:2960–2967.

20. Donnelly SC, Strieter RM, Kunkel SL, Walz A, Robertson CR, Carter DC, Grant IS, Pollok AJ, Haslett C. Interleukin-8 and development of adult respiratory distress syndrome in at-risk patient groups. Lancet 1993; 341:643–647.

21. Rampart M, Van Damme J, Zonnekeyn L, Herman AG. Granulocyte chemotactic protein-interleukin-8 induces plasma leakage and neutrophil accumulation in rabbit skin. Am J Pathol 1989; 1345:21–30.

22. Miller EJ, Cohen AB, Nagao S, Griffith D, Maunder RJ, Martin TR, Wiener-Kronish JP, Sticherling M, Christophers E, Matthay MA. Elevated levels of NAP-1/interleukin-8 are present in the airspaces of patients with the adult respiratory distress syndrome and are associated with increased mortality. Am Rev Respir Dis 1992; 146:427–436.

23. Pittet JF, Mackersie RC, Martin TR, Matthay MA. Biological markers of acute lung injury: prognostic and pathogenetic significance. Am J Respir Crit Care Med 1997; 155:1187–1205.

24. Sherry B, Horii Y, Manogue KR, Widmer M, Cerami A. Macrophage inflammatory proteins 1 and 2: an overview. Cytokine 1992; 4:127–130.

25. VanOtteren GM, Strieter RM, Kunkel SL, Paine R, Greenberger MJ, Danforth JM, Burdick MD, Standiford TJ. Compartmentalized expression of RANTES in a murine model of endotoxemia. J Immunol 1995; 154:1900–1908.

26. Strieter RM, Kunkel SL, Showell HJ, Marks RM. Monokine-induced gene expression of human endothelial cell-derived neutrophil chemotactic factor. Biochem Biophys Res Comm 1988; 156:1340–1345.

27. Strieter RM, Kunkel SL, Showell H, Remick DG, Phan SH, Ward PA, Marks RM. Endothelial cell gene expression of a neutrophil chemotactic factor by TNF, LPS, and IL-1. Science 1989a; 243:1467–1469.

28. Strieter RM, Phan SH, Showell HJ, Remick DG, Lynch JP, Genard M, Raiford C, Eskandari M, Marks RM, Kunkel SL. Monokine-induced neutrophil chemotactic factor gene expression in human fibroblasts. J Biol Chem 1989b; 264:10621–10626.

29. Thornton AJ, Strieter RM, Lindley I, Baggiolini M, Kunkel SL. Cytokine-induced gene expression of a neutrophil chemotactic factor/interleukin-8 by human hepatocytes. J Immunol 1990; 144:2609–2613.

30. Brown Z, Strieter RM, Chensue SW, Ceska P, Lindley I, Nield GH, Kunkel SL, Westwick J. Cytokine activated human mesangial cells generate the neutrophil chemoattractant – interleukin 8. Kidney Int 40:86–90.

31. Rolfe MW, Kunkel SL, Standiford TJ, Chensue SW, Allen RM, Evanoff HL, Phan SH, Strieter RM. Pulmonary fibroblast expression of interleukin-8: a model for alveolar macrophage-derived cytokine networking. Am J Respir Cell Mol Biol 1991; 5:493–501.

32. Thornton AJ, Ham J, Kunkel SL. Kupffer cell–derived cytokines induce the synthesis of a leukocyte chemotactic peptide, interleukin-8, in human hepatoma and primary hepatocyte cultures. Hepatol 1991; 14:1112–1122.

33. Chensue SW, Terebuh PD, Remick DG, Scales WE, Kunkel SL. In vivo biologic and immunohistochemical analysis of interleukin-1 alpha, beta and tumor necrosis factor during experimental endotoxemia. Am J Pathol 1991; 138:395–402.

34. Baker CC, Chaudry IH, Gaines HO, Baue AE. Evaluation of factors affecting mortality rate after sepsis in a murine cecal ligation puncture model. Surgery 1983; 94:331–335.

5

Pulmonary Pathophysiology in ARDS

Keith R. Walley and James A. Russell

Introduction

It is worthwhile to consider briefly the transport of oxygen from the air we breathe to the mitochondria. The first step of transport is just bulk flow of air into the lungs and ultimately into the alveoli so that oxygen is delivered to the alveolar capillary membrane. This bulk flow of oxygen is achieved by ventilation of the lungs. The next step in transport is diffusion of oxygen from the alveoli into blood contained within the pulmonary capillary bed. The pulmonary capillaries are different from the tubelike capillaries of the systemic circulation. Pulmonary capillaries are instead like sheets of blood surrounding air-filled alveoli, maximizing surface area for diffusion. Oxygen diffuses down a pressure gradient from the alveoli to the capillary blood where, for the most part, oxygen is bound to hemoglobin in red blood cells. The next step in gas transport is again bulk flow, accomplished by pumping blood by the heart from the lungs to the systemic capillary bed. Then oxygen diffuses from capillary blood across the capillary wall into the tissues. Oxygen content in many tissues is increased by the presence of oxygen-carrying molecules such as myoglobin. These molecules decrease the resistance to oxygen flow in the tissue beds and therefore facilitate diffusion of oxygen to even the most distant cells. Oxygen in the tissues then readily diffuses to the mitochondria where it acts as an electron acceptor for the electron transport chain at the final stage of ATP production.

The lungs perform the first two steps in this chain of oxygen transport. Thus, the

James A. Russell and Keith R. Walley, eds. *Acute Respiratory Distress Syndrome*. Printed in the United States of America. Copyright © 1999. Cambridge University Press. All rights reserved.

two main functions of the lungs are (1) ventilation, and (2) to provide a surface for diffusion of oxygen into, and carbon dioxide out of, the blood.

This chapter discusses pulmonary physiology and approaches to monitoring of the respiratory system of patients who have ARDS. First, transport of oxygen from the alveolus to pulmonary capillary blood is discussed. Then we review causes of arterial hypoxemia. Measurements that can be made in the ICU to assess adequacy of oxygenation are examined. Then we discuss oxygen measurements to assess lung function versus assessment of oxygen delivery. We then present the effects of PEEP on oxygenation. Next we review ventilation, its unique relation to arterial PCO_2, the causes of hypoventilation, and measurements that can be made in the ICU to assess adequacy of ventilation. Patients with ARDS have substantial changes in pulmonary mechanics that are directly or indirectly related to impaired gas exchange. Therefore, we then discuss pulmonary mechanics and measurements of compliance, resistance, pressure-volume relationships, and intrinsic PEEP. Respiratory muscle function is required to drive the respiratory system so we next discuss measures of respiratory muscle strength and endurance. Finally, we consider respiratory muscle drive and bedside physiologic measures to assess this.

Gas Transport across the Alveolar–Capillary Membrane

Fick's law states that diffusion across the alveolar-capillary membrane depends on the oxygen partial pressure difference across the membrane, the area of the membrane (A), the diffusivity of the gas in the membrane (D), and depends inversely on membrane thickness (T). Thus, Fick's law is as follows:

$$\text{Oxygen flux} = (P_AO_2 - P_{cap}O_2) \times A \times D/T \qquad \text{(Eq. 1)}$$

where P_AO_2 is the alveolar partial pressure of oxygen and $P_{cap}O_2$ is the pulmonary capillary partial pressure of oxygen. Diffusivity of a gas is a physical constant proportional to the solubility of the gas in the membrane divided by the square root of its molecular weight. The area for diffusion and the thickness of the membrane depend on anatomy. Thus, in the lung, transport of oxygen from the alveoli to the capillaries depends heavily on the pressure gradient across the alveolar-capillary membrane. At partial pressure gradients observed in the lung, oxygen diffuses into the capillary and fully loads hemoglobin within approximately one-quarter of a second. The normal red blood cell transit time through the pulmonary capillaries is approximately three-quarters of a second.[1] Therefore, there is ample time for fully loading hemoglobin with oxygen.

Fick's law also applies to carbon dioxide elimination across the alveolar-capillary membrane. Carbon dioxide is more soluble than oxygen in the membrane so diffusion limitation is essentially never a problem with carbon dioxide. As a result, carbon dioxide elimination depends heavily on ventilation and, as discussed later, P_aCO_2 becomes an important marker of effectiveness of ventilation.

Arterial Hypoxemia

The important mechanisms contributing to arterial hypoxemia include (1) low alveolar PO_2 from a number of different causes including hypoventilation, (2) shunt of venous blood into the arterial circulation, and (3) ventilation-perfusion mismatching. Limitation of (4) oxygen diffusion is rarely a clinically important cause of arterial hypoxemia. Finally, in ARDS patients, (5) mixed venous oxygen desaturation can contribute substantially to arterial hypoxemia.

Decreased Alveolar PO_2 and Hypoventilation

Alveolar PO_2 can be decreased in a number of different ways. Alveolar PO_2 can be low due to a low inspired oxygen partial pressure, for example, at high altitudes where normal humans have significantly lower arterial PO_2 than humans living at sea level. In unusual instances people are exposed to gases with low oxygen partial pressure such as the air in an enclosed fire. This is a rare cause of arterial hypoxemia. Most frequently a low alveolar PO_2 is caused by hypoventilation.

Because nitrogen uses up almost four-fifths of the atmosphere by volume, only one-fifth remains for oxygen and carbon dioxide. The simplified alveolar gas equation describes how oxygen and carbon dioxide partition the non-nitrogen component of alveolar gas. Alveolar oxygen partial pressure, P_AO_2, is reduced as a result of elevated alveolar carbon dioxide partial pressure as follows:

$$P_AO_2 = P_iO_2 - P_aCO_2/R \qquad \text{(Eq. 2)}$$

where P_AO_2 is the partial pressure of oxygen in the alveolus. P_iO_2 is the partial pressure of oxygen in fully water-saturated inspired gas (partial pressure of water at body temperature is 47 mmHg) so that P_iO_2 equals $FiO_2 \times$ (barometric pressure – 47) mmHg. P_aCO_2 is the arterial partial pressure of carbon dioxide. R is the respiratory quotient (equals rate of carbon dioxide production divided by rate of oxygen consumption). Thus, when P_aCO_2 rises, P_AO_2 must decrease. A decrease in alveolar PO_2 results in a decrease in arterial PO_2 (P_aO_2). P_aCO_2 is inversely proportional to alveolar ventilation. Thus, hypoventilation results in an elevated P_aCO_2 and, according to the alveolar gas equation, a decrease in alveolar PO_2. This effect can be overcome in a number of ways. Steps can be taken to increase alveolar ventilation, including using assisted mechanical ventilation. In addition, inspired gas with a lower partial pressure of nitrogen means a greater fraction of barometric pressure is available to accommodate both oxygen and carbon dioxide within the alveolus. Hence, high FiO_2 can be used in selected cases as an adjunct to mechanical ventilation in treating alveolar hypoventilation. For example, all else being equal, increasing the inspired oxygen fraction from 21% to 100% increases alveolar ventilation by oxygen by about five times. However, excessively high inspired oxygen concentrations may detrimentally increase dead space, decrease the drive to breathe, and have an adverse impact on patients with chronically elevated P_aCO_2.

Shunt

Shunting of mixed venous blood directly into the pulmonary veins can be an important contributor to arterial hypoxemia. Significant shunt occurs in ARDS where pulmonary arterial blood shunts past flooded and collapsed alveoli into pulmonary veins. Direct shunt of poorly oxygenated pulmonary arterial blood into pulmonary veins has a particularly dramatic effect on arterial PO_2 due to the nonlinear oxygen-hemoglobin dissociation curve. Consider a 50% mixture of oxygenated blood from functioning alveoli having an oxygen saturation (SO_2) of 100% being combined with deoxygenated venous blood having SO_2 of 60%. This half-and-half mixture will result in arterial blood with S_aO_2 very close to 80%. Because of the curvilinear oxygen-hemoglobin dissociation curve, a reduction in S_aO_2 by 20% results in far greater than a 20% reduction in P_aO_2. The PO_2 of 80% saturated blood is approximately 40 mmHg. Thus, shunting of the poorly oxygenated venous blood into the arterial circulation is often a significant contributor to arterial hypoxemia in ARDS.

The physiologic shunt fraction (Q_S/Q_T, where Q_T is cardiac output), which includes true shunt and the effective shunt due to V/Q mismatch (see later), can be calculated from arterial oxygen content (C_aO_2) and mixed venous oxygen content (C_vO_2):

$$Q_S/Q_T = (C_AO_2 - C_aO_2)/(C_AO_2 - C_vO_2) \qquad \text{(Eq. 3)}$$

where C_AO_2 is oxygen content of maximally saturated alveolar end-capillary blood. C_vO_2 measurement is possible when a pulmonary artery catheter is placed so that mixed venous oxygen saturation can be measured using reflectance oximetry, or mixed venous blood can be sampled and oxygen saturation measured directly.

Because almost all of the oxygen in the blood is carried by hemoglobin (there is a small fraction of dissolved oxygen), oxygen contents can be replaced by oxygen saturations to give a rapid rough approximation of the shunt fraction:

$$Q_S/Q_T \sim (1 - S_aO_2)/(1 - S_vO_2) \qquad \text{(Eq. 4)}$$

V/Q Mismatch

The most important cause of clinically significant arterial hypoxemia is V/Q mismatch. That is, oxygen ventilation of alveoli does not adequately match blood perfuson of adjacent alveolar capillaries. As a result some regions have ventilation in excess of perfusion and other regions have perfusion in excess of ventilation. The regions with excess ventilation contribute to dead space; the regions with excess perfusion in relation to ventilation contribute to physiologic shunt. Physiologic shunt contributes in exactly the same way to arterial hypoxemia as true shunt. V/Q mismatch occurs in areas of diseased lung evident on chest radiographs and also occurs in apparently normal areas. For example, in lobar pneumonia significant V/Q mismatch occurs in radiographically normal areas of the lung. V/Q mismatch is similarly a very important cause of arterial hypoxemia in ARDS.

Diffusion Limitation

A potential theoretical cause of arterial hypoxemia is diffusion limitation due to decreased lung surface area for gas exchange, increased thickness of the alveolar-capillary membrane, or exceedingly short pulmonary capillary transit times. However, in practice this mechanism of hypoxemia is rarely clinically significant and, in particular, diffusion limitation is not a cause of hypoxemia in ARDS. Carbon monoxide or nitric oxide can be used to measure the diffusing capacity of lungs of patients having ARDS. Diffusing capacity reflects the surface area for diffusion and, to a much lesser extent, the thickness of the alveolar capillary membrane. Although significant reductions can be found in the diffusing capacity of the lungs of patients with ARDS,[2] diffusion limitation of oxygen transport from alveoli to blood only becomes the limiting step to overall gas transport in exceptional circumstances. During maximal exercise at high altitude the transit time of blood through the pulmonary capillaries can become shorter than the loading time of oxygen onto hemoglobin, resulting in diffusion limitation.[3] Similarly, when transit times of red cells in pulmonary capillaries are short in the setting of lung disease it is possible that diffusion limitation contributes to arterial hypoxemia.[4] However, in almost all other circumstances, diffusion does not limit gas transport as demonstrated by studies using gases with very high diffusivity compared to oxygen. Thus, diffusion limitation is not generally an important mechanism of arterial hypoxemia.

Mixed Venous Oxygen Desaturation

A final important cause of arterial hypoxemia in ARDS patients is mixed venous oxygen desaturation. If mixed venous oxygen saturation is decreased in the setting of a high shunt fraction (both true shunt and physiologic shunt from V/Q mismatch), then desaturated venous blood mixing with oxygenated blood from functioning lung units can decrease arterial saturation substantially (see Figure 6.8 in Chapter 6). The corollary is that increasing mixed venous oxygen saturation can be a very effective approach to improving arterial oxygen saturation in hypoxemic ARDS patients.

Mixed venous oxygen saturation is set by the difference between whole body oxygen delivery and the fraction of whole body oxygen delivery that is consumed by the body (see Chapter 6). In shock, decreased oxygen delivery and unchanged oxygen consumption cause a decrease in mixed venous oxygen saturation because of increased oxygen extraction by peripheral tissue (Figure 5.1). Conversely, increasing whole body oxygen delivery means that oxygen consumption is a smaller fraction of the total resulting in a higher mixed venous oxygen saturation. That is, increasing whole body oxygen delivery decreases the oxygen extraction ratio (Figure 5.1) so that mixed venous oxygen saturation increases. In addition, minimizing whole body oxygen consumption can increase mixed venous oxygen saturation. Clinical approaches to correcting mixed venous oxygen desaturation, in order to improve arterial hypoxemia, include a combination of increasing cardiac output and oxygen-carrying capacity of the blood (e.g., transfusion) together with minimizing whole body oxygen consumption using sedation and paralysis if necessary.

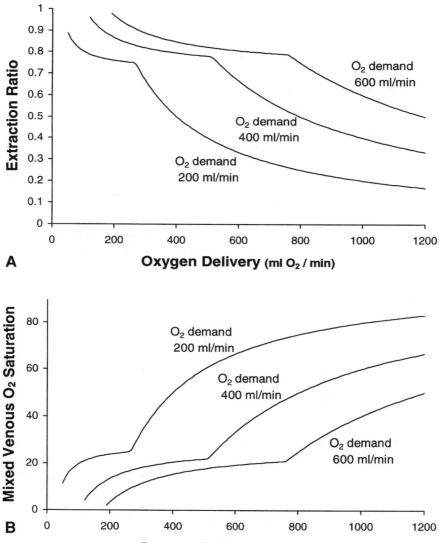

Figure 5.1. (A) illustrates that as oxygen delivery (= cardiac output × oxygen saturation × oxygen-carrying capacity of the blood) decreases, the fraction of oxygen extracted (extraction ratio) increases to maintain whole body oxygen consumption at the level of oxygen demand. Above an extraction ratio of approximately 0.75, the oxygen extraction ratio cannot increase sufficiently for oxygen consumption to be sufficient to meet oxygen demand, resulting in the onset of anaerobic metabolism. (B) illustrates that mixed venous oxygen saturation decreases as oxygen delivery decreases. At greater values of oxygen demand, the oxygen extraction ratio increases and mixed venous oxygen saturation decreases so that the onset of anaerobic metabolism (notch in the curves) occurs at an increased oxygen delivery.

Clinical Assessment of Oxygenation

In early, severe ARDS, difficulties in oxygenation can be the major physiologic change that requires careful assessment, titration of therapy, and assiduous monitoring.

Pulse and Reflectance Oximetry

Continuous oximetry has become the fifth vital sign in critically ill patients because it is noninvasive, readily available, and used in ERs, ORs, ICUs, and even on cruise ships. Measurement of two or more wavelengths of reflected or transmitted light through the skin allows estimation of arterial oxygen saturation. Lightweight probes attached to a finger or earlobe measure transmitted infrared light at wavelengths appropriate for delineation of the hemoglobin absorption spectrum. The pulsatile component of absorption corresponds to arterial blood and hence arterial oxygen saturation can be deduced. Current oximeters determine arterial oxygen saturation to within a few percentage points when arterial oxygen saturation is greater than approximately 80%. At lower oxygen saturations, transmission oximeters are less accurate. Inaccurate values of oxygen saturation may be caused by shock, where very limited peripheral perfusion may result in low capillary and venous oxygen saturation falsely decreasing the estimate of arterial oxygen saturation; by carboxyhemoglobin, methemoglobinemia, or in sickle-cell disease where shifts of the oxygen-hemoglobin dissociation curve invalidate the mathematical assumptions made by the oximeter computer in calculating oxygen saturation from light absorption; by some clinically used dyes that absorb wavelengths of light used by cooximeters (e.g., methylene blue); and by deep skin pigmentation.

Continuous oximetry results in rapid detection of periods of arterial oxygen desaturation. When clinically significant, a simultaneous arterial blood gas determination is useful in confirming the oximeter finding. Continuous oximetry can reduce the frequency of arterial blood gas sampling by eliminating the need for "routine" arterial blood gas sampling.[5] Because hypoxemia is difficult to detect clinically, continuous oximetry greatly increases detection of episodes of hypoxemia and leads to fewer adverse sequela of hypoxemia, including myocardial ischemia postoperatively.[6]

Arterial Blood Gas Analysis

Arterial blood gas analysis is one of the cornerstones of assessment and management of ARDS patients. Key features to be kept in mind in obtaining accurate and useful results include anaerobic collection and transport of blood samples, recording the FiO_2 at the time of sampling, rapid analysis with a calibrated blood gas machine, transporting blood gas samples on ice if there is any significant time delay, and temperature correction of the blood gas results where appropriate. Arterial blood gas samples should be taken only after 15 to 20 minutes of equilibration on current ventilator settings if the blood gas analysis is expected to reflect those ventilator settings.

Blood gas analysis measures PO_2, PCO_2, and pH. All other values reported in addition to these measured values are calculated and are therefore based on assumptions that frequently are incorrect in critically ill patients. For example, oxygen saturation is often estimated from PO_2 based on the oxygen-hemoglobin dissociation curve corrected for pH, PCO_2 and temperature. This estimate is reasonably accurate for oxygen saturations > 80% but makes significant errors at lower oxygen saturations. Therefore, this is not an appropriate method for determining mixed venous oxygen saturation or for measuring arterial oxygen saturation in profoundly hypoxemic patients.

Oxygen Saturation Measurement

Arterial blood samples can also be sent for cooximeter measurement of oxygen saturation, carboxyhemoglobin saturation, and methemoglobin saturation where these measurements are clinically appropriate. Cooximeters measure absorption by the blood of approximately four different wavelengths of light to distinguish between different hemoglobin species. Thus, cooximeter measurements yield values for total hemoglobin and the fraction of hemoglobin that is oxygenated, reduced, carboxyhemoglobin, and methemoglobin. Oxygen saturation measurement is particularly important when low arterial saturations are anticipated or for mixed venous samples, as indicated earlier. In this setting oxygen saturations fall within the steep midportion of the oxygen-hemoglobin dissociation curve (Figure 5.2) so that small shifts in the curve can result in significant errors in estimating oxygen saturation from P_aO_2. Shifts in the oxygen-hemoglobin dissociation curve occur commonly in critically ill patients. Therefore, direct cooximeter measurement of oxygen saturation is necessary.

Effect of Increasing FiO_2

An important difference between true and physiologic shunt is that true shunt does not respond to increasing the inspired oxygen fraction because blood that does not come close to alveolar gas with high FiO_2 will not benefit by increasing inspired FiO_2. Thus, increasing FiO_2, possibly to toxic levels, is of little or no benefit in ARDS patients with high true shunt fractions. The diagnostic corollary is that when changes in FiO_2 that are reliably delivered to the lungs in hemodynamically stable patients do not substantially increase S_aO_2, the presence of a high right-to-left shunt fraction should be suspected. However, in the setting of V/Q mismatch when FiO_2 is increased, the alveolar ventilation of oxygen increases (total alveolar ventilation is unchanged but the fraction that is oxygen increases) so that many lung units with previously low V/Q ratios now normalize their oxygen ventilation-perfusion ratios, resulting in improvement of physiologic shunt. Thus, contrasting these two causes of hypoxemia, true shunt is not responsive to changes in FiO_2, whereas V/Q mismatch is very responsive.

True shunt can be estimated therefore by placing patients on 100% FiO_2. However, an adverse effect of ventilation with very high FiO_2 is that the partial pressure

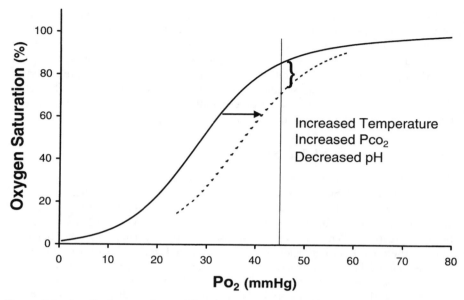

Figure 5.2. A stylized oxygen-hemoglobin dissociation curve is illustrated as a solid curve. At high PO_2 (> 60 mmHg) further increases in PO_2 do not result in substantial increases in oxygen saturation because oxygen saturation is already high. At low PO_2 (< 50 mmHg) the oxygen-hemoglobin dissociation curve is steep so that small changes in PO_2 can substantially alter oxygen saturation.

The oxygen-hemoglobin dissociation curve can be shifted by a number of factors common in critically ill patients. For example, hyperthermia, hypercapnia, and acidosis shift the curve to the right. This is particularly important for the steep middle section of the curve (low PO_2) because the same low PO_2 (e.g., 45 mmHg, thin vertical line) can indicate a range of oxygen saturations (curved bracket) that range from low but acceptable to fatal. It follows that at low PO_2, oxygen saturation must be directly measured using a cooximeter.

of nitrogen in the blood decreases so the ensuing absorption of nitrogen from alveoli results in absorption atelectasis, which can increase physiologic and true shunt.

Which Measures Reflect Lung Function and Which Reflect Blood Oxygenation?

P_aO_2 is often interpreted as a measure of lung function – a low P_aO_2 is interpreted as impaired gas transport in the lung. However, P_aO_2 is also frequently used as a measure of adequacy of arterial oxygenation and, by inference, a measure of adequacy of tissue oxygenation. It is important to recognize that these two uses are distinct. It is even more important to recognize that P_aO_2 has serious limitations in both cases and that other measures should be used in ARDS patients.

Depending on the degree of V/Q mismatch and shunt, P_aO_2 varies with FiO_2 in a variable way. Therefore, clinicians tend to use the alveolar-arterial oxygen partial pressure difference ($AaDO_2$) or the P_aO_2/FiO_2 ratio to assess oxygen exchange across the lungs in ventilated patients. Indeed, all recent multicenter randomized controlled trials of new therapy for ARDS use the P_aO_2/FiO_2 ratio as the oxygenation inclusion criterion. Also, the European-American Consensus Conference definition[7] of ARDS uses the P_aO_2/FiO_2 ratio as follows:

	Mild	Moderate abnormality	Acute lung injury	ARDS	Severe ARDS
P_aO_2/FiO_2 Ratio	< 500	< 400	< 300	< 200	< 100

Adequate delivery of oxygen to the tissues depends on cardiac output, oxygen-carrying capacity of the blood (i.e., hemoglobin concentration), and arterial oxygen saturation.[8] Thus, arterial oxygen saturation is a key clinically useful component of oxygen delivery. P_aO_2 is less useful than arterial oxygen saturation to assess blood oxygenation because the oxygen-hemoglobin dissociation curve can shift substantially in critically ill patients (Figure 5.2). As a result, large changes in P_aO_2 when P_aO_2 is relatively high have little or no clinical significance because S_aO_2 does not change much. In contrast, a P_aO_2 of 50 mmHg can represent adequate arterial oxygen saturation when the oxygen-hemoglobin dissociation curve is left-shifted, whereas the same P_aO_2 can represent serious arterial oxygen desaturation when the oxygen-hemoglobin dissociation curve is right-shifted (e.g., by hypercapnia, acidosis, or hyperthermia) (Figure 5.2).

What Is the Target P_aO_2 or S_aO_2 in ARDS Patients?

Surprisingly, the lower limits for acceptable oxygen saturation are not known. Many intensivists seem to accept $S_aO_2 > 90\%$ or $P_aO_2 > 60$ mmHg as a lower limit below which they would increase FiO_2, increase PEEP, or intervene in other ways. It is important to recognize that S_aO_2 and P_aO_2 do not stand alone as clinical endpoints. P_aO_2 is not as useful as S_aO_2, as discussed earlier. Adequate tissue oxygenation depends on adequate oxygen delivery, which is the product of cardiac output, oxygen-carrying capacity of the blood (i.e., hemoglobin concentration), and S_aO_2. Therefore, a low S_aO_2 in the setting of low cardiac output and anemia (oxygen delivery would be very low) has a much greater clinical significance than when cardiac output and hemoglobin concentration are normal or high (oxygen delivery would be somewhat low or normal).

Acute reductions in S_aO_2 have more severe physiologic consequences than do chronic reductions in S_aO_2, which are often surprisingly well tolerated. In the setting of normal cardiac output and hemoglobin, acute reduction in S_aO_2 below 70% results in sudden death in animal studies.[9] With this in mind, our current clinical practice is to maintain $S_aO_2 > 90\%$ as our oxygenation goal during initial evaluation and management of ARDS patients. When the patient has been stabilized and more clinical data is available, we then balance the need for high FiO_2 and high ventilatory pressures with the possible detriment of these interventions. When cardiac output and hemoglobin are not low we accept $S_aO_2 > 85\%$ when necessary to avoid toxic FiO_2 ($> 60\%$) and to reduce ventilator pressures to avoid barotrauma and ventilator-induced worsening of lung injury. We do not make this our oxygenation goal in all patients – only in those where very significant risk is incurred by persisting with high FiO_2 and high ventilator pressures. Very occasionally in patients with prolonged severe ARDS we have accepted lower S_aO_2 goals when safe alternative approaches were not available. In all of these instances careful attention to oxygen delivery (including cardiac output and hemoglobin concentration) is essential.

PEEP

The clinical application of PEEP is discussed in Chapter 7. Positive end-expiratory pressure prevents alveolar pressure from falling to atmospheric pressure during exhalation so that functional residual capacity (FRC) is increased. PEEP is helpful in ARDS because ARDS is characterized by low FRC due to flooded and collapsed alveoli. In ARDS patients FRC is increased by positive airway pressure largely by recruitment of previously flooded alveoli. PEEP results in redistribution of alveolar edema fluid to the corners between the walls of the alveoli – because the radius of curvature is shortest at the corners so that surface tension is highest.[10] This means that on PEEP, alveolar walls are exposed for gas exchange. PEEP does not by itself reduce pulmonary edema. As discussed later, the lower inflection point on the pressure-volume curve of the lung (Figure 5.3) gives an estimate of the pressure at which most recruitable alveoli are open. Thus, one ventilator strategy chooses a tidal volume of around 6 mL/kg and PEEP to equal or slightly exceed the pressure at the lower inflection point.[11]

Similar to the application of PEEP, increasing airway pressure throughout the respiratory cycle can increase arterial oxygenation by recruiting flooded and collapsed alveoli. This can be accomplished by increasing the inspiratory fraction of the respiratory cycle (i.e., inspiratory time : total time = T_I/T_{TOT}) associated with increased airway pressure. Increasing the inspiratory fraction decreases the time for exhalation, which contributes to the development of intrinsic PEEP (see later). However, note that externally applied PEEP, intrinsic PEEP, and high inspiratory pressures are all associated with barotrauma and impaired venous return. Therefore, the beneficial effects of increasing airway pressures on arterial oxygenation must be balanced by the detrimental effects. Thus, another reasonable strategy for managing PEEP in ARDS patients is to choose a tidal volume of 6 to 8 mL/kg and the lowest PEEP that results in adequate arterial oxygenation and adequate cardiac output at a nontoxic FiO_2.

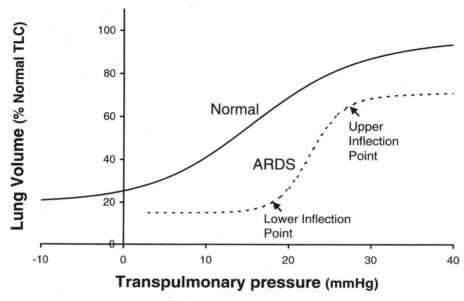

Figure 5.3. Pressure-volume curves of the normal lung and the lung in ARDS are illustrated. Transpulmonary pressure is the difference between airway opening pressure (mouth pressure in normals) and pleural pressure. In the mechanically ventilated patient pleural pressure is often not measured, and airway opening pressure serves as a surrogate of transpulmonary pressure. The relationship is curvilinear, characterized by a slope (a measure of compliance), a lower inflection point, and an upper inflection point. ARDS results in stiffer lungs (right-shifted relationship) with a decreased total lung capacity (TLC). In ARDS the lower inflection point occurs at an airway pressure of 15 to 20 mmHg. The compliance (slope) is low below the lower inflection point because alveoli are flooded and collapsed. The compliance is low above the upper inflection point because alveoli are fully open and distended so that the lung is stiff. One ventilator strategy is to choose PEEP at the lower inflection point value and to limit tidal volumes so that the upper inflection point is not exceeded on inspiration. This is usually accomplished by tidal volumes of 6 to 8 ml/kg.

Hypercapnia and Hypoventilation

In early severe ARDS when hypoxemia is marked, patients can go through a phase of hyperventilation and increased work of breathing. If sustained, respiratory muscle fatigue can complicate the primary parenchymal lung injury and lead to secondary hypoventilation, hypercapnia, and respiratory acidosis. This is an ominous sign that is often followed in short order by respiratory arrest. During the ICU course of ARDS, abrupt changes in P_aCO_2 while on mechanical ventilation must trigger a search for the complicating cause. Later in ARDS, increased work of breathing due to stiff lungs can impede weaning from mechanical ventilation. Thus, a rational clinical approach to hypercapnia and hypoventilation is fundamental in managing ARDS patients.

Breathing results in tidal ventilation of the lungs, which brings oxygen to the alveoli and eliminates carbon dioxide. In normal humans a typical tidal volume is 500 mL ($\sim$ 6 mL/kg) at a rate of 10 to 15 breaths/minute. The important physiologic component of ventilation is alveolar ventilation. Ventilation of upper airways does not contribute to gas exchange and therefore is referred to as dead space. Anatomic dead space of the upper airways is approximately 150 mL. In addition, ventilation of poorly perfused and non-perfused alveoli results in physiologic dead space so that total dead space (V_D) is approximately one-third of the total tidal volume (V_T) in normal humans. Total dead space is the sum of anatomic and physiologic dead space. Anatomic dead space does not change appreciably so that at higher respiratory rates and lower tidal volumes the dead space fraction (V_D/V_T) increases. Conversely, at higher tidal volumes the dead space fraction decreases. ARDS patients can develop an increase in physiologic dead space such that V_D/V_T can exceed 60%. This change is characteristic of the later (2 to 3 week) phase of ARDS when oxygenation is often not a major problem. Indeed, a V_D/V_T greater than 0.6 requires an increased total minute ventilation to maintain P_aCO_2 and is therefore predictive of difficulty in weaning from mechanical ventilation.

Carbon dioxide is much more diffusible than oxygen, and inspired carbon dioxide partial pressure is approximately zero (zero inspired PCO_2 for carbon dioxide elimination is, in a way, analogous to an FiO_2 of 100% for oxygen uptake). Therefore diffusion limitation and V/Q mismatch have little effect on carbon dioxide transfer across the lungs. As a result arterial PCO_2 (P_aCO_2) is very dependent on alveolar ventilation so that:

$$P_aCO_2 = k \times VCO_2/V_A \qquad \text{(Eq. 5)}$$

where VCO_2 is whole body carbon dioxide production, V_A is alveolar ventilation, and k is a proportionality constant. Alveolar ventilation can be written as

$$V_A = (1 - V_D/V_T) \times V_T \times \text{respiratory rate} \qquad \text{(Eq. 6)}$$

Thus, the alveolar equation for CO_2 becomes

$$P_aCO_2 = k \times VCO_2/([1 - V_D/V_T] \times V_T \times \text{respiratory rate}) \qquad \text{(Eq. 7)}$$

This indicates that P_aCO_2 increases with increases in whole body carbon dioxide production, P_aCO_2 increases as the ratio of dead space to tidal volume increases, and P_aCO_2 increases with decreasing tidal volume and respiratory rate. These are clinically useful observations to make during physical examination of the patient and when adjusting ventilatory settings. For the clinician, it is relevant to remember that P_aCO_2 can be increased because of increased CO_2 production or decreased CO_2 elimination, or both. Decreased CO_2 elimination is caused by decreased alveolar ventilation.

Fever, ICU interventions (such as suctioning, turning, physiotherapy), seizures, and agitation can all increase CO_2 production by 10% to 20%. However, VCO_2 generally does not change much acutely in the hemodynamically stable patient. An important exception to this is that a sudden decrease in cardiac output from any cause decreases carbon dioxide delivery to the lungs so that VCO_2, end-tidal PCO_2, and P_aCO_2 can all decrease. Note however that mixed venous PCO_2 will increase.

Thus, based on the preceding discussion, an elevated PCO_2 is generally due to alveolar hypoventilation. To determine the cause of elevated P_aCO_2 due to alveolar hypoventiltion, follow a stepwise approach considering (1) central control of ventilation, (2) neuromuscular transmission of the drive-to-breathe signal, (3) the chest wall and ventilatory muscles, (4) the airways, and (5) the lungs (Table 5.1).

Central Hypoventilation

Central hypoventilation is clinically characterized by decreased respiratory effort (e.g., not triggering the ventilator) and a low respiratory rate (e.g., apnea alarm triggered when spontaneous breathing modes of mechanical ventilation are chosen) without evidence of increased ventilatory drive (e.g., anxiety and use of accessory muscles absent) and without the associated evidence of increased sympathetic tone (e.g., tachycardia and diaphoresis absent). These clinical features are in sharp contrast to clinical features of other causes of hypercapnia described later where ventilatory drive and sympathetic tone are greatly increased. Central hypoventilation can result from CNS disease, CNS depressant drugs, and hypothyroidism. In ARDS patients in the ICU, CNS depressant drugs, including narcotics and benzodiazepines, impair the normal ventilatory response to elevated PCO_2 or decreased pH and are very frequent contributors to respiratory acidosis due to central hypoventilation.

The central response to hypoventilation depends on PCO_2 and pH in blood and in the fourth ventricle, which superfuses the brainstem respiratory drive centers. Acute increases in P_aCO_2 or acute decreases in pH trigger substantial increases in ventilatory drive. In contrast, chronic respiratory or metabolic acidosis may not increase ventilatory drive to the same extent because equilibration of PCO_2 and pH with brainstem respiratory centers occurs over the course of days.

Metabolic alkalosis blunts central drive in response to an elevated P_aCO_2. This effect is minor in young previously healthy patients, but metabolic alkalosis can contribute significantly to central hypoventilation in many critically ill patients, particularly those with preexisting cardiopulmonary disease. Whether and when metabolic alkalosis should be treated with bicarbonate wasting diuretics like acetazolamide is unclear. Certainly underlying causes and contributors, such as hypokalemia and hypomagnesemia,[12] should be corrected. A modest degree of metabolic alkalosis, and the compensatory hypercapnia, has not been shown to adversely affect outcome. Metabolic alkalosis has the interesting effect of decreasing the ventilatory requirement for a given whole body CO_2 production rate (VCO_2) which, in some instances, can be beneficial.

Table 5.1. Causes of and contributors to hypoventilation

Central drive

CNS disease, sedatives, hypothyroidism, obesity-hypoventilation syndromes, Ondine's curse

Neuromuscular transmission

Cervical spine injury
Motor neuron
    Phrenic nerve injury, polio, amyotrophic lateral sclerosis
Demyelinating diseases
    Guillain-Barré
Neuromuscular junction
    Neuromuscular blocking agents, myasthenia gravis, Eaton-Lambert syndrome, amino-
    glycoside antibiotics, botulism, tetanus

Chest wall and respiratory muscles

Chest wall
    Emphysema, kyphoscoliosis, obesity, chest wall edema, flail chest
Respiratory muscles
    Polymyositis, steroid myopathy, hypokalemia, hypomagnesemia, hypophospatemia, mal-
    nutrition, sepsis, shock, hypercapnia, acidosis, fatigue

Airways

Endotracheal tube
    Inadequate diameter, dried secretions or blood, kinking
Large airways
Laryngeal edema, bilateral vocal cord paralysis, tracheal edema, extratracheal compression by
    hematoma or mass
Peripheral airways
    Asthma, COPD, Airway edema

Lungs

Decreased compliance
    Pulmonary fibrosis, pulmonary edema, pneumonia
Increased dead space
    Late phase ARDS, hypovolemia, pulmonary embolism
Ineffective ventilation
    Pneumothorax, right mainstem intubation

Increased CO_2 production requiring increased ventilation

Excessive muscle work, seizures, fever, sepsis, overfeeding

Neuromuscular Causes

Transmission of the drive-to-breathe signal from the brain to the respiratory muscles is the next step in the normal regulation of ventilation. A cervical spine injury or bilateral phrenic nerve injury can result in significant hypoventilation even though central drive to breathe is unimpaired. Polio and amyotrophic lateral sclerosis affect motor neuron transmission. Demyelinating diseases such as Guillain-Barré syndrome and (rarely) multiple sclerosis also affect motor neuron transmission. Transmission of the signal from nerve to muscle across the motor end plate is another potential site of impairment. Myasthenia gravis can impair signal transmission, an effect that can be exacerbated by the use of aminoglycoside antibiotics and by delayed clearance of neuromuscular blocking drugs. Botulism and tetanus can similarly impair normal transmission at the neuromuscular junction of the drive to breathe to respiratory muscles.

The Chest Wall and Respiratory Muscles

The next step in the ventilatory pathway that needs to be considered is the chest wall. A stiff or deformed chest wall can make ventilation difficult. Patients with emphysema have low flat diaphragms which are no longer in an anatomic configuration that allows them to ventilate the lungs easily. Patients with marked chest wall deformity (such as severe kyphoscoliosis) or significant emphysema frequently develop chronic respiratory acidosis with metabolic compensation. Obesity results in restriction of chest wall movement and is an important contributor to the work of breathing and hypoventilation.

The respiratory muscles themselves can be the cause of hypoventilation. Polymyositis, steroid myopathy, the myopathy associated with the combinations of neuromuscular blockers and steroids, and other diseases can contribute to respiratory muscle weakness. As discussed in Chapter 9, the muscle weakness syndromes associated with use of neuromuscular blockers can cause prolonged, severe muscle weakness that can complicate the course of ARDS and significantly prolong ventilation. Muscular dystrophy and other inherited myopathies likewise can contribute. Electrolyte abnormalities, including sometimes missed hypomagnesemia and hypophosphatemia, should be looked for. Malnutrition is among the most important reversible causes of respiratory muscle weakness in the ICU. Sepsis and the associated inflammatory response can decrease respiratory muscle strength. Shock may decrease respiratory muscle strength when oxygen delivery is inadequate to meet metabolic needs or when metabolic or respiratory acidosis develop. When respiratory muscles become fatigued by an excessive load, respiratory muscle function remains impaired for as long as 12 to 24 hours of rest.

The Airways

Airway obstruction due to asthma or reactive airways disease, airway edema in patients with congestive heart failure, upper airways obstruction, and obstruction of the endotracheal tube with secretions or by kinking all contribute to increased ventilatory load which, when it exceeds ventilatory capacity, can lead to hypoventilation. Physical examination reveals evidence of high central ventilatory drive with high respiratory rate, anxiety, tachycardia, diaphoresis, accessory muscle use, intercostal indrawing, and paradoxical inspiratory abdominal movement. Clinically significant pulsus paradoxus is observed because highly negative intrathoracic pressure during inspiration lowers both systolic and diastolic arterial pressure. Polyphonic expiratory wheezes over multiple lung fields suggest asthma, reactive airways disease, and small airway edema. Inspiratory stridor suggests extrathoracic upper airways obstruction. Inspiratory stridor and a monophonic expiratory wheeze suggests a fixed large airway obstruction. A monophonic wheeze only on expiration over central airways suggests variable intrathoracic large airway obstruction possibly due to dynamic central airway collapse during forceful expiration. Difficulty passing a suction catheter should prompt further evaluation of the endotracheal tube (e.g., bronchoscopy).

The Lungs

Finally, lung disease needs to be considered as a cause of elevated P_aCO_2. Diseases that increase V_D/V_T mean that increased total ventilation is required to maintain the same alveolar ventilation. Diseases that increase work of breathing put extra load on the respiratory muscle so that hypoventilation ensues. Late-phase ARDS does both. After the acute phase of ARDS, progressive fibrosis replaces the normal alveolar architecture. The result is increased dead space and decreased pulmonary compliance. To maintain a normal P_aCO_2 high minute ventilation is required, which is difficult to achieve in the face of decreased pulmonary compliance. Other pulmonary causes of ineffective ventilation and increased P_aCO_2 to be considered in ARDS patients include pneumothorax and right mainstem intubation.

Measures of Ventilation

From Equation 7 it can be seen that important measures in assessing P_aCO_2 and ventilation include respiratory rate, tidal volume (their product which is minute ventilation), V_D/V_T, and VCO_2. Respiratory rate, tidal volume, and minute ventilation are values that are almost always displayed by the mechanical ventilator. These values can be confirmed by measurements at the bedside using a watch and hand-held spirometer.

By collecting exhaled gas, V_D/V_T can be calculated as follows. Gas in the alveolar dead space has a PCO_2 of approximately zero, and this gas mixes with alveolar gas on exhalation so that mixed exhaled gas has a lower PCO_2 than alveolar PCO_2 depending on the dead space to tidal volume ratio.

$$V_D/V_T = (P_aCO_2 - P_ECO_2)/P_aCO_2 \qquad \text{(Eq. 8)}$$

where P_ECO_2 is PCO_2 in mixed exhaled gas. Exhaled gas is collected in a compliant balloon (Douglas bag) over multiple breaths (e.g., 5 minutes) to provide a sample of mixed exhaled gas. P_ECO_2 is measured in this gas, for example, by using a blood gas machine. Together with a simultaneous arterial blood gas measurement V_D/V_T is calculated using Equation 8. Because V_T is known, V_D can be calculated.

Oxygen Consumption and Carbon Dioxide Production

Oxygen consumption and carbon dioxide production can be measured at the bedside using analysis of expired gas. Metabolic carts compute the difference in oxygen and CO_2 delivered from inhaled gases to that removed in exhaled gas. Minute-by-minute oxygen consumption and CO_2 production can be displayed at the bedside. In most patients, oxygen consumption is very stable. In very hemodynamically unstable patients with clinical evidence of shock, oxygen consumption can be reduced when whole body oxygen delivery is so low that metabolic needs for oxygen are not met (see Chapter 6). When oxygen consumption is reduced in this way, oxygen delivery to the whole body must be restored immediately; otherwise death ensues within minutes to hours.[13] More often, oxygen consumption measurements in the ICU are used to estimate metabolic demand so that caloric requirements in feeds can be reasonably accurately calculated. Estimates of CO_2 production and the calculation of RQ (RQ = VCO_2/VO_2) can be used to identify overfeeding. When RQ is greater than 1, then some CO_2 production must come from nonenergy producing metabolic pathways such as lipogenesis as a result of overfeeding.

End tidal CO_2 measurement is another common bedside measurement that can contribute to noninvasive estimates of arterial CO_2 concentrations. Using a capnograph, CO_2 concentration in exhaled air is measured. At the end of expiration, the CO_2 in exhaled gas is alveolar gas, which is approximately in equilibrium with arterial CO_2 in patients with normal lungs. Thus, end tidal CO_2 measurement is a noninvasive estimate of P_aCO_2. End tidal CO_2 measurement is a less useful tool in estimating P_aCO_2 in ARDS patients with significant V/Q mismatch and dead space. V/Q mismatch decreases end tidal CO_2 measurement because alveolar CO_2 from well-perfused alveoli is mixed with CO_2 from nonperfused alveoli (physiologic dead space) even at the end of exhalation. Sudden reductions in end tidal CO_2 may occur with acute reduction in cardiac output due to pulmonary embolism, pneumothorax, or cardiac arrest.

Respiratory Mechanics in ARDS

Figure 5.3 illustrates the static pressure-volume relationships of the lung and chest wall. In nonventilated patients, transpulmonary pressure is positive because pleural pressure is negative so that alveolar pressure exceeds pleural pressure throughout the respiratory cycle. In the ventilated patient, transpulmonary pressure is kept positive primarily by positive airway pressure transmitted to alveoli. In the mechanically ventilated patient, pleural pressure can be negative during spontaneous respiratory efforts but can be positive at higher lung volumes and when the chest wall is relaxed.

The pressure-volume relationship is characterized by a slope, Δ volume/Δ pressure, which is equal to compliance. The relationship is curvilinear with a sigmoid shape characterized by a lower concave-up inflection and an upper concave-down inflection. At low volumes below the "lower inflection point," the slope of the pressure-volume relationship is low, indicating stiff lungs. At this lung volume, alveoli are collapsed. Surface tension maintaining the collapsed state of alveoli makes these lung regions noncompliant and difficult to open. When the majority of alveoli are recruited and open, the pressure-volume relationship has its greatest slope. At higher lung volume, alveoli become overdistended and stiff so that once again the slope of the pressure-volume relationship is decreased. The transition to stiff, overdistended alveoli is termed the "upper inflection point."

In patients with ARDS, the pressure-volume relationship is shifted to the right and has, in general, a decreased slope indicating decreased lung compliance. Decreased compliance measured in patients with ARDS is initially mainly related to loss of the surface tension lowering effect of surfactant. There is little evidence of increased tissue elastance, although changes in chest wall mechanics can also contribute to decreased overall respiratory system compliance. Later in ARDS pulmonary fibrosis can contribute substantially to decreased compliance.

Note that when assessing airway pressure and tidal volumes clinically using the mechanical ventilator, the relationship of tidal volume to delivered airway pressure reflects total respiratory system compliance. Total respiratory system compliance includes both chest wall and lung compliance. Therefore a relatively low total respiratory system compliance can be caused by a stiff chest wall (e.g., abdominal distension, obesity, pneumothorax) and/or by stiff lungs. To separate the chest wall and lung components, an esophageal pressure measurement is necessary. Esophageal pressure is used as an indirect estimate of pleural pressure. However, this is not usually done for clinical purposes because it is rather cumbersome, somewhat invasive, and requires attention to technical detail to obtain accurate measurements of esophageal pressure.

Measurement of Compliance at the Bedside

Many current ventilators display breath-by-breath estimates of resistance and compliance derived from internal ventilator measurements of flow and airway pressure. Respiratory system and lung compliance and airways resistance can be calculated using similar principles at the bedside.

Compliance is defined by $\Delta V/\Delta P$. Because the pressure-volume relationship of the lung is curvilinear, any measurement of compliance depends very much on the start-

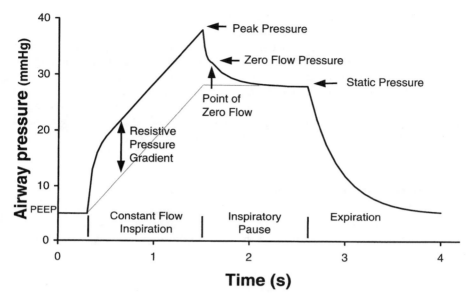

Figure 5.4. Contributions to airway pressure during constant flow positive pressure inspiration are shown. During constant flow inspiration the increase in pressure from the end-expiratory PEEP level is due to increased elastic recoil of the lungs and chest wall (light line) plus a resistive pressure gradient due to flow through the resistive airways and lung viscoelastance. Soon after an inspiratory pause is applied, flow falls to zero. The difference between peak pressure and zero flow pressure (i.e., 38 − 32 = 6 mmHg) is the pressure gradient across the airways resistance. Then pressure decays more slowly at zero flow to the static pressure. The difference between zero flow pressure and static pressure (i.e., 32 − 28 = 4 mmHg) is the pressure gradient during inspiration due to lung viscoelastance. Static pressure is the pressure due to the elastic recoil of the lungs and chest wall. All of these measurements are easily made by applying a pause during inspiration – usually at end-inspiration.

ing volume and the tidal volume (ΔV) chosen. The corresponding measurement of ΔP requires static measurements of airway pressures (i.e., no gas movement) because airway resistance and lung viscoelastance can contribute to a difference between airway opening pressure and alveolar pressure during inspiration; intrinsic PEEP can contribute to a difference between airway opening pressure and alveolar pressure at end-expiration (Figure 5.4). Ohm's law states that a pressure drop is equal to flow times resistance. Thus, when there is no airflow, the pressure drop across the airways is zero so that airway opening pressure approximates alveolar pressure. Inspiratory pressure (P_I) is determined during an end-inspiratory pause, and end-expiratory pressure (P_E) is determined during an end-expiratory pause. Then total compliance of the respiratory system (C) is calculated as follows:

$$C = V_T/(P_I - P_E) \qquad \text{(Eq. 9)}$$

It is important to recognize that this calculation assumes that pleural pressure is equal at end-inspiration and end-expiration. This is not strictly true and, in particular, is not even approximately true when the patient is making active respiratory efforts. Therefore, accurate calculation of compliance requires measurement of pleural pressure, which is reasonably well approximated by measuring esophageal pressure using an esophageal balloon catheter. When pleural pressure is subtracted from P_I and P_E, Equation 9 gives compliance of the lungs.

Measurement of Resistance at the Bedside

Airways with resistance require increased airway opening pressure, above that required to overcome elastic recoil of the lung, to drive air flow. Again, Ohm's law states that

$$\text{resistance} = \Delta P/\text{flow} \qquad \text{(Eq. 10)}.$$

Inspiratory flow can be set at a constant value using the assist control and several other ventilator modes. When this is done, ΔP is measured as the difference between airway pressure during constant flow inflation and airway pressure after an inspiratory pause is applied. Resistance is then calculated using Equation 10. Like compliance, resistance is also a nonlinear function so that the measured value of resistance depends on the flow rate. Calculated resistance increases as flow increases. Part of the increase in resistance is due to the increasing component of turbulent flow that occurs at higher flow rates.

During an end-inspiratory pause, the decay of airway pressure down to a static inspiratory pressure does not occur along a single exponential. At least two components can frequently be resolved so that there is a very rapid fall to an intermediate pressure at zero airway flow and then a slower exponential decay to the static inspiratory pressure. The rapid initial fall in airway pressure has been attributed to airways resistance, and the slower exponential decay in pressure has been attributed to pulmonary viscoelastance.[14] Total pulmonary resistance is the sum of airways resistance and pulmonary viscoelastance.

The endotracheal tube can contribute substantially to airways resistance. The resistance of the endotracheal tube depends on the length and cross-sectional area of the tube. The cross-sectional area of the tube can be reduced by inspissated secretions, blood, and by bending or kinking of the endotracheal tube. Endotracheal tubes with a diameter less than 7.5 are associated with very significant pressure drops of more than 5 cm H_2O pressure. During weaning from mechanical ventilation, this can have significant impact on the patient's work of breathing.

Measurement of Pressure-Volume Relationships at the Bedside

Pressure-volume relationships of the lung can be determined in heavily sedated or paralyzed mechanically ventilated patients in several ways. One approach at the bedside is to use a large (2L) air- or oxygen-filled syringe connected to the airway opening to measure semistatic airway pressure at a series of volumes above FRC. An alternative approach is to measure airway pressure during a brief end-inspiratory pause for a range of tidal volumes. The end-inspiratory pressure-volume points approximately define the pressure-volume relationship. Alternatively, during assist control ventilation, the dynamic pressure-volume relationship can be displayed on the bedside monitor. Although these dynamic measurements include resistive pressure gradients, evidence of excessively large tidal volumes can be visually derived. In the airway pressure versus time display, concave upward patterns at the end of inspiration suggest that volumes and pressures above the upper inflection point have been exceeded.

A rational ventilator strategy is to choose a level of PEEP approximately at the lower inflection point so that alveoli are not repeatedly opened and closed during the respiratory cycle.[11] A tidal volume is chosen small enough so that volumes and pressures do not exceed the upper inflection point. This strategy ventilates patients along the pressure-volume relationship where pulmonary compliance is highest. This approach attempts to avoid overdistending alveoli by ventilating at lung volumes below the upper inflection point and to avoid excessive closing and opening of collapsible alveoli by ventilating above the lower inflection point.

Intrinsic PEEP

The decrease in transpulmonary pressure during expiration occurs along approximately an exponential relationship. The decay half-life of this relationship depends on the product of airways resistance and pulmonary compliance. It follows that when expiratory resistance is high, when compliance is high, or at high respiratory rates, expiratory time is insufficient for complete exhalation to FRC. Incomplete exhalation is termed *dynamic hyperinflation,* and the positive end expiratory pressure in the alveoli due to dynamic hyperinflation is termed *intrinsic PEEP* or *auto PEEP.*

Intrinsic PEEP has exactly the same complications as externally applied PEEP.[15] Unrecognized intrinsic PEEP can contribute to barotrauma because airway pressure measurements do not adequately reflect elevated alveolar pressures which may lead to barotrauma. Intrinsic PEEP also acts in an identical manner to externally applied PEEP in impeding venous return to the heart and thus may contribute to decreased cardiac output and hypotension. On the positive side, intrinsic PEEP also improves oxygenation in the same way that externally applied PEEP does. In the spontaneously breathing patient with intrinsic PEEP, the patient's work of breathing can be greatly increased, even on a mechanical ventilator. First, the patient must reduce alveolar pressure further, from the intrinsic PEEP level to airway opening pressure, before any inspiratory airflow can occur, and then the patient must reduce alveolar pressures below airway opening pressure to draw in a normal tidal breath. The extra work in reducing alveolar pressure from the intrinsic PEEP level to airway opening pressure can contribute very substantially to the workload. In patients who have intrinsic PEEP who are taking spontaneous breaths on a mechanical ventilation mode such as assist-control or pressure-control, the patient must lower pressure to below the set sensitivity trigger value of the ventilator. So, if a patient has 10 cm of intrinsic PEEP, the externally applied PEEP is zero, and the sensitivity is set at −2 cm H_2O, then the patient must lower airway pressure from 10 to −2 cm H_2O, a difference of 12 cm H_2O, to open the inspiratory valve to obtain a tidal volume. Therefore, one clue to the presence of intrinsic PEEP in patients taking spontaneous breaths is increased work of breathing during inspiration. Addition of externally applied PEEP or CPAP reduces the amount of work the patient has to do to decrease the end-expiratory alveolar pressure to the externally applied airway pressure, and this can markedly decrease the work of breathing and increase patient comfort.

Intrinsic PEEP should be suspected when positive flow persists to the very end of exhalation. Intrinsic PEEP should also be suspected in patients breathing at high rates, patients with high airways resistance, or patients with increased lung compliance, for example, in patients with COPD. Total PEEP (which includes intrinsic PEEP and externally applied PEEP) can be measured at the bedside by applying an end-expiratory pause and measuring the airway pressure during zero airflow during this pause (Figure 5.5). Many current ventilators have built-in automated procedures to estimate total PEEP. When the patient is breathing spontaneously, esophageal pressure and airflow at the mouth can be measured, and intrinsic PEEP is determined by measuring the decrease in esophageal pressure needed to initiate inspiratory flow.

In patients who have ARDS, intrinsic PEEP is minimized by the decreased lung compliance, but can occur because of high respiratory rates, short expiratory times (when inspiratory to expiratory ratios are increased or inversed, i.e., > 1), increased airways resistance (e.g., underlying COPD, secretions), and because of increased airways resistance and lung viscoelastance that can accompany ARDS. In COPD patients with intrinsic PEEP due to dynamic expiratory airway collapse in the distal trachea, application of low or moderate levels of external PEEP does not result in an increase in alveolar pressure because positive airway pressure is not transmitted beyond the site of dynamic flow limitation. In contrast, in ARDS patients only part of the intrinsic PEEP that can develop may be due to flow limitation, as in COPD. Some, or all, of the intrinsic PEEP may be due to short expiratory time and linear airway resistance so that externally applied PEEP may be transmitted to the alveoli. Therefore, the only truly clinically relevant PEEP measurement is total PEEP, which includes externally applied PEEP and intrinsic PEEP.

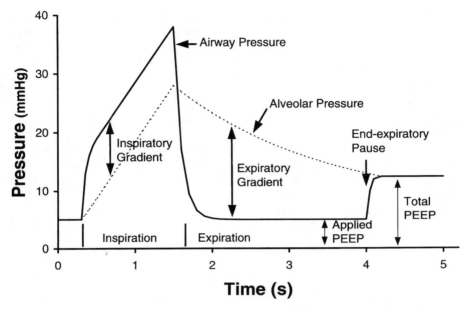

Figure 5.5. Airway pressure measured during an end-expiratory pause demonstrates the presence of intrinsic PEEP. At the onset of expiration airway pressure at the mouth (solid line) rapidly falls to the level of applied PEEP. However, if there is significant obstruction to expiratory flow, alveolar pressure does not fall quickly (light dashed line). Even at the end of expiration (at 4-second time point in this example) alveolar pressure has not decreased back to the externally applied PEEP level. As a result, when an end-expiratory pause is applied (the airway is rapidly occluded just outside the mouth), there is no flow through the pulmonary airways so that the airway pressure at the mouth quickly equilibrates with alveolar pressure. The jump up in airway pressure at the mouth indicates the presence of intrinsic PEEP – incomplete exhalation. The measured value is total PEEP, which is the clinically relevant value to record.

Respiratory Muscle Strength

To sustain unassisted ventilation, the load on the respiratory muscles must be less than 30% to 40% of the maximal pressure that the respiratory muscles can generate. Therefore, either respiratory muscle strength must be high compared to load or the load must be low compared to respiratory muscle strength.

Measurements reflecting respiratory muscle strength are notoriously variable even within the same patient over fairly brief periods of time. Muscle strength measurements depend very much on central drive, which is difficult to maintain constant. The most reproducible measure of respiratory muscle strength is maximal inspiratory pressure. Maximal inspiratory pressure should be measured at approximately FRC to standardize the measurement and also to put the inspiratory muscles at a reasonable mechanical advantage. A one-way valve at the airway allows exhalation and increasing inspiratory effort over the course of several breaths. Maximum inspiratory pressure in healthy young adults can easily exceed 100 mm of mercury. In most patients on mechanical ventilation, maximum inspiratory pressure is more negative than –40 mmHg. Although the muscle strength required to maintain spontaneous ventilation depends very much on muscle load, a number of studies have shown that maximum inspiratory pressures more negative than –25 mmHg are predictive of successful extubation.

Measurement of tidal volume reflects respiratory dive, respiratory muscle strength, and pulmonary mechanics. Rapid shallow breathing characterized by a ratio of respiratory rate to tidal volume greater than 100 predicts failure of spontaneous ventilation within several hours. Measurement of vital capacity is more useful than measurement of tidal volume but is not as specific as measurements of maximum inspiratory pressure (MIP) in assessing respiratory muscle strength. A decreased vital capacity can be caused by poor effort (e.g., obtundation, confusion, indifference), decreased muscle strength, decreased lung compliance, or increased airways resistance. An analogy is that if one is unable to lift a given weight, it is either because of lack of effort, weakness, or excessive weight. A low vital capacity and low MIP in a cooperative patient suggest respiratory muscle weakness. Conversely, a low vital capacity and a very good MIP in a cooperative patient suggest ongoing decreased lung compliance or increased airways resistance.

Respiratory Drive

Ventilation is regulated by respiratory drive. Decreased respiratory drive leading to inadequate alveolar ventilation and elevated P_aCO_2 was discussed in the central hypoventilation section. When central nervous system function is adequate but other causes lead to alveolar hypoventilation, respiratory drive is increased. Thus, measures of respiratory drive are adjunct measures of alveolar hypoventilation because they may be sensitive indicators of a high respiratory workload relative to muscle strength. This is clinically important because patients with elevated drive to breathe frequently fail to wean from mechanical ventilation.

Measures of inspiratory flow and diaphragm EMG signals have been used to measure respiratory drive but are limited by their marked dependence on the measurement conditions. In the ICU the airway occlusion pressure at 100 msec after the start of an inspiratory effort ($P_{0.1}$) is a useful measure of respiratory drive.[16] Although special equipment to occlude the airway at the start of inspiration is often used to measure $P_{0.1}$, in the ICU a simple modified technique provides similar information. Airway pressure is plotted on a chart recorder at the bedside and the trigger sensitivity of the mechanical ventilator is decreased from a typical value of around –2 to around –4 cm H_2O. This results in a brief occlusion of the airway at the start of inspiration.

The decrease in airway pressure on the strip chart 100 msec after the start of inspiration (the start of inspiration is estimated as the time when pressure first starts to decrease from the end-expiratory value) is a reasonable estimate of $P_{0.1}$, which depends on respiratory drive and also on respiratory muscle strength. Therefore this measurement is only useful if repeated over relatively short time intervals in an individual patient.[17] For example, if $P_{0.1}$ increases over the course of a 1-hour trial of spontaneous ventilation then, following extubation at that point, successful sustained spontaneous ventilation is unlikely.

References

1. Hogg JC, Coxson HO, Brumwell ML, Beyers N, Doerschuk CM, MacNee W, Wiggs BR. Erythrocyte and polymorphonuclear cell transit time and concentration in human pulmonary capillaries. J Appl Physiol 1994; 77:1795–1800.
2. Macnaughton PD, Evans TW. Measurement of lung volume and DLCO in acute respiratory failure. Am J Respir Crit Care Med 1994; 150:770–775.
3. Torre-Bueno JR, Wagner PD, Saltzman HA, Gale GE, Moon RE. Diffusion limitation in normal humans during exercise at sea level and simulated altitude. J Appl Physiol 1985; 58:989–995.
4. Wagner PD, West JB. Effects of diffusion impairment on O_2 and CO_2 time courses in pulmonary capillaries. J Appl Physiol 1972; 33:62–71.
5. Bierman MI, Stein KL, Snyder JV. Pulse oximetry in the postoperative care of cardiac surgical patients. A randomized controlled trial. Chest 1992; 102:1367–1370.
6. Moller JT, Johannessen NW, Espersen K, Ravlo O, Pedersen BD, Jensen PF, Rasmussen NH, Rasmussen LS, Pedersen T, Cooper JB, et al. Randomized evaluation of pulse oximetry in 20,802 patients: II. Perioperative events and postoperative complications. Anesthesiology 1993; 78:445–453.
7. Bernard GR, Artigas A, Brigham KL, et al. The American-European Consensus Conference on ARDS. Am J Respir Crit Care Med 1994; 149:818–824.
8. Schumacker PT, Cain SM. The concept of a critical oxygen delivery. Intensive Care Med 1987; 13:223–229.
9. Walley KR, Becker CJ, Hogan RA, Teplinsky K, Wood LD. Progressive hypoxemia limits left ventricular oxygen consumption and contractility. Circ Res 1988; 63:849–859.
10. Pare PD, Warriner B, Baile EM, Hogg JC. Redistribution of pulmonary extravascular water with positive end-expiratory pressure in canine pulmonary edema. Am Rev Respir Dis 1983; 127:590–593.
11. Amato MB, Barbas CS, Medeiros DM, Magaldi RB, Schettino GP, Lorenzi-Filho G, Kairalla RA, Deheinzelin D, Munoz C, Oliveira R, Takagaki TY, Carvalho CR. Effect of a protective-ventilation strategy on mortality in the acute respiratory distress syndrome. N Engl J Med 1998; 338:347–354.
12. Dhingra S, Solven F, Wilson A, McCarthy DS. Hypomagnesemia and respiratory muscle power. Am Rev Respir Dis 1984; 129:497–498.
13. Ronco JJ, Fenwick JC, Tweeddale MG, Wiggs BR, Phang PT, Cooper DJ, Cunningham KF,

Russell JA, Walley KR. Identification of the critical oxygen delivery for anaerobic metabolism in critically ill septic and nonseptic humans JAMA 1993; 270:1724–1730.

14. Eissa NT, Ranieri VM, Corbeil C, Chasse M, Robatto FM, Braidy J, Milic-Emili J. Analysis of behavior of the respiratory system in ARDS patients: effects of flow, volume, and time. J Appl Physiol 1991; 70:2719–2729.

15. Romand JA, Suter PM. Dynamic hyperinflation and intrinsic PEEP during mechanical ventilation. Europ J Anaesthesiol 1994; 11:25–28.

16. Alberti A, Gallo F, Fongaro A, Valenti S, Rossi A. $P_{0.1}$ is a useful parameter in setting the level of pressure support ventilation. Intensive Care Med 1995; 21:547–553.

17. Sassoon CS, Mahutte CK. Airway occlusion pressure and breathing pattern as predictors of weaning outcome. Am Rev Respir Dis 1993; 148:860–866.

6

Cardiovascular Management of ARDS

Keith R. Walley and James A. Russell

Introduction

ARDS is often thought of as primarily a pulmonary disease. However, ARDS has a profound effect on the cardiovascular system, and cardiovascular management can have a profound impact on physiologic status and outcome in ARDS for several reasons. First, oxygen delivery to the whole body is a product of arterial oxygen saturation, oxygen-carrying capacity of the blood, and cardiac output. It follows that management of cardiac output and hemoglobin are just as important as achieving high arterial oxygen saturations by ventilator management. Second, ARDS is characterized by a large intrapulmonary shunt and therefore is a setting where mixed venous oxygen saturation has a direct impact on arterial oxygenation. Cardiac output, as a component of oxygen delivery and oxygen consumption, plays a key role in determining mixed venous oxygen saturation – emphasizing the importance of cardiovascular management. Third, in the early exudative phase of ARDS, a low pulmonary capillary wedge pressure can decrease the rate of edema formation and thus have an impact on oxygenation and outcome. Therefore, finding the lowest pulmonary capillary wedge pressure that gives an adequate cardiac output is a focus of cardiovascular management of ARDS.

Conversely, ventilator strategy can have a profound impact on cardiovascular function. For example, ARDS can be associated with significant pulmonary hypertension, which can be exacerbated by positive airway pressures. This effect, plus the direct transmission of high airway pressures to right atrial pressure, can significantly decrease venous return. Thus, ARDS is a pulmonary disease where cardiopulmonary interaction is exceedingly important and where cardiovascular management is fundamental to excellent care.

Cardiovascular Physiology Essential for Management of ARDS

Cardiac Function

Starling function curves, or cardiac function curves, for the heart relate the input of the heart to output. Most frequently we use right atrial pressure (CVP) or left atrial pressure (approximated by pulmonary wedge pressure) as clinically measurable inputs to the heart. Cardiac output is a common measure of output of the heart. As the filling pressure of the heart increases, cardiac output also increases. The relationship is curvilinear (Figure 6.1). Increased ventricular contractility is associated with a shift up and to the left of this cardiac function curve so that, at the same filling pressures, a greater cardiac output is achieved. Conversely, decreased ventricular contractility is associated with a shift down and to the right of the cardiac function curve and so cardiac output is lower at a given filling pressure. However, it is important to recognize that other factors, such as ventricular compliance and afterload, have a profound influence on cardiac function curves. Understanding the underlying mechanisms requires consideration of pressure-volume relationships of the ventricle.[1]

Ventricular Pressure-Volume Relationships

Figure 6.2 illustrates that during diastole the heart fills at quite low pressures along the normally compliant diastolic pressure-volume relationship of the ventricle. With the onset of isovolumic systole the ventricle contracts, raising intraventricular pressure at constant volume (in the absence of valvular heart disease). When ventricular pressure exceeds aortic pressure, the aortic valve opens and ejection occurs and continues to an end-systolic pressure-volume point. Intraventricular pressure decreases during the isovolumic relaxation phase, and the cardiac cycle starts again. It is not surprising that at high afterloads the ventricle is not able to eject far, whereas at lower afterloads the ventricle is able to eject further. End-systolic points for differently loaded ejections all fall along an approximately linear end-systolic pressure-volume relationship. The slope, Emax, of the end-systolic pressure-volume relationship is an excellent measure of ventricular contractility.[2] That is, if Emax increases it can be seen (Figure 6.2) that the ventricle is able to eject further (to a smaller end-systolic volume) at the same afterload.

The pressure-volume loops of a cardiac cycle as described earlier are directly related to cardiac function curves (Figure 6.3). Stroke volume, determined as the difference between end-diastolic volume and end-systolic volume multiplied by heart rate, yields cardiac output. It follows that cardiac function curves are affected by more than just changes in systolic contractility. For example, decreasing afterload results in increased systolic ejection, particularly in the failing heart. This results in increased stroke volume and cardiac output so that decreased afterload shifts the

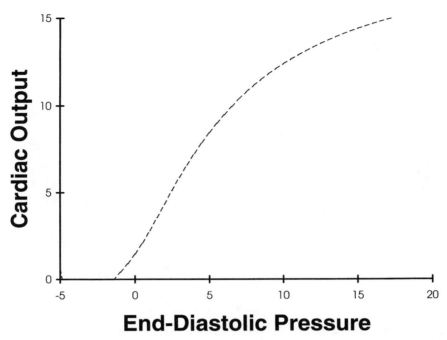

Figure 6.1. The cardiac function curve relates an input to the heart, such as end-diastolic pressure (abscissa) to an output of the heart, such as cardiac output (ordinate). As end-diastolic pressure increases, cardiac output increases. However, this relationship is curvilinear so that at high end-diastolic pressure, further increases cause less increase in cardiac output.

cardiac function curve up and to the left. Conversely, decreased compliance (increased stiffness) of the diastolic left ventricle decreases stroke volume because end-diastolic volume is decreased at the same filling pressure. A decrease in stroke volume decreases cardiac output and therefore shifts the cardiac function curve down and to the right – similar to a decrease in systolic contractility. This observation is particularly important in ARDS because diastolic filling can become an important issue, as indicated later.

In sepsis, ventricular function is decreased.[3] Identical changes in diastolic and systolic ventricular mechanics have been reported in patients with ARDS.[4] For example, left ventricular ejection fraction measured in humans is decreased during ARDS and sepsis.[3,4] In those patients who survive, ejection fraction increases back to the normal range within approximately 10 days.[3] End-systolic volumes increase at comparable end-systolic pressures indicating a decrease in systolic contractility.[5] In addition, survivors have dilated end-diastolic ventricles compared to nonsurvivors.[5] The dilated diastolic ventricles of patients with sepsis also return to normal within approximately

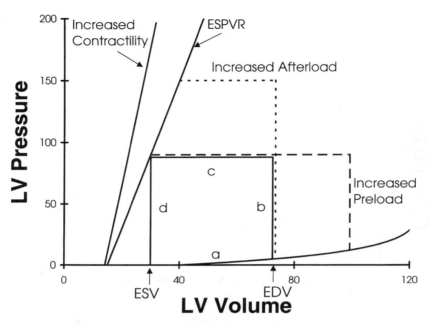

Figure 6.2. Left ventricular pressure-volume relationships are illustrated. A single cardiac cycle pressure-volume loop is illustrated as a, b, c, d. During diastole the ventricle fills along a diastolic pressure-volume relationship (a) to end-diastolic volume (EDV). At the onset of systole, left ventricular pressure rises with no change in volume (b). When left ventricular pressure exceeds aortic pressure, the aortic valve opens and the left ventricle ejects blood (c) to an end-systolic pressure-volume point. The ventricle then relaxes isovolumically (d).

At increased pressure afterload the left ventricle is not able to eject as far (short interrupted lines). Conversely, at a lower afterload the left ventricle is able to eject further so that all end-systolic points lie along and define the end-systolic pressure volume relationship (ESPVR). Increased preload (long interrupted lines) results in increased stroke volume from the larger EDV to an end-systolic volume (ESV) that lies on the same ESPVR. The slope of the ESPVR is Emax. An increase in contractility results in an increase in Emax so that the ventricle ejects to a smaller ESV at the same afterload.

10 days. Dilation of end-diastolic ventricles appears to be an appropriate and normal compensatory mechanism to maintain stroke volume in the face of the dilated end-systolic ventricle. When the diastolic ventricle fails to dilate, stroke volume and cardiac output are decreased. Failure of the diastolic ventricle to dilate in the face of decreased systolic contractility appears to be the pathologic event associated with nonsurvival in patients with sepsis.[6]

The changes in systolic contractility and the impaired diastolic compliance of sepsis and ARDS appear to be caused by multiple mediators associated with the inflammatory response observed in these states.[7] Endotoxins and other bacterial products have minimal direct effects on ventricular contractility, but early inflammatory medi-

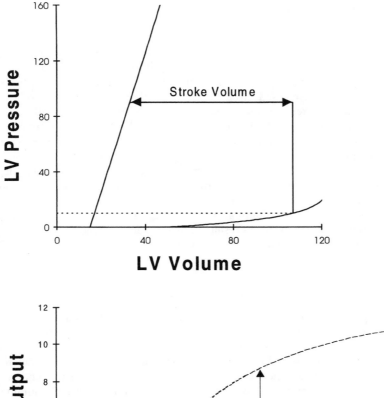

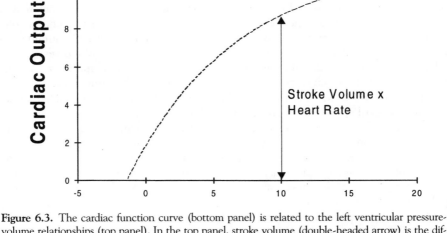

Figure 6.3. The cardiac function curve (bottom panel) is related to the left ventricular pressure-volume relationships (top panel). In the top panel, stroke volume (double-headed arrow) is the difference between end-systolic volume and end-diastolic volume. End-diastolic volume is determined by the diastolic pressure-volume relationship and end-diastolic pressure (equals 10 mmHg in this example). End-systolic volume is determined by the end-systolic pressure-volume relationship and end-systolic pressure. Therefore, for any end-diastolic pressure, cardiac output can be calculated if heart rate is known. An increase in end-diastolic pressure increases end-diastolic volume, stroke volume, and cardiac output in the bottom panel. Factors that can decrease cardiac function in the bottom panel are therefore factors that can decrease stroke volume in the upper panel. These include a decrease in contractility, which decreases stroke volume by increasing end-systolic volume; a decrease in diastolic compliance, which decreases stroke volume by decreasing end-diastolic volume; and an increase in afterload, which decreases stoke volume by increasing end-systolic volume.

ators, such as TNF-alpha and interleukin-6, play key roles in mediating a subsequent decrease in systolic contractility.[8,9] TNF-alpha and IL-6, potentiated by IL-1,[10] cause release of nitric oxide from leukocytes, endothelial cells, and cardiac myocytes. Nitric oxide then mediates decreased myocardial contractility by stimulating cyclic GMP, which results in a decrease in intracellular calcium. Nitric oxide may also combine with oxygen free radicals to form the peroxynitrite radical, which is histotoxic and also appears to mediate decreased ventricular contractility.[11] Finally, nitric oxide can combine with key heme proteins of oxygen metabolism and electron transport, providing a potential further mechanism for nitric oxide–mediated myocardial depression. In addition, leukocytes are important contributors to myocardial tissue damage and decreased ventricular contractility.[12] Leukocytes may contribute by release of oxygen free radicals, pro-inflammatory cytokines, and nitric oxide. Damage to endothelium and cardiac myocytes results in tissue edema,[13] which, in part, accounts for decreased diastolic compliance in nonsurvivors compared to survivors of ARDS and sepsis.

Hemodynamic Features of Right Heart Failure

In ARDS, pulmonary artery pressure may be elevated, in part, as a consequence of increased pulmonary vascular resistance caused by various pro-inflammatory mediators, hypoxia, acidosis, or thrombi and, in part, by increased airway pressures due to positive pressure ventilation. Increased pulmonary artery pressure results in increased right ventricular afterload. Increased afterload increases right ventricular end-systolic volume. In order to maintain cardiac output, stroke volume must be maintained so that right ventricular end-diastolic volume must also increase. When severe, the dilated right heart may distend the pericardium to its elastic limit, and the right ventricle may shift the intraventricular septum from right to left during diastole. When this happens, left ventricular diastolic filling is limited, decreasing left-sided stroke volume and cardiac output. In this setting pulmonary vasodilators can result in significant hemodynamic improvement. Inhaled nitric oxide can be particularly helpful in decreasing pulmonary vascular resistance. Inhaled nitric oxide is very rapidly bound to tissues and hemoglobin and therefore has the least effect on the systemic circulation of the many pulmonary vasodilators that have been studied. Because the right heart is essentially a flow pump that is not good at developing high pressures, pulmonary vasodilators initially may cause almost no change in pulmonary artery pressure and may instead almost exclusively increase cardiac output. Calculated pulmonary vascular resistance is decreased.

In health, cardiac output does not change as heart rate increases from 50 to 150 beats per minute because increased heart rate decreases diastolic filling so that stroke volume is reduced in inverse proportion to the increase in heart rate. Here, artificially increasing heart rate is of no benefit. However, in the setting of a greatly dilated right ventricle, diastolic filling is limited by the pericardium and surrounding structures. Consequently, filling during late diastole may be greatly reduced or almost zero. Prolonged diastolic filling time is of no benefit. Therefore, increased heart rate is not associated with a reduction in diastolic filling, so that increased heart rate increases cardiac output. In general, benefit can be observed in this situation by increasing heart rate from the 60 to 80 range to approximately 100 beats per minute. Further increases in heart rate rarely increase cardiac output even in right ventricular failure states.

The Arterial Circulation and SVR

ARDS is accompanied by characteristic hemodynamic changes that, importantly, are indistinguishable from the hemodynamic changes of sepsis.[14] These include a relatively high cardiac output in comparison to mean arterial pressure so that systemic vascular resistance (SVR), calculated as the difference between mean arterial pressure and central venous pressure divided by cardiac output, is decreased. Vascular resistance is decreased by a number of vasodilator inflammatory mediators including endogenous production of nitric oxide. Pro-inflammatory mediators released as part of the initiating inflammatory stimulus of ARDS cause stimulation of inducible nitric oxide synthase resulting in excessive nitric oxide production.[15] The arterial circulation is also characterized by a diminished response to infused vasopressors. Function of adrenergic receptors can be further diminished by the relative adrenal insufficiency that appears commonly in ARDS and sepsis.[16] Clinically significant adrenal insufficiency can be detected using an ACTH stimulation test where baseline cortisol levels of more than 250 nmol/L double after ACTH stimulation. When the response is significantly less than normal, steroid administration can dramatically potentiate the effect of infused catecholamines.

Control of Cardiac Output by Factors Governing Venous Return

In animal experiments, Guyton and colleagues[17] sought to determine the importance of the systemic vessels in controlling cardiac output. They replaced the heart with a pump that simply regulated its own flow in order to maintain right atrial pressure constant. In control animals with a normally functioning heart, they found that an adrenaline infusion approximately doubled cardiac output. In their experimental preparation where the heart was removed they found that infusion of a similar amount of adrenaline resulted in a similar doubling of cardiac output. These data demonstrate that cardiac output is largely determined by factors governing venous return and not by the heart. A healthy heart has multiple mechanisms that allow it to respond to changes in venous return over a wide range, but the heart does not primarily determine venous return (which equals cardiac output in steady state).

The factors governing venous return are illustrated in Figure 6.4.[18] When right atrial pressure equals mean systemic pressure there is no driving pressure gradient for blood flow, thus venous return is zero. As right atrial pressure is reduced, the impediment to venous return decreases so that venous return rises approximately linearly. The slope of this venous return curve has units that are the inverse of a resistance – termed *resistance*

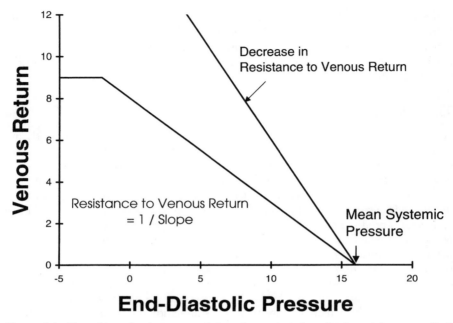

Figure 6.4. The relationship between end-diastolic pressure (equal right atrial pressure, Pra) and venous return is illustrated. When end-diastolic pressure equals mean systemic pressure (Pms), there is no pressure gradient (Pms-Pra) driving the blood flow back to the heart, so venous return is zero. As end-diastolic pressure decreases the gradient from the veins to the heart to drive blood flow back to the heart increases, so that venous return increases. At very low end-diastolic pressures (Pra <0), central veins collapse and act as Starling resistors, so that further decreases in EDP do not increase venous return. "Resistance to venous return" is just the inverse of the slope of the venous return curve. A decrease in resistance to venous return increases slope so that venous return increases for any end-diastolic pressure.

to venous return. When right atrial pressure is reduced to approximately zero, the central veins collapse at the level of the diaphragm – limiting venous flow. Further reduction in right atrial pressure below this low value does not increase venous return.

It can be seen that venous return at any right atrial pressure can be increased by increasing mean systemic pressure or by decreasing resistance to venous return. Mean systemic pressure is a vascular compartment pressure that arises from venous blood volume distending the systemic veins. If the volume of the distensible venous compartment is increased, then mean systemic pressure increases. Alternatively, if the compliance of the venous compartment decreases, say by catecholamine infusion or increased sympathetic tone, then the pressure within the venous compartment can increase without a change in volume. Adrenaline also causes a reduction in resistance to venous return. Adrenaline does this by redistributing arterial blood flow from vascular beds with long

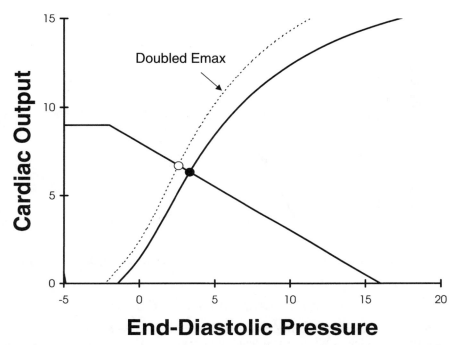

Figure 6.5. The cardiac function curve and the venous return curve are drawn on the same axes (continuous lines). The intersection of the cardiac function curve and the venous return curve (solid circle) defines the operating point of the circulation, here at an end-diastolic pressure of approximately 3 mmHg and a cardiac output of approximately 6 L/minute. The interrupted cardiac function curve illustrates increased cardiac function due to a doubling of Emax (increased ventricular contractility). It can be seen that increases in normal ventricular contractility have little effect on cardiac function.

transit times and high resistance to venous return (e.g., the gastrointestinal circulation) to vascular compartments with short transit times and low resistance to venous return (e.g., skeletal muscle).[19] The average resistance to venous return therefore decreases. Thus, strategies for increasing venous return include increasing intravascular volume to increase mean systemic pressure, decreasing compliance of the venous compartment to increase mean systemic pressure, and reducing resistance to venous return.

In steady state, the amount of blood returning to the heart must equal the amount of blood leaving the heart so that venous return must equal cardiac output. Therefore, as illustrated in Figure 6.5, the cardiac function curve and venous return curve can be plotted on the same set of axes. The intersection of the cardiac function curve and venous return curve give the value of steady-state cardiac output and the value of steady-state right atrial pressure. In health, the cardiac function curve is already steep so that an

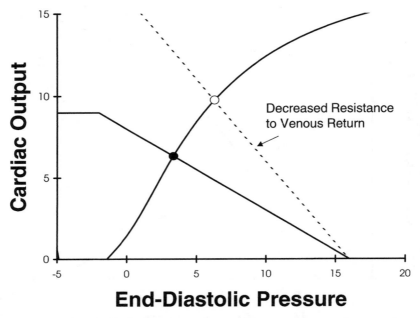

Figure 6.6. The cardiac function curve and the venous return curve are drawn on the same axes (continuous lines). When venous return is increased (in this example by a decrease in the resistance to venous return), cardiac output increases substantially. Thus, in normal humans and most patients, factors that govern venous return are primarily responsible for changes in cardiac output.

increase in slope has little impact on cardiovascular function, whereas small changes in the venous return curve can have very significant effects on cardiac output (Figure 6.6).

In ARDS and sepsis, the cardiac function curve can be somewhat depressed but the venous return curve is steeper than in healthy patients, reflecting a decrease in the resistance to venous return. In this setting the main approach to altering cardiac output is to focus on the factors governing venous return. Fluid infusion in ARDS patients can increase mean systemic pressure and therefore increase venous return. Infusion of sympathomimetic agents such as dopamine, adrenaline, or noradrenaline decrease venous compliance so that mean systemic pressure increases, increasing venous return. In addition, these catecholamines also decrease resistance to venous return, resulting in increased cardiac output. Whether the redistribution of blood flow with catecholamines is advantageous or disadvantageous has not been fully elucidated. However, evidence indicates that dopamine infusions can impair the gut's ability to extract oxygen,[20] illustrating that drugs that improve measures of hemodynamic function do not necessarily result in a beneficial physiologic effect.

In occasional patients with other causes of decreased cardiac function, the cardiac

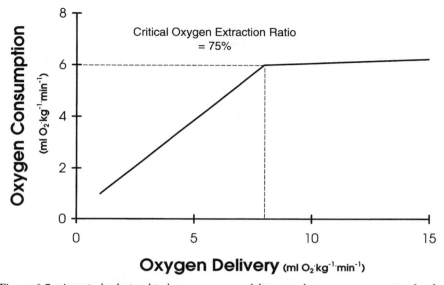

Figure 6.7. A typical relationship between oxygen delivery and oxygen consumption for the whole body and many noncardiac organs is shown. Oxygen consumption is set by oxygen demand at high oxygen deliveries so that oxygen consumption is independent of oxygen delivery and relatively constant. Because oxygen consumption cannot exceed oxygen delivery, at some low oxygen delivery, oxygen consumption must decrease, and this is associated with evidence of tissue hypoxia and anaerobic metabolism. The oxygen extraction ratio (oxygen consumption divided by oxygen delivery) at the transition from plateau to downslope is the critical oxygen extraction ratio and a measure of the ability of tissues to extract oxygen.

function curve is greatly depressed. Then changes in the venous return curve no longer have as great an impact on cardiac output. In this circumstance changes in the cardiac function curve can result in significant increases in cardiac output.

Oxygen Delivery–Consumption Relationships

The amount of oxygen delivered to the body each minute is the product of arterial oxygen saturation, the oxygen-carrying capacity of the blood, and cardiac output.[21] Oxygen dissolved in plasma contributes only a small fraction. Oxygen consumption by the whole body at rest is a reasonably constant value, determined by basal metabolic needs. If oxygen delivery decreases, as it may in disease states including ARDS, the basal metabolic needs remain constant and therefore oxygen consumption remains constant. However, it is impossible to consume more oxygen than is delivered, so that, at some point, whole body oxygen consumption must decrease as oxygen delivery decreases (Figure 6.7). A decrease in oxygen consumption due to a low oxygen delivery is associated with the onset of anaerobic metabolism, rising lactate levels, and evidence of organ system dysfunction. Patients die soon after the onset of this supply dependence of oxygen consumption.

The exact features of biphasic oxygen consumption and oxygen delivery relationships are determined by the ability of peripheral tissues to extract oxygen.[22] Many of the same mechanisms that limit gas exchange in the lungs also limit gas exchange by the peripheral tissues. These include diffusion limitation, shunt, mismatching of oxygen supply to demand, and lack of a pressure gradient to drive oxygen diffusion from capillaries to tissues.

Diffusion limitation of oxygen transfer from red blood cells to the peripheral tissues may be exacerbated in edematous tissue due to fluid resuscitation and generalized endothelial damage seen in ARDS and sepsis. The limit to diffusion appears to occur in the unloading of oxygen from red blood cells. Once oxygen is within tissues a number of mechanisms, including myoglobin binding, aid transfer of oxygen into metabolizing mitrochrondria. Schumacker and Samsel have examined the theoretical oxygen extraction in a simple model of oxygen diffusion.[23] To predict experimentally measured values of the critical oxygen extraction ratio, a significant shunt of arterial blood into veins has to be included.

Shunting of oxygen from small arteries to veins past metabolizing tissues has been demonstrated notably in circulations where the feeding arteries and veins lie in close approximation,[24] such as in villi of the gut. Oxygen can diffuse directly from artery to vein, bypassing the capillaries and tissues. However, much of the measured physiologic shunt may be due to mismatching of oxygen supply to demand.[25] A theoretical model examining the effect of mismatching of oxygen supply to demand demonstrated that reasonable estimates of maximum oxygen extraction capacity by the gut could be predicted from measures of heterogeneity of capillary blood flow.[25] In sepsis and ARDS microvascular function is impaired so that perfused capillary density is no longer tightly regulated by tissue hypoxia sensors.[26] This leads to mismatch of oxygen supply to demand and may result in patchy areas of relatively hypoperfused tissue. For example, the myocardial dysfunction that occurs following endotoxin infusion is associated with patchy subendocardial damage.

Oxygen Delivery–Consumption Relationships in ARDS

Adequate oxygen delivery is ultimately the goal of physiologic management of the cardiovascular system in ARDS, and understanding oxygen delivery is important in recognizing that cardiac output and hemoglobin contribute just as much as arterial oxygen saturation to total oxygen delivery.

Initial studies of patients with ARDS suggested that whole body oxygen uptake was directly correlated with whole body oxygen delivery.[27] This suggested that patients may be functioning on the "down slope" of the oxygen delivery–consumption relationship illustrated in Figure 6.7. If this were true, then these results suggest that either overt or occult tissue hypoxia was occurring in these patients. More recent studies using appropriate measurement methods do not demonstrate a correlation between whole body oxygen uptake and oxygen delivery in patients with ARDS and sepsis.[28]

Abnormal dependence of oxygen consumption on oxygen delivery observed in early studies of patients with ARDS may be flawed by methodologic problems. One problem is that oxygen demand of critically ill patients can vary considerably. An increase in oxygen demand can secondarily increase in oxygen delivery, for example, during exercise.[29–33] Indeed, oxygen demand of critically ill patients varies considerably with sedation,[30] with changes in mechanical ventilation,[31] and with changes in body temperature.[29] Conversely, primary changes in oxygen delivery can increase oxygen demand in some organs. The heart is the organ that most clearly manifests increased oxygen demand when oxygen delivery is increased because delivering oxygen (i.e., cardiac output) requires cardiac work. Similarly, increased renal blood flow increases metabolic work of reabsorption and thus increases oxygen consumption.[34] Similarly, increased hepatic blood flow augments the delivery of metabolic substrates to the liver and increases oxygen consumption.[35] The relationship between oxygen delivery and oxygen consumption for the heart, kidney, and liver is a linear slope. This may be misinterpreted as pathologic dependence of oxygen consumption on oxygen delivery but, in fact, does not represent tissue hypoxia.

If oxygen availability is reduced, metabolic activity may also be downregulated in tissues, called *oxygen conforming*. Cultured hepatocytes and cardiac myocytes reduce their metabolic activity and oxygen demand without cellular injury during reductions of oxygen availability.[36,37] This appears to be a normal adaptive response to states of decreased oxygen availability that protects cells from hypoxic injury. Patients with stable aortic stenosis who do not appear to have tissue hypoxia increase both oxygen delivery and consumption after aortic valvuloplasty.[38] Reversal of oxygen-conforming behavior has been proposed as the mechanism. Furthermore, stable patients with COPD and obstructive sleep apnea increase their oxygen consumption when oxygen delivery is increased by passive leg elevation.[39] These patients do not have tissue hypoxia but rather could have reversal of oxygen-conforming behavior.

The second problem in many of the studies of oxygen consumption and oxygen delivery that potentially confounds the interpretation of the results is the problem of mathematical coupling of shared measurement error.[28,40] In many clinical studies of oxygen consumption and oxygen delivery, oxygen consumption (VO_2) and oxygen delivery (DO_2) were calculated from a common set of variables:

$$DO_2 = Q \times (Hg \times 1.36 \times [SaO_2] \quad\quad + [PaO_2])$$

$$VO_2 = Q \times (Hg \times 1.36 \times [SaO_2 - SvO_2] + [PaO_2 - PvO_2])$$

where Q is cardiac output, SaO_2 and SvO_2 are the arterial and mixed venous oxygen saturations, respectively, Hg is hemoglobin concentration, 1.36 is the binding constant of O_2 to Hg, and PaO_2 and PvO_2 are the arterial and mixed venous oxygen tensions, respectively. It is evident that the two equations share many variables. Therefore, errors in the measurement of any one of these variables will result in similar directional errors in oxygen delivery and oxygen consumption calculations. As a result, an artifactual relationship exists between oxygen delivery and oxygen consumption that is explained by the coupling of shared measurement error rather than by the presence of pathologic dependence of oxygen consumption and oxygen delivery, and covert oxygen debt.

Mathematical coupling of shared measurement error can be avoided by determining oxygen consumption and oxygen delivery by independent techniques.[41–46] Specifically, oxygen consumption is measured by analysis of respiratory gases, and oxygen delivery has been calculated using thermodilution cardiac output and arterial oxygen content. When this is done oxygen consumption is not dependent on oxygen delivery until just prior to death at an oxygen delivery less than 4 mL O_2/kg/minute[47] – a state easily detected by clinical evidence of shock. Thus, the observation that oxygen consumption changes in response to changes in oxygen delivery is not particularly useful in detecting occult tissue hypoxia. Rather, effort to detect local tisue hypoxia may be more beneficial.

Principles of Cardiovascular Management in ARDS

Maintenance of an Adequate Cardiac Output

Oxygen Delivery

It is crucial to maintain whole body oxygen delivery above the critical level where whole body oxygen consumption decreases[47] – hence the focus on maintaining adequate arterial PO_2 in patients with ARDS. However, it is important to note that two further degrees of freedom remain. That is, if arterial oxygen saturation has been increased to the greatest extent possible by changes in FiO_2 and by ventilator management, it is still possible to increase oxygen delivery by increasing arterial oxygen-carrying capacity and cardiac output. Indeed, these terms are multiplied to give oxygen delivery so that, to some extent, if arterial oxygen saturation is 10% lower than a "desired" level this can be compensated for by either a 10% increase in cardiac output or a 10% increase in oxygen-carrying capacity. The limit to this strategy is that some tissues, such as the metabolically active heart, depend more on arterial PO_2 than on arterial oxygen saturation,[48] so that excessively low PO_2s cannot be fully compensated for by increasing cardiac output or oxygen-carrying capacity. Nevertheless, it is clear that the management of severe hypoxemia should not focus exclusively on arterial oxygen saturation. Attention to cardiac output and oxygen carrying capacity are equally important.

It is helpful to consider the normal physiologic responses to primary threats to oxygen delivery to establish priorities for management of oxygen delivery. If one examines the components of oxygen delivery, oxygen delivery can be decreased by hypoxia, anemia, or decreased cardiac output. If hypoxia develops, for example, by a decrease of arterial oxygen saturation from 100% to 80%, then the organism can easily adapt acutely by increasing cardiac output and chronically by increasing hemoglobin concentration (secondary polycythemia) to maintain oxygen delivery. In healthy humans, cardiac output can increase four to five times so that a 20% increase in cardiac output is easily achieved to maintain oxygen delivery constant. If the primary threat to oxygen delivery is anemia, say hemoglobin drops by 20%, then the healthy individual can maintain oxygen delivery only by increasing cardiac output. Arterial oxygen saturation cannot be increased beyond 100%. Finally, if hemorrhagic shock develops and cardiac output drops 20%, then the healthy human cannot maintain oxygen delivery because hemoglobin concentration and arterial oxygen saturation cannot be increased. Therefore, oxygen delivery will decrease 20% if cardiac ouput decreases 20%. These examples illustrate the fundamental importance of control of cardiac output and maintenance of cardiac output to global oxygen delivery.

Inotropes and Vasopressors

Infused vasopressors and positive inotropic agents are frequently used to increase an excessively low arterial blood pressure or increase an excessively low cardiac output. At very low mean arterial pressure, the regulation of distribution of cardiac output is impaired so that regional tissue hypoxia can occur despite a normal or high cardiac output. The minimum value for mean arterial pressure differs from patient to patient and changes over time and with severity of disease in individual patients. In young patients, a mean arterial pressure 55 or even 50 mmHg may be sufficient to prevent evidence of organ system hypoperfusion. In contrast, in older patients with significant vascular disease, a mean arterial pressure of 75 mmHg or higher may be required for adequate perfusion. A minimum value for cardiac output depends very much on arterial oxygen saturation and hemoglobin concentration. However, a cardiac index (cardiac index is cardiac output indexed to body size by dividing cardiac output by estimated body surface area) much less than 2 L/minute/m^2 is usually associated with inadequate oxygen delivery and clinical evidence of organ system dysfunction. In all patients the goal arterial pressure and cardiac output depend on physiologic evidence of adequate organ system function – a physiologic end point, not a numerical goal. Tachycardia, tachypnea, poor peripheral perfusion, impaired mentation, a decreasing urine output, rising creatinine, rising metabolic acidosis, elevated lactate, and evidence of coronary ischemia are important signs to consider that may be due to organ system hypoperfusion. The lower limit of mean arterial pressure and cardiac output are clearly defined when a trial of increased blood pressure or cardiac output reverses these signs of inadequate perfusion.

The use of vasopressor and inotropic medications should follow adequate fluid resuscitation (see later). In inadequately fluid resuscitated patients these drugs will not have their intended effect. Beta adrenergic agents used to increase ventricular contractility in hypovolemic patients will usually cause significant hypotension because cardiac output is limited by venous return so that the vasodilating effects of these drugs become all too evident. Alpha adrenergic agents used to increase mean arterial pressure in hypovolemic patients will further decrease cardiac output, and the "acceptable" numeric value of blood pressure may inappropriately reassure caregivers.

The hemodynamic changes of ARDS are indistinguishable from those of sepsis and septic shock.[14] These include decreased systemic vascular resistance associated with a high cardiac output hyperdynamic circulation, the possibility of significant hypovolemia with a low cardiac output, and decreased systolic contractility and decreased diastolic compliance (increased stiffness) contributing to inadequate cardiac output. Therefore, the use of vasopressors and positive inotropic agents is common. Initial management of hypotension may include a nonspecific agent such as dopamine or occasionally epinephrine (Table 6.1). Dopamine has beta adrenergic effects at lower doses and increasing alpha adrenergic effects at higher doses. When more data become available, such as thermodilution cardiac output from a pulmonary artery catheter, a more appropriate combination of agents can be chosen. For example, if cardiac output is high but mean arterial pressure is excessively low, then norepinephrine is a useful vasopressor. Phenylephrine is an alternative choice in this setting. When high doses of these alpha agonists are ineffective and adrenal insufficiency has been ruled out or treated, then a vasopressin infusion may be effective. The beta agonist dobutamine can be added to a norepinephrine infusion if cardiac output is excessively low despite an adequate cardiac filling pressure. Dopexamine is a reasonable alternative agent. When beta agonists are no longer effective, phosphodiesterase inhibitors such as amrinone may beneficially increase ventricular contractility. These agents are summarized in Table 6.1.

Trials of Supranormal Oxygen Delivery

Although some evidence indicates that increasing oxygen delivery may improve outcome of critically ill patients, this has not been confirmed in randomized controlled trials of supranormal oxygen delivery and there is also evidence that increasing oxygen delivery may be detrimental.

Shoemaker and colleagues demonstrated fewer single organ failures in patients who received supranormal oxygen delivery compared to controls.[49] Similarly, mortality was lower in high-risk surgical patients who were randomized to supranormal oxygen delivery.[50] In contrast, Hayes and colleagues[51] randomized a heterogeneous group of critically ill patients to either standard therapy or to supranormal oxygen delivery (cardiac index > 4.5 L/minute/m², oxygen delivery > 600 mL/minute/m², and oxygen consumption > 170 mL/minute/m² using fluid and dobutamine). ICU mortality was 30% in the control group and 50% in the supranormal oxygen delivery group. Interestingly, although high doses of dobutamine were used, the excess deaths in the treatment group were not due to cardiac events, but were attributed to development of multiple organ failure.[51]

The largest study so far of supranormal oxygen delivery is reported by Gattinoni and colleagues.[52] This was a multicenter study of 762 heterogeneous critically ill patients randomly allocated to one of the three groups designed to achieve different hemodynamic goals: (1) a normal cardiac index (between 2.5 and 3.5 L/minute/m², the control group); (2) supranormal cardiac index (> 4.5 L/minute/m², the cardiac index group); and (3) a normal mixed venous oxygen saturation (> 70%, the oxygen saturation group). Volume expansion, transfusion, inotropes, vasodilators, and vasopressors aimed at achieving the study target for 5 days. There were no differences in ICU mortality (48%, 49%, and 52%, respectively) or 6-month mortality (62%, 62%, and 64%, respectively) between the three groups. Importantly, there were also no differences in

Table 6.1. Some common vasopressor and inotropic agents

Agent	Mechanism	Dose	HR	Cont	SVR	CO	MAP
Dopamine	Dopaminergic agonist at 1–5 µg/kg/min, β agonist above 5 µg/kg/min, α agonist above 10 µg/kg/min	1–20 µg/kg/min	↑	↑	↑	↑	↑
Epinephrine	Combined strong α and β agonist	1–10 µg/min	↑	↑↑↑	↑↑↑	↑	↑↑↑
Norepinephrine	α agonist primarily, weak β agonist	1–20 µg/min	↔	↔↑↑	↑↑↑↑	↓	↑↑↑
Phenylephrine	α agonist primarily	20–200 µg/min	↔	↕	↑↑↑↑	↓	↑↑↑
Vasopressin	Vasopressin receptor agonist	1–10 units/hr	↔	↕	↑↑↑	↓	↑↑↑
Dobutamine	β agonist primarily	1–20 µg/kg/min	↑↑↑	↑↑↑↑	↓	↑↑	↓↔↓
Amrinone	Phosphodiesterase III inhibitor	5–15 µg/kg/min	↑↑↑	↑↑↑↑	↓	↑↑	↓↔↓

the number of organ failures between the groups. Even post hoc analysis of diagnostic subgroups of patients failed to show benefit from supranormal oxygen delivery.[52]

Timing of intervention may be important in explaining why some studies of supranormal oxygen delivery have shown benefit whereas others have not. One interpretation of the results of all studies combined is that early aggressive resuscitation of shock or prevention of shock is beneficial. In contrast, supranormal goals in already resuscitated patients are of no benefit. This is supported by a recent meta-analysis showing a relative risk of death of 0.20 (95% confidence intervals 0.07 to 0.55) if therapy was initiated preoperatively compared to relative risk of 0.98 (95% confidence intervals 0.79 to 1.22) if therapy was initiated after ICU admission.[53]

Ventilation Strategies Affect Cardiac Output

Pulmonary management can have a substantial impact on cardiac function. The most important feature of this aspect of cardiopulmonary interaction is limitation of venous return caused by increased pulmonary airspace pressures compressing the right atrium and superior vena cava. In addition, pulmonary vascular resistance is frequently increased as a component of the inflammatory response triggered in ARDS. Early on this is partly accounted for by increased thromboxane A_2 production in the lungs, increased endothelin production, and impaired endothelium-mediated relaxation. High pulmonary artery pressures result in increased right ventricular end-systolic and end-diastolic volumes. Increased right ventricular end-diastolic volumes associated with increased right atrial pressure directly reduce the driving pressure for venous return. Furthermore, very high right ventricular diastolic pressures can shift the intraventricular septum from right to left so that left ventricular diastolic filling is impaired. This can decrease stroke volume and hence, cardiac output.

An important ventilator strategy in early exudative ARDS is to recruit and maintain alveoli open. Positive end-expiratory pressure (PEEP) prevents alveolar collapse and redistributes pulmonary edema away from the alveolar-capillary surface to the corners between alveolar walls where the radius of curvature is smallest and surface tension effects are greatest. Indeed, increasing mean airway pressure by other means (inspiratory pauses, decelerating inspiratory wave form, pressure-control ventilation with increased I:E ratio) also aids in improving arterial oxygenation in the same way. This increase in airspace pressure can add to the resistance to pulmonary blood flow but, more importantly, airspace pressures can be directly transmitted to other organs in the thorax so that mean intrathoracic pressure and right atrial pressure increase, directly reducing the pressure gradient driving venous return. A decrease in venous return in steady state is equivalent to a decrease in cardiac output. Even though the addition of positive airway pressure may have increased arterial oxygen saturation, the associated decrease in cardiac output may reduce whole body oxygen delivery.

Least PEEP Consistent with an Adequate Cardiac Output

From our discussion it can be seen that PEEP has both beneficial and detrimental effects. The correct amount of PEEP that should be applied in an individual patient has not yet been determined in clinical studies. A recent exciting approach is to measure the lower inflection point of pulmonary volume-pressure curves and apply this amount of PEEP.[54] The rationale is that at this point PEEP will prevent opening and closure of alveoli during the ventilatory cycle, a process thought to be detrimental and potentially injurious to alveoli. This approach may reduce cytokine expression by lungs in experimental animals.[55] However, lower inflection point PEEP levels are generally in the range of 15 or more centimeters H_2O. These high levels of PEEP may impede venous return.

To strike a balance between the beneficial and detrimental effects of PEEP in an individual patient, our clinical approach is to use the least PEEP that provides adequate arterial oxygenation at a nontoxic FiO_2. In general, we also do not reduce PEEP below 5 cm H_2O because some degree of PEEP prevents atelectasis and prevents some of the opening and closure of alveoli. For example, if a PEEP of 10 provides an SaO_2 of 90% on an FiO_2 of 0.5, then we would not increase the PEEP further even though a lower inflection point measurement in the patient may be a pressure of 15 cm H_2O.

Fluid Management

Pulmonary Wedge Pressure and Edema Formation

Edema formation in the lungs is reasonably well described by the Starling equation:

$$\text{Edema flux} = K_f \left([P_c - P_i] - \sigma [\pi_c - \pi_i] \right)$$

where K_f is the filtration coefficient, P_c is the pulmonary capillary hydrostatic pressure, P_i is pulmonary interstitial hydrostatic pressure, π_c is plasma oncotic pressure, π_i is interstitial oncotic pressure, and σ is the reflection coefficient for protein by the pulmonary capillary endothelium. Normally, P_c exceeds P_i so that hydrostatic pressure in the capillaries drives fluid out of the proximal end of pulmonary capillaries. This effect is countered by plasma oncotic pressure, which exceeds interstitial oncotic pressure so that water is brought back into the pulmonary capillaries, particularly toward the distal end of the pulmonary capillaries (where the hydrostatic pressure gradient is smallest and the plasma oncotic pressure of the blood is the highest). The effect of oncotic pressure differences relative to hydrostatic pressure differences is governed by the reflection coefficient σ, which, in health, ranges from approximately 0.6 to 0.8. Early in ARDS the alveolar-capillary membrane becomes leaky. That is, σ is reduced to approximately zero. Loss of the oncotic pressure gradient, which tends to keep the lungs dry, leads to early pulmonary edemagenesis. Because σ is effectively zero, the second term in the Starling equation drops out so that efforts to reduce edema flux depend almost entirely on changes in P_c, the pulmonary capillary hydrostatic pressure.

Pulmonary capillary hydrostatic pressure can be approximated by pulmonary wedge pressure in most clinical settings. Thus, cardiovascular management aimed at reducing edemagenesis depends on strategies to reduce pulmonary wedge pressure. However, Starling function curves of the heart demonstrate that cardiac output depends on preload. Thus, excessively low pulmonary wedge pressures will reduce cardiac output. Excessive reduction in pulmonary wedge pressure and cardiac output will lead to organ hypoperfusion. Total oxygen delivery will decrease even though reduced edema formation may have improved arterial oxygen saturation. Clearly, achieving the most beneficial physiologic state depends on a balance.

Our approach is to maintain patients at the lowest pulmonary wedge pressure that results in an adequate cardiac output. We test for adequacy of cardiac output by checking lactate when indicated and by monitoring organ system function including following urine output, measuring creatinine, and following level of consciousness. If there is no evidence of inadequate cardiac output, we aim for a slightly lower pulmonary wedge pressure and retest our measures. When any measure suggests the potential for inadequate cardiac output, we reinfuse a small volume or, in select cases, adjust inotrope management, and repeat the measurement. In this way we titrate pulmonary wedge pressure to maintain an adequate cardiac output.

Although this approach is fundamental to managing the early stages of ARDS, later, during the fibroproliferative phase, the alveolar-capillary membrane may no longer be excessively leaky, and increasing dead space may become an important clinical issue. In this setting, reducing the pulmonary wedge pressure will increase the proportion of West's zone 1 lung. In West's zone 1 lung, alveolar pressure exceeds pulmonary capillary pressure so that these lung regions are hypoperfused and act as dead space. This further impairs CO_2 clearance by the lungs. Thus, it is important to recognize that low pulmonary wedge pressures improve oxygenation best when employed early in the exudative phase of ARDS and become progressively less important, and can become detrimental, by impairing CO_2 elimination, later in the fibroproliferative phase of ARDS.

Crystalloid versus Colloid

There is no firm clinical evidence that choosing crystalloid versus colloid as a volume resuscitation agent in ARDS results in a significant difference in outcome. Inadequate or excessive fluid administration causes more frequent and more severe complications than the choice of crystalloid or colloid. The cost of crystalloid solutions is many fold less than the cost of colloid solutions. For the majority of patients this may be the most important deciding factor when no other medical indication favors one approach versus the other.

A number of important differences exist between crystalloid and colloid administration that, in some patients, may be very important considerations. An infusion of one liter of normal saline results in approximately one-quarter of this volume being retained in the intravascular compartment. In contrast, a similar volume infusion of albumin, or a synthetic colloid such as pentastarch, results in more than double this fraction of the infused volume being retained in the intravascular compartment. Thus, when vascular access is very limited and the intravascular volume must be expanded rapidly, colloid is an appropriate choice. Side effects of the administered solution also must be considered. Large volumes of normal saline can cause a dilutional non-anion gap acidosis. However, appropriate crystalloid substitutes that contain bicarbonate or bicarbonate equivalents, such as Ringer's lactate, can avoid this problem. Some colloid preparations can affect platelet function and, in individual patients, this may become a significant concern.

Crystalloid resuscitation is clearly most appropriate in a number of clinical settings. In cardiogenic shock where total plasma protein and albumin may be completely normal there is no benefit to colloid use. Crystalloid in this setting has the additional benefit that, if overly aggressive volume expansion occurs resulting in pulmonary edema, in a few minutes the crystalloid will redistribute and the pulmonary edema will subside to some extent. Similarly, in hypovolemia without protein loss, or in the early volume resuscitation of hypovolemia of any cause, crystalloid solutions are appropriate. In early volume resuscitation, expansion of both the intravascular and extravascular compartments, including the intracellular compartment, needs to occur.

Colloids are possibly of benefit in the clinical setting of intravascular hypovolemia with interstitial edema and severe hypoproteinemia.[56] Colloid may also potentially be of benefit in states where edema formation may be detrimental such as in wound healing, burns, and sepsis. In these clinical settings large-volume crystalloid resuscitation results in tissue edema and more capillary narrowing compared to colloid infusions. The increased tissue edema may conceivably result in impaired oxygen extraction.

There are no large randomized controlled trials of crystalloid versus colloid in ARDS.

Effect of Mixed Venous Oxygen Saturation on Arterial PO_2

When we think of the causes of arterial hypoxemia, it usually suffices to consider (1) V/Q mismatch, (2) shunt, (3) low alveolar PO_2 states due to hypoventilation or low FiO_2, and, to a lesser extent, (4) diffusion limitation. However, in critically ill ARDS patients with high physiologic shunt fractions, (5) mixed venous oxygen saturation becomes a critically important variable. Figure 6.8 illustrates that if mixed venous oxygen saturation is increased in the setting of a high physiologic shunt fraction, arterial oxygen saturation can increase dramatically. Conversely, a low mixed venous oxygen saturation has an increasingly important effect on decreasing arterial oxygen saturation as shunt fraction increases. Mixed venous oxygen saturation depends on the balance of whole body oxygen delivery (DO_2) and whole body oxygen consumption (VO_2)

$$S_VO_2 = SaO2 \times (DO_2 - VO_2)/DO_2.$$

If whole body oxygen delivery is increased, oxygen consumption becomes a smaller fraction of the total so that mixed venous oxygen saturation increases. Alternatively, if whole body oxygen consumption is minimized, mixed venous oxygen saturation increases. Successful strategies to increase mixed venous oxygen saturation include a combination of increasing cardiac output and oxygen-carrying capacity of the blood. Possibly more important is decreasing whole body oxygen consumption to a minimum value by sedating, and, if necessary, paralyzing the very hypoxemic patient.

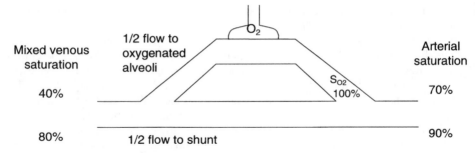

Figure 6.8. The effect of mixed venous oxygen saturation on arterial oxygen saturation, in the presence of shunt, is illustrated. Oxygen in a stylized alveolus increases oxygen saturation (SO_2) to 100%. In this example a mixed venous oxygen saturation of 40% in the setting of a 50% shunt results in an arterial saturation of approximately 70% – severe arterial hypoxemia. Without altering the lungs, increasing mixed venous oxygen saturation to 80% increases arterial oxygen saturation to 90%.

Best Hemoglobin

Previously it was common for clinicians to transfuse patients when they fell below an arbitrary numerical threshold value of hemoglobin, for example, a hemoglobin of 100 g/L. Yet many patients, such as chronic renal failure patients (before recombinant erythropoiten), usually had hemoglobin concentrations well below this level. Therefore, a number of investigators are comparing the effect of transfusing to higher hemoglobins versus leaving hemoglobin at the relatively low values that are frequently encountered in critically ill patients with ARDS. Initial reports indicate that patients with cardiovascular risk factors may benefit from increased hemoglobin levels.[57] Increasing benefit was found as hemoglobin increased to 100 g/L. Even higher hemoglobin levels may be of benefit in this subset of patients. In addition, in patients with cardiovascular risk factors, higher hemoglobin levels in hypoxemic ARDS patients with very low mixed venous oxygen saturations may help prevent severe arterial hypoxemia. As discussed earlier, low mixed venous oxygen saturations have a significant impact on arterial oxygen saturation so that an increase in oxygen-carrying capacity can improve arterial hypoxemia by its effect on mixed venous oxygen saturation. Marik and Sibbald[58] have demonstrated the important caveat that red blood cells which have been stored for prolonged periods of time do not appear to have the same oxygen-carrying capacity as fresh red blood cells. Recent results show that a strategy of maintaining a high hemoglobin concentration (i.e., 100–120 g/L) regardless of physiologic need using stored blood transfusions is detrimental.[59] Hébert and colleagues[59] compared a liberal (Hg 100–120 g/L) to a conservative (Hg 70–90 g/L) transfusion strategy in the critically ill and found higher mortality (28% vs. 22%, $p < 0.05$) and less transfusion (2.6 units vs. 4.6 units of packed erythrocytes) in the liberal transfusion group. Given the current evidence for and against transfusion, we

reserve red blood cell transfusion for those patients where a strong physiologic rationale suggests increasing oxygen-carrying capacity will be beneficial.

Tools and Tests to Assess and Manage Cardiovascular Function

Lactate

Although hyperlactatemia is a very useful global marker of anaerobic metabolism,
there are also several nonhypoxic mechanisms of hyperlactatemia. High circulating
lactate levels are associated with increased morbidity and mortality so that lactate is
a useful indicator of poor prognosis even though it is not specific for tissue hypoxia,
especially in patients with sepsis. However, some studies find a poor relationship
between lactate levels and multiple organ failure.[60]

There are several nonhypoxic mechanisms of hyperlactatemia. Because liver and
kidney are the major organs of lactate clearance and because dysfunction of these
organs is so prevalent in the critically ill, delayed clearance of lactate may be a frequent contributor to the hyperlactatemia of critical illness.[61,62] Another nonhypoxic
mechanism of hyperlactatemia is increased protein breakdown (catabolism) in critical illness. Catabolism causes release of amino acids that are converted to pyruvate
and lactate. A normal lactate/pyruvate ratio indicates aerobic metabolism.[63] During
volume resuscitation, increased flow could "flush" lactate from the periphery to the
central circulation. Thus a "lactate hangover" could occur during reversal of tissue
hypoxia.

Sepsis can cause lactic acidosis in the absence of tissue hypoxia.[64,65] Dysfunction
of pyruvate dehydrogenase (PDH) occurs in sepsis. PDH converts pyruvate to
oxaloacetate, permitting pyruvate to enter the Kreb's cycle. Dysfunction of PDH
causes accumulation of pyruvate and lactate – but the lactate/pyruvate (L/P) ratio
remains normal indicating aerobic metabolism. PDH activity is decreased in muscle
of septic rats and can be partially reversed by dichloracetate.[66] Endotoxin increases
mRNA and protein synthesis of a glucose transporter protein on the cell membrane.
This increases cellular glucose uptake and release of lactate and pyruvate.[67]
Increased glucose transporter protein and increased release of pyruvate and lactate
have been described in muscle and liver of septic rats.[68]

Respiratory alkalosis, metabolic alkalosis,[69,70] and the administration of
bicarbonate[71] increase lactate levels due to increased peripheral lactate production.
Similarly, accelerated aerobic glycolysis due to catecholamines causes pyruvate to
accumulate and convert to lactate and alanine. Again the lactate/pyruvate ration is
normal. Adrenaline infusion in healthy volunteers increases carbohydrate metabolism
and causes a small rise in plasma lactate.[72] Increased skeletal muscle glycogenolysis
increases peripheral lactate production. Splanchnic glucose production and lactate
extraction are also increased probably secondary to increases in hepatic glycogenolysis

and gluconeogenesis.[73] However, worsening tissue perfusion and deleterious effects on tissue oxygenation in response to adrenaline infusion cannot be excluded in critically ill patients. Adrenaline infusion decreased portal venous and total hepatic blood flow and increased mesenteric vascular resistance and lactate levels in experimental models of sepsis and caused lactic acidosis in critically ill patients with severe sepsis.[74,75]

When to Use a Pulmonary Artery Catheter

One study[76] and subsequent investigator workshops have suggested that pulmonary artery catheters are not universally beneficial. Based on these reports we now restrict our pulmonary artery catheter use to situations where the information obtained from the pulmonary artery catheter will directly influence patient management. This scenario most frequently occurs when severe hypoxia is accompanied by cardiovascular dysfunction. In this setting the clinician would like to increase intravascular volume to improve cardiac output and mean arterial pressure to levels adequate to perfuse organ systems to maintain function. However, further fluid resuscitation will worsen already severe arterial hypoxemia with potentially fatal consequences. We also use a pulmonary artery catheter when cardiac function is impaired and high doses of inotropic or vasopressor drugs are used. In this setting alpha agonists may further decrease a low cardiac output, reducing oxygen delivery to oxygen-starved tissues. Conversely, if cardiac output is relatively high with a low calculated systemic vascular resistance, as is typical of ARDS, the use of unopposed beta agonists may result in excessive hypotension and worsened organ system dysfunction. Measures of ventricular filling pressures, mixed venous oxygen saturation, and cardiac output in these settings are invaluable in balancing the beneficial and detrimental aspects of fluid and vasopressor therapy.

Gastric Tonometry

Tissue PCO_2 changes with changes in tissue blood flow. Gastric mucosal CO_2 can readily diffuse into a salt solution or gas in a gas-permeable balloon attached to a nasogastric tube. Thus, gastric mucosal PCO_2 can be easily measured by instilling fluid or gas into a tonometer nasogastric tube, allowing enough time for PCO_2 to equilibrate, and measuring PCO_2 in the fluid or gas. A similar tonometer approach to measuring tissue PCO_2 can be applied at other sites such as small bowel, colon, bladder, and CSF.

Tonometric measurement of gastric PCO_2[77] is an attractive clinical measurement for several reasons. A greatly elevated tonometer PCO_2 measurement, and by inference tissue PCO_2, suggests the presence of tissue anaerobic metabolism,[78,79] resulting in proton formation[80] and titration of bicarbonate-based buffer systems to produce CO_2. A less severely elevated gastric tonometer PCO_2 suggests a relative imbalance between local tissue perfusion and metabolic demands.[79] That is, during steady state, gastric mucosal PCO_2 reflects the balance between CO_2 production by tissue and CO_2 removal by gastric blood flow. Therefore, gastric PCO_2 can increase because of decreased gastric blood flow (stagnant flow) without implying anaerobic production of CO_2. Thus, clinically an increase in tonometer PCO_2 is useful in detecting inadequate tissue perfusion even if it has not progressed to frank anaerobic metabolism.[81] These potentially important measurements have generated a great deal of enthusiasm because they are easily measured clinically using a device no more invasive than the ubiquitous nasogastric tube in critically ill patients. Several important studies have shown potential for significant clinical benefit using gastric tonometry.[82–87]

Part of the reason measures of gut perfusion, such as tonometer PCO_2, may be useful is that the gut may be an organ particularly sensitive to systemic hypoperfusion.[88] For example, several investigators have found that the onset of oxygen supply dependency occurred earlier in the gut than in the whole body in animal models.[88] In addition, gut ischemia may be important in the pathogenesis of a systemic inflammatory response.[89,90] Intestinal permeability increases after gut ischemia resulting in leakage of bacteria and bacterial products into the portal circulation. This results in activation of hepatic Kupffer cells and circulating leukocytes. The subsequent systemic inflammatory response results in distal organ damage and dysfunction. Thus, there is a strong physiologic rationale for monitoring gut perfusion in critically ill patients.

Initial investigators estimated gastric intracellular pH using the Henderson-Hasselbalch equation, substituting arterial HCO_3^- concentration for the unknown equivalent intracellular base concentration. Calculation of pH_i is important for interpretation of early clinical studies, but calculation of pH_i is not necessary and makes erroneous assumptions. The assumption that HCO_3^- of the gastric mucosa is in equilibrium with the systemic arterial HCO_3^- is not always true. For example, when gastric mucosal blood flow decreases in shock, the effective gastric tissue HCO_3^- may be significantly lower than the systemic arterial HCO_3^-.

A number of studies demonstrate that tonometry may be a useful clinical tool. Gutierrez and colleagues found that, in critically ill patients with an initial gastric tonometer $pH_i > 7.35$, if tonometer-derived pHi subsequently fell below 7.35, then resuscitation with fluids and dobutamine significantly improved survival.[83] Mohsenifar and colleagues have demonstrated that a low pHi, calculated from gastric juice PCO_2, predicts failure of spontaneous ventilation at the time of extubation in critically ill patients.[87] Studies by Marik[85] and by Maynard and colleagues[86] suggest that gastric tonometer-derived pH_i is a more robust predictor of outcome in critically ill patients than hemodynamic measurements and other common predictors. Similarly, Mohsenifar and colleagues[84] found that pHi was a better predictor of outcome than all other presently used parameters in hemodynamically stable, mechanically ventilated patients. A pH_i less than 7.25 had a sensitivity of 86% and a specificity of 83% in predicting mortality.[84] Thus, tonometry has the potential to play an important role in the ICU, adding to other hemodynamic and physiologic data in assessing adequacy of perfusion and enhancing prognostic measures, including severity of illness scoring systems such as APACHE II.

Problems have been identified with gastric tonometer measurements. Gastric mucosal acid-base balance is complex so that the relationship between pH_i and tissue perfusion may not be straightforward. Reflux of alkaline duodenal contents into the acidic stomach or back diffusion of gastric mucosal bicarbonate produces a significant amount of CO_2 unrelated to tissue hypoperfusion. Therefore, H_2 antagonist treatment has been used when gastric tonometric measurements are to be made. This recommendation is based on studies performed in healthy volunteers,[91] but recent studies in critically ill patients contradict those in healthy volunteers.[92] In critically ill patients the use of H_2 blockers may have no effect on calculated gastric pH_i. Function of the gastric mucosa may be disturbed and the acid secretion defect may explain the lack of need of H_2 blockers in the critically ill. It is possible, however, that the use of H_2 blockers modifies normal values for pH_i, although this has not been confirmed in critically ill patients. Enteral feeding decreases gastric pH_i by stimulating secretion of hydrogen ions, which are then buffered by bicarbonate secreted by the nonparietal gastric cells generating CO_2. Therefore, discontinuation of enteral feeding for at least 1 hour before measurements are taken has been recommended when measuring gastric pH_i.

In addition, gastric intramural PCO_2 may not be an accurate reflection of the more important gut intramural PCO_2 because the gastric arterial blood supply is more extensive than the blood supply of the gut, which is predominantly via the superior mesenteric artery. Thus, gut ischemia does not necessarily indicate gastric ischemia.

Problems common to all tonometry include that tonometer-measured PCO_2 requires a prolonged equilibration time so that a correction factor must be introduced to account for incomplete CO_2 equilibration. Gastric mucosal CO_2 and arterial bicarbonate HCO_3^- (representing gastric mucosal HCO_3^-) are needed for the calculation of pH_i. The technique relies heavily on the correct sampling technique, a short time between sampling and testing, and calibration and maintenance of the blood gas analyzer used. At present, we do not use gastric tonometry for routine clinical care; however, gastic tonometry may be useful in specific clinical settings such as high-risk vascular (i.e., aortic) surgery to detect and correct gut ischemia.

Summary

Cardiovascular management recognizes that oxygen delivery to the whole body and specific organs is of primary importance. Thus, arterial oxygen saturation, oxygen-carrying capacity, and cardiac output or regional flow are equally important. Mixed venous oxygen saturation is both an important measure of adequacy of oxygen delivery and a modulator of arterial oxygen saturation. That is, a low mixed venous oxygen saturation also contributes significantly to decreased arterial oxygen saturation in the high pulmonary shunt state of ARDS. Pulmonary edemagenesis is worsened by excessive fluid administration so cardiovascular management aims at a balance between adequate volume resuscitation of the circulation versus dry lungs. In very hypoxemic patients this balance is difficult to achieve, and the goal-oriented clinical hypothesis–driven use of a pulmonary artery catheter is valuable. In specific settings the use of a gut tonometer catheter may be helpful in judging the adequacy of resuscitation.

References

1. Sagawa K. End-systolic pressure-volume relationship in retrospect and prospect. Fed Proc 1984; 43:2399–2401.

2. Kass DA, Maughan WL, Guo ZM, Kono A, Sunagawa K, Sagawa K. Comparative influence of load versus inotropic states on indexes of ventricular contractility: experimental and theoretical analysis based on pressure-volume relationships. Circulation 1987; 76:1422–1436.

3. Parker MM, Shelhamer JH, Bacharach SL, Green MV, Natanson C, Frederick TM, Damske BA, Parrillo JE. Profound but reversible myocardial depression in patients with septic shock. Ann Int Med 1984; 100:483–490.

4. Russell JA, Ronco JJ, Lockhat D, Belzberg A, Kiess M, Dodek PM. Oxygen delivery and consumption and ventricular preload are greater in survivors than in nonsurvivors of the adult respiratory distress syndrome. Am Rev Respir Dis 1990; 141:659–665.

5. Parker MM, Shelhamer JH, Natanson C, Alling DW, Parrillo JE. Serial cardiovascular variables in survivors and nonsurvivors of human septic shock: heart rate as an early predictor of prognosis. Crit Care Med 1987; 15:923–929.

6. Parker MM, Suffredini AF, Natanson C, Ognibene FP, Shelhamer JH, Parrillo JE. Responses of left ventricular function in survivors and nonsurvivors of septic shock. J Crit Care 1989; 4:19–25.

7. Walley KR. Mechanisms of decreased cardiac function in sepsis. In Yearbook of intensive care and emergency medicine, ed JL Vincent, Springer, Berlin, 1997, pp. 243–255.

8. Walley KR, Hebert PC, Wakai Y, Wilcox PG, Road JD, Cooper DJ. Decrease in left ventricular contractility after tumor necrosis factor-alpha infusion in dogs. J Appl Physiol 1994; 76:1060–1067.

9. Finkel MS, Oddis CV, Jacob TD, Watkins SC, Hattler BG, Simmons RL. Negative inotropic effects of cytokines on the heart mediated by nitric oxide. Science 1992; 257:387–389.

10. Kumar A, Thota V, Dee L, Olson J, Uretz E, Parrillo JE. Tumor necrosis factor alpha and interleukin 1 beta are responsible for in vitro myocardial cell depression induced by human septic shock serum. J Exp Med 1996; 183:949–958.

11. Schulz R, Dodge KL, Lopaschuk GD, Clanachan AS. Peroxynitrite impairs cardiac contractile function by decreasing cardiac efficiency. Am J Physiol 1997; 272:H1212–H1219.

12. Granton JT, Goddard CM, Allard MF, van Eeden S, Walley KR. Leukocytes and decreased left-ventricular contractility during endotoxemia in rabbits. Am J Respir Crit Care Med 1997; 155:1977–1983.

13. Goddard CM, Allard MF, Hogg JC, Walley KR. Myocardial morphometric changes related to decreased contractility after endotoxin. Am J Physiol 1996; 270:H1446–H1452.

14. Ronco JJ, Belzberg A, Phang PT, Walley KR, Dodek PM, Russell JA. No differences in hemodynamics, ventricular function, and oxygen delivery in septic and nonseptic patients with the adult respiratory distress syndrome. Crit Care Med 1994; 22:777–782.

15. Curzen NP, Jourdan KB, Mitchell JA. Endothelial modification of pulmonary vascular tone. Intensive Care Med 1996; 22:596–607.

16. Briegel J, Schelling G, Haller M, Mraz W, Forst H, Peter K. A comparison of the adrenocortical response during septic shock and after complete recovery. Intensive Care Med 1996; 22:894–899.

17. Guyton AC, Lindsey AW, Abernathy B, Langston JB. Mechanism of increased venous return and cardiac output caused by epinephrine. Am J Physiol 1958; 192:126–130.

18. Goldberg HS, Rabson J. Control of cardiac output by systemic vessels. Circulatory adjustments to acute and chronic respiratory failure and the effect of therapeutic interventions. Am J Cardiol 1981; 47:696–702.

19. Mitzner W, Goldberg H. Effects of epinephrine on resisitive and compliant properties of the canine vasculature. J Appl Physiol 1975; 39:272–280.

20. Segal JM, Phang PT, Walley KR. Low-dose dopamine hastens onset of gut ischemia in a porcine model of hemorrhagic shock. J Appl Physiol 1992; 73:1159–1164.

21. Schumacker PT, Samsel RW. Oxygen supply and consumption in the adult respiratory distress syndrome. Clinics Chest Med 1990; 11:715–722.

22. Walley KR. Heterogeneity of oxygen delivery impairs oxygen extraction by peripheral tissues: theory. J Appl Physiol 1996; 81:885–894.

23. Schumacker PT, Samsel RW. Analysis of oxygen delivery and uptake relationships in the Krogh tissue model. J Appl Physiol 1989; 67:1234–1244.

24. Piiper J, Meyer M, Scheid P. Dual role of diffusion in tissue gas exchange: blood-tissue equilibration and diffusion shunt. Respir Physiol 1984; 56:131–144.

25. Humer MF, Phang PT, Friesen BP, Allard MF, Goddard CM, Walley KR. Heterogeneity of gut capillary transit times and impaired gut oxygen extraction in endotoxemic pigs. J Appl Physiol 1996; 81:895–904.

26. Drazenovic R, Samsel RW, Wylam ME, Doerschuk CM, Schumacker PT. Regulation of perfused capillary density in canine intestinal mucosa during endotoxemia. J Appl Physiol 1992; 72:259–265.

27. Danek SJ, Lynch JP, Weg JG, Dantzker DR. The dependence of oxygen uptake on oxygen delivery in the adult respiratory distress syndrome. Am Rev Respir Dis 1980; 122:387–395.

28. Ronco JJ, Phang PT, Walley KR, Wiggs B, Fenwick JC, Russell JA. Oxygen consumption is independent of changes in oxygen delivery in severe adult respiratory distress syndrome. Am Rev Respir Dis 1991; 143:1267–1273.

29. Manthous CA, Hall JB, Olson D, Singh M, Chatila W, Pohlman A, Kushner R, Schmidt GA, Wood LDG. Effect of cooling on oxygen consumption in febrile critically ill patients. Am J Respir Crit Care Med 1995; 151:10–14.

30. Boyd O, Grounds M, Bennett D. The dependency of oxygen consumption on oxygen delivery in critically ill postoperative patients is mimicked by variations in sedation. Chest 1992; 101:1619–1624.

31. Manthous CA, Hall JB, Kushner R, Schmidt GA, Russo G, Wood LDG. The effect of mechanical ventilation on oxygen consumption in critically ill patients. Am J Respir Crit Care Med 1995; 151:210–214.

32. Weissman C, Kemper M. The oxygen uptake–oxygen delivery relationship during ICU interventions. Chest 1991; 99:430–435.

33. Weissman C, Kemper BA, Elwyn DH, Askanazi J, Hyman AI, Kinney JM. The energy expenditure of the mechanically ventilated critically ill patients. Chest 1986; 89:254–259.

34. Schlichtig R, Kramer DJ, Boston R, Pinsky MR. Renal O_2 consumption during progressive hemorrhage. Am Appl Physiol 1991; 70:1957–1962.

35. Samsel RW, Cherqui D, Pietrabissa A, Sanders WM, Roncella M, Edmond JC, Schumacker PT. Hepatic oxygen and lactate extraction during stagnant hypoxia. J Appl Physiol 1991; 17:186–193.

36. Arai AE, Pantely GA, Anselone CG, Bristow J, Bristow JD. Active downregulation of myocardial energy requirements during prolonged moderate ischemia in swine. Circ Res 1991; 69:1458–1469.
37. Schumacker PT, Chandel N, Agusti AGN. Oxygen conformance of cellular respiration in hepatocytes. Am J Physiol 1993; 265:L395–L402.
38. Schumacker PT, Soble JS, Feldman T. Oxygen delivery and uptake relationships in patients with aortic stenosis. Am J Respir Crit Care Med 1994; 149:1123–1131.
39. Albert RK, Schrijen F, Poincelot F. Oxygen consumption and transport in stable patients with chronic obstructive pulmonary disease. Am Rev Respir Dis 1986; 134:678–682.
40. Stratton HH, Feustel PJ, Newell JC. Regression of calculated variables in the presence of shared measurement error. J Appl Physiol 1987; 62:2083–2093.
41. Carlile PV, Gray BA. Effect of opposite changes in cardiac output and arterial PO_2 on the relationship between mixed venous PO_2 and oxygen transport. Am Rev Respir Dis 1989; 140:891–898.
42. Lutch JS, Murray JF. Continuous positive-pressure ventilation: effects on systemic oxygen transport and tissue oxygenation. Ann Intern Med 1972; 76:193–202.
43. Ronco JJ, Fenwick JC, Wiggs BR, Phang PT, Russell JA, Tweeddale MG. Oxygen consumption is independent of increases in oxygen delivery by dobutamine in septic patients who have normal or increased plasma lactate. Am Rev Respir Dis 1993; 147:25–31.
44. Manthous CA, Schumacker PT, Pohlman A, Schmidt GA, Hall JB, Samsel RW, Wood LDH. Absence of supply dependence of oxygen consumption in patients with septic shock. J Crit Care 1993; 8:203–211.
45. Marik PE, Sibbald WJ. Effect of stored-blood transfusion on oxygen delivery in patients with sepsis. JAMA 1993; 269:3024–3029.
46. Mira JP, Fabre JE, Baigorri F, Coste J, Annat G, Artigas A, Nitemberg G, Dhainaut JF. Lack of oxygen supply dependence in patients with severe sepsis. A study of oxygen delivery increased by military antishock trouser and dobutamine. Chest 1994; 106:1524–1531.
47. Ronco JJ, Fenwick JC, Tweeddale MG, Wiggs BR, Phang PT, Cooper DJ, Cunningham KF, Russell JA, Walley KR. Identification of the critical oxygen delivery for anaerobic metabolism in critically ill septic and nonseptic humans. JAMA 1993; 270:1724–1730.
48. Walley KR, Collins RM, Cooper DJ, Warriner CB. Myocardial anaerobic metabolism occurs at a critical coronary venous PO_2 in pigs. Am J Respir Crit Care Med 1997; 155:222–228.
49. Shoemaker WC, Appel PL, Kram HB, Waxman K, Lee TS. Prospective trial of supranormal values of survivors as therapeutic goals in high-risk surgical patients. Chest 1988; 94:1176–1186.
50. Tuchschmidt J, Fried J, Astiz M, Rackow E. Elevation of cardiac output and oxygen delivery improves outcome in septic shock. Chest 1992; 102:216–220.
51. Hayes MA, Timmins AC, Yau EHS, Palazzo M, Hinds CJ, Watson D. Elevation of systemic oxygen delivery in the treatment of critically ill patients. N Engl J Med 1994; 330:1717–1722.
52. Gattinoni L, Brazzi L, Pelosi P, Latini R, Tognoni G, Pesenti A, Fumagalli R. A trial of goal-oriented hemodynamic therapy in critically ill patients. SvO_2 Collaborative Group. N Engl J Med 1995; 333:1025–1032.
53. Heyland DK, Cook DJ, King D, Kernerman P, Brun-Buisson C. Maximizing oxygen delivery in critically ill patients: a methodologic appraisal of the evidence. Crit Care Med 1996; 24:517–524.

54. Amato MB, Barbas CS, Medeiros DM, Magaldi RB, Schettino GP, Lorenzi-Filho G, Kairalla RA, Deheinzelin D, Munoz C, Oliveira R, Takagaki TY, Carvalho CR. Effect of a protective-ventilation strategy on mortality in the acute respiratory distress syndrome. N Engl J Med 1998; 338:347–354.
55. Tremblay L, Valenza F, Ribeiro SP, Li J, Slutsky AS. Injurious ventilatory strategies increase cytokines and c-fos m-RNA expression in an isolated rat lung model. J Clin Invest 1997; 99:944–952.
56. Mazzoni MC, Borgstrom P, Intaglietta M, Arfors KE. Capillary narrowing in hemorrhagic shock is rectified by hyperosmotic saline-dextran reinfusion. Circ Shock 1990; 31:407–418.
57. Hébert PC, Wells G, Tweeddale M, Martin C, Marshall J, Pham B, Blajchman M, Schweitzer I, Pagliarello G. Does transfusion practice affect mortality in critically ill patients? Transfusion Requirements in Critical Care (TRICC) Investigators and the Canadian Critical Care Trials Group. Am J Respir Crit Care Med 1997; 155:1618–1623.
58. Marik PE, Sibbald WJ. Effect of stored-blood transfusion on oxygen delivery in patients with sepsis. JAMA 1993; 269:3024–3029.
59. Hébert PC, Wells G, Blajchman MA, et al. Transfusion requirements in critical care: a multicentre randomized controlled clinical trial. N Engl J Med (in press).
60. Marik PF. Gastric intramucosal pH: a better predictor of multiorgan dysfunction syndrome and death than oxygen-derived variables in patients with sepsis. Chest 1993; 104:225–229.
61. Rowell LB, Kraning KK, Evans TO. Splanchnic removal of lactate and pyruvate during prolonged exercise in man. J Appl Physiol 1966; 21:1773–1783.
62. Levraut J, Ciebieva JP, Chave S, et al. Mild hyperlactatemia in stable septic patients is due to impaired lactate clearance rather than overproduction. Am J Resp Crit Care Med 1998; 157:1021–1026.
63. Garber AJ, Karl IE, Kipnis DM. Alanine and glutamine synthesis and release from skeletal muscle. J Biol Chem 1976; 251:836–843.
64. Jepson MM, Cox M, Bates PC, Rothwell NJ, Stock MJ, Cady EB, Millward DJ. Regional blood flow and skeletal muscle energy status in endotoxemic rats. Am J Physiol 1987; 252:E581–E587.
65. Jacobs DO, Maris J, Fried R, Settle RG, Rolandelli RR, Korunda MJ, Chance B, Rombeau JL. In vivo phosphorus 31 magnetic spectroscopy of rat hind limb, skeletal muscle during sepsis. Arch Surg 1988; 123:1425–1428.
66. Curtis SE, Cain SM. Regional and systemic oxygen delivery uptake relations and lactate flux in hyperdynamic endotoxin-treated dogs. Am Rev Respir Dis 1992; 145:348–354.
67. Zeller WP, The SM, Sweet M. Altered glucose transporter in RNA abundance in a rat model of endotoxic shock. Biochem Biophys Res Comm 1991; 176:535–540.
68. Hotchkiss RS, Karl IE. Reevaluation of the role of cellular hypoxia and bioenergetic failure in sepsis. JAMA 1992; 267:1503–1510.
69. Huckabee WE. Relationships of pyruvate and lactate during anaerobic metabolism: I. Effects of infusion of pyruvate or glucose and of hyperventilation. J Clin Invest 1958; 37:244–254.
70. Goldstein PJ, Simmons DH, Tashkin DP. Effect of acid-base alterations on hepatic lactate utilization. J Physiol (London) 1972; 223:261–278.
71. Morris LR, Murphy MB, Kitabchi AE. Bicarbonate therapy in severe diabetic ketoacidosis. Ann Intern Med 1986; 105:836–840.

72. Ensinger H, Lindner K, Dirks B, Kilian J, Grunert A, Ahnefeld F. Adrenaline: relationship between infusion rate, plasma concentration, metabolic and haemodynamic effects in volunteers. Eur J Anaesthesiol 1992; 9:435–446.

73. Bearn A, Billing B, Sherlock S. The effect of adrenaline and noradrenaline on hepatic blood flow and splanchnic carbohydrate metabolism in man. J Physiol 1951; 115:430–441.

74. Cheung P-Y, Barrington KL, Pearson RJ, Bigam DL, Finer NN, van Aerde JE. Systemic, pulmonary and mesenteric perfusion and oxygenation effects of dopamine and epinephrine. Am J Respir Crit Care Med 1997; 155:32–37.

75. Day NPJ, Phu NH, Bethell DP, Mai NTH, Chau TTH, Hien TT, White NJ. The effects of dopamine and adrenaline infusions on acid-base balance and systemic haemodynamics in severe infection. Lancet 1996; 348:219–223.

76. Connors AF Jr, Speroff T, Dawson NV, Thomas C, Harrell FE Jr, Wagner D, Desbiens N, Goldman L, Wu AW, Califf RM, Fulkerson WJ Jr, Vidaillet H, Broste S, Bellamy P, Lynn J, Knaus WA. The effectiveness of right heart catheterization in the initial care of critically ill patients. JAMA 1996; 276:889–897.

77. Fiddian-Green RG, McGough E, Pittenger G, Rothman E. Predictive value of intramural pH and other risk factors for massive bleeding from stress ulceration. Gastroenterology 1983; 85:613–620.

78. Brown SD, Gutierrez G. Does gastric tonometry work? Yes. Controversies Crit Care Med 1996; 12:569–585.

79. Schlichtig R, Bowles SA. Distinguishing between aerobic and anaerobic appearance of dissolved CO_2 in intestine during low flow. J Appl Physiol 1994; 76:2443–2451.

80. Hotchkiss RS, Karl IE. Reevaluation of the role of cellular hypoxia and bioenergetic failure in sepsis. JAMA 1992; 267:1503–1510.

81. Vallet B. In Yearbook of intensive care and emergency medicine, ed JL Vincent, Springer-Verlag, Berlin, 1997, pp. 669–676.

82. Doglio GR, Pusajo JF, Egurrola MA, Bonfigli GC, Parra C, Veterre L, Hernandez MS, Fernandez S, Palizas F, Gutierrez G. Gastric mucosal pH as a prognostic index of mortality in critically ill patients. Crit Care Med 1991; 19:1037–1040.

83. Gutierrez G, Palizas F, Doglio G, Wainsztein N, Gallesio A, Pacin J, Dubin A, Schiavi E, Jorge M, Pusajo J, Klein F, San Roman E, Dorfman B, Shottlender J, Giniger R. Gastric intramucosal pH as a therapeutic index of tissue oxygenation in critically ill patients. Lancet 1992; 339:195–199.

84. Mohsenifar Z, Coolier J, Koerner SK. Gastric intramural pH in mechanically ventilated patients. Thorax 1996; 51:606–610.

85. Marik PF. Gastric intramucosal pH: a better predictor of multiorgan dysfunction syndrome and death than oxygen-derived variables in patients with sepsis. Chest 1993; 104:225–229.

86. Maynard N, Bihari D, Beale R, Smithies M, Baldock G, Mason R, McColl I. Assessment of splanchnic oxygenation by gastric tonometry in patients with acute circulatory failure. JAMA 1993; 270:1203–1210.

87. Mohsenifar Z, Hay A, Hay J, Lewis MI, Koerner SK. Gastric intramural pH as a predictor of success or failure in weaning patients from mechanical ventilation. Ann Intern Med 1993; 119:794–798.

88. Nelson DP, King CE, Dodd SL, Schumacker PT, Cain SM. Systemic and intestinal limits of O_2 extraction in the dog. J Appl Physiol 1987; 63:387–394.

89. Fiddian-Green RG. Splanchnic ischaemia and multiple organ failure in the critically ill. Ann Royal Coll Surg Engl 1988; 70:128–134.
90. Fink MP. Gastrointestinal mucosal injury in experimental models of shock, trauma, and sepsis. Crit Care Med 1991; 19:627–641.
91. Heard SO, Helsmoortel CM, Kent JC, Shahnarian A, Fink PM. Gastric tonometry in healthy volunteers: effects of ranitidine on calculated intramural pH. Crit Care Med 1991; 19:271–274.
92. Baigorri F, Calvet X, Duarte M, Saura P, Jubert P, Royo C, Joseph D, Artigas A. Effect of ranitidine treatment in gastric intramucosal pH determinations in critical patients. Intensive Care Med 1994; 20(Suppl 2):S2.

7

Mechanical Ventilation

Gregory A. Schmidt

Introduction

In many patients mechanical ventilation simply supports tidal breathing, for example, patients under general anesthesia or patients with trauma, drug overdose, sepsis, shock, or COPD. However, in ARDS patients, appropriate adjustment of mechanical ventilation may sometimes choose to support tidal breathing inadequately (permissive hypercapnia) to achieve more important goals. Mechanical ventilation of ARDS patients is complex and requires consideration of underlying pulmonary and cardiovascular physiology (Chapters 5 and 6), oxygen transport, beneficial and detrimental effects of positive pressure ventilation, the time course of airway pressure changes (e.g., assist-control mode vs. pressure control or other modes), cardiopulmonary interaction, and the effect of other nonpulmonary therapies (e.g., diuresis, inotropes). In this chapter the issue of mechanical ventilation of ARDS patients is approached from the perspective of the clinician – stepwise from the beginning. Issues that must be addressed in all patients, such as tidal volume, PEEP, and ventilator mode, are addressed first. This is then followed by "what if." What if hypoxemia is still a problem? What if hypotension is a problem? Finally, important complications of mechanical ventilation are addressed.

Initiating Mechanical Ventilation

In patients with significant ARDS, one of two fundamental derangements typically leads the intensivist to begin mechanical ventilation: either hypoxemia no longer responds to oxygen (due to intrapulmonary shunt) or the work of breathing becomes

Table 7.1. Indications for mechanical ventilation

Hypoxemia refractory to oxygen or mask CPAP
Excessive work of breathing unresponsive to mask ventilation
Hemodynamic instability
Rapidly deteriorating clinical course
Inability to maintain and protect the airway

excessive and unsustainable (due to reduced lung compliance, often compounded by a high minute ventilation). A subset of patients may be candidates for noninvasive ventilation, described later. Most will require endotracheal intubation (see Table 7.1). When signs point to impending respiratory failure (SaO_2 below 0.9 despite high flow oxygen, respiratory rate > 40, increasing patient agitation or delirium), the patient should be semielectively intubated before progression to full-blown respiratory failure. It is probably better to subject a few patients to an early, possibly unnecessary, but well-planned intubation than to risk aspiration, anoxia, or myocardial ischemia by waiting for the occasional patient to recover.

Noninvasive Ventilation

Noninvasive positive pressure ventilation (NIPPV) is finding increasing application in the management of acute respiratory failure in the postoperative setting and in patients with COPD or CHF. There is little published experience with NIPPV in patients with ARDS, however. Although it would often be an inappropriate choice due to hemodynamic instability, severe hypoxemia, or a rapidly progressive course, one might predict that it would be successful in carefully chosen patients by recruiting alveoli and reducing shunt (through expiratory positive airway pressure, EPAP) and unloading the respiratory muscles (through inspiratory positive airway pressure, IPAP). Reasonable initial noninvasive ventilatory settings are EPAP = 7 to 10 cm H_2O, adjusted to maintain SaO_2 > 0.9 and IPAP = 15, adjusted according to patient comfort. A good response to NIPPV is usually apparent within 30 minutes of its initiation (often sooner), signaled by a falling respiratory rate, less tachycardia, improved pulse oximeter readings, and less patient distress. What role NIPPV will find in ARDS, if any, remains to be defined.

Intubation Technique

Patients with evolving ARDS are at risk for severe hypoxemia during intubation, related to their typically reduced FRC and compounded by the often elevated VO_2. Additional risks derive from concomitant hemodynamic instability and a potentially full stomach. Reasonable cautions include preoxygenation and correction of hypovolemia followed by rapid securing of the airway by the most experienced operator available. In the majority of patients who are not severely hemodynamically unstable,

Table 7.2. Principles of ventilator management

1. Use the lowest PEEP (with a lower limit of 7.5 cm H_2O) that effects an adequate arterial oxygen saturation on an $FiO_2 < 0.6$.
2. If PEEP > 15 cm H_2O or $FiO_2 > 0.6$ are needed to maintain the $SaO_2 > 0.90$, attempt to reduce VO_2, raise SvO_2, or consider novel methods to aid oxygenation (unconventional modes of ventilation, nitric oxide, positional maneuvers).
3. Use the lowest tidal volume that maintains adequate CO_2 elimination.
4. If the plateau airway pressure exceeds 30 cm H_2O despite small tidal volumes, lower the Vt further; then attempt to lower VCO_2, reduce dead space, or allow the PCO_2 to rise (permissive hypercapnia).

an awake orotracheal intubation is preferred, using topical anesthesia. Mild to moderate sedation with a benzodiazepine, narcotic, or barbiturate may facilitate the procedure. Advantages of this approach over a rapid-sequence intubation include better airway protection and better gas exchange in the time before the tube is positioned. In an urgent crisis, succinylcholine along with anesthetic doses of a rapid-acting barbiturate or propofol is given while cricoid pressure is applied.

Changing of the endotracheal tube later in response to cuff failure or luminal obstruction is similarly fraught with risk. The loss of PEEP may cause severe and rapid (less than 15 seconds) desaturation from which the patient may not recover fully for over a half hour. When possible, the airway should be changed by two operators, one to remove the old tube and another to insert the replacement.

Goals of Mechanical Ventilation

Mechanical ventilation is merely supportive, allowing time for treatment of the underlying cause of ARDS and for healing of the lung. Its goals are to provide adequate oxygenation and ventilation while minimizing complications. The past several years have seen the evolution of two fundamental concepts that have changed the way ARDS patients are ventilated: (1) alveolar overdistension must be avoided by limiting tidal volumes or inspiratory pressures, and (2) a level of PEEP should be chosen which is sufficiently high to prevent excessive derecruitment at end-expiration. The particular mode of ventilation is probably less important than the general goals of preventing both overdistension and derecruitment. The principles that guide the ventilatory management of ARDS derive from these "lung protection" goals, combined with attempts to avoid toxic concentrations of oxygen ($FiO_2 > 0.6$), and are summarized in Table 7.2 and elaborated in the sections to follow.

Choosing the Tidal Volume

It is increasingly believed that large tidal volume ventilation (10–15 cc/kg) of patients with ARDS is dangerous.[1] Our picture of the acutely injured lung has improved, based in part on CT scanning of patients with ARDS (see Chapter 2), and it is now recognized that the lesion is remarkably inhomogeneous, with some alveoli normally compliant and fragile while others are flooded or collapsed. This loss of functional alveoli necessitates that the tidal volume be distributed to many fewer aerated alveoli than in a healthy lung. Indeed, the apparent stiff lungs of ARDS may be better understood as gross overdistension of a few relatively normal alveoli than as due to generalized parenchymal "stiffness." Even healthy animals ventilated with high tidal volumes (e.g., volumes corresponding to a peak airway pressure of only 30 cm H_2O) for several hours develop pulmonary edema that is histologically identical to ARDS. Lung injury is caused by excessive lung volume (so-called volutrauma), rather than high airway pressure per se,[2] and is seen across a large spectrum of animal species. Further, in animals with acute lung injury, large tidal volumes increase edema accumulation[3] and pulmonary cytokine production.[4] Although confirmatory human data are lacking, it is likely that large tidal volume ventilation results in similar amplification of injury, and the guidelines of a recent ACCP Consensus Conference on Mechanical Ventilation reflect this belief.[5]

The pressure-volume curve in ARDS has a sigmoidal shape, with a lower and an upper inflection point (UIP) (see Figure 7.1 and Chapter 5). The UIP, seen at a pressure between 20 and 35 cm H_2O (mean value 26[6]), indicates that further increases in pressure result in less volume change, presumably because some alveoli are maximally stretched. It has been proposed that the UIP be used in individual patients to select the maximum end-inspiratory volume. In one study of severe ARDS, when patients were initially ventilated at Vt of 10 cc/kg, the Pplat rose above UIP in 80% of cases,[6] necessitating a reduction in mean Vt to 7 to 8 cc/kg. Because it is somewhat cumbersome to perform a pressure-volume study daily in ARDS patients, most authorities advocate simply using a tidal volume appropriate to the loss of alveoli (such as 7–8 cc/kg) and adjusting it downward as necessary to keep the Pplat below 30. Alternatively, one can use a pressure-cycled mode of ventilation with an inspiratory pressure no higher than 30 cm H_2O. A common consequence of limiting the tidal volume in this manner is that the PCO_2 is permitted to rise above 40 mmHg. This approach, termed permissive hypercapnia, is further described later.

Choosing the Level of PEEP

The second area of change in the approach to ventilating ARDS patients is the titration of the level of PEEP, reflecting a new understanding that PEEP can protect the lung. In experiments showing the damaging effect of alveolar overdistension referred to earlier, the addition of PEEP had a striking effect – small amounts could dramatically reduce gross and histologic injury. It is quite likely that lung inflation and deflation past the lower inflection point (LIP) generates huge shearing stresses. If PEEP is applied to keep the lung above the LIP at end-expiration, these damaging forces can be avoided, limiting the progression of lung injury. CT scanning during the progressive addition of PEEP has shown that the volume of reopening-collapsing tissue is significantly reduced with PEEP.[7]

Applying this knowledge clinically, however, is far from simple. For one thing, the lower inflection point is really an inflection zone, across which there is progressive

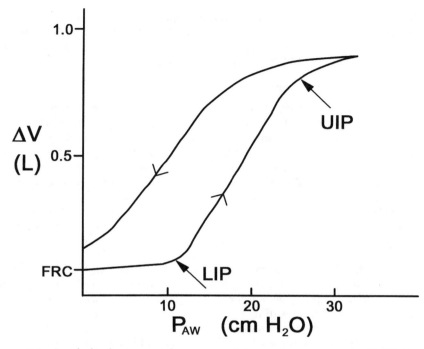

Figure 7.1. An idealized pressure-volume curve of the respiratory system in ARDS. During inflation the airway opening pressure (P_{AW}) initially rises with little increment in lung volume (V). Subsequently V increases much more for a given rise in P_{AW}. This change in behavior indicates the recruitment of previously flooded or atelectatic alveoli and is signaled by the lower inflection point (LIP), a point that tends to be seen at P_{AW} of about 10 cm H_2O. The slope of the inflation curve flattens at the upper inflection point (UIP), signifying the overdistension of alveoli. This UIP is seen at a mean P_{AW} of 26 cm H_2O and a lung volume only 850 mL above FRC and 610 mL above PEEP[5]

recruitment with progressively higher PEEP. When the pressure-volume relationship is measured in ARDS, the LIP is in the range of 8 to 15 cm H_2O. In the aforementioned CT study, the amount of reopening-collapsing tissue became insignificant only when PEEP reached 20 cm H_2O (although the greatest reduction was seen between 10 and 15 cm H_2O PEEP). Such an attempt to prevent ventilation across the LIP in dependent alveoli necessitates that nondependent alveoli are overdistended, due to the substantial gradient of pleural pressure in edematous lungs. The clinical importance of avoiding ventilation across the LIP remains unknown. Many intensivists who follow a "lung protection" strategy of ventilating between the LIP and UIP do not perform pressure-volume curves routinely, instead simply choosing a minimum PEEP level that is likely to limit tidal cycling across the LIP in much, but not all, of the lung, such as 10 cm H_2O. The end result of this approach is not much different, in practice, than an alternative strategy to use the "least PEEP" that effects adequate arterial saturation on $FiO_2 < 0.6$ because most patients with significant ARDS will be on at least 10 cm H_2O PEEP just for oxygenation needs.

Choosing the Mode of Ventilation

Confronted with a bewildering array of ventilatory styles, the intensivist is best served by focusing on the fundamental goals – limiting alveolar overdistension, avoiding derecruitment, preventing oxygen toxicity – rather than troubling about the specific ventilatory mode. These goals can all be achieved using volume-cycled modes (assist control, IMV), pressure-cycled modes (pressure support, pressure control), or less conventional modes (inverse ratio ventilation, high-frequency ventilation, airway pressure release ventilation, BIPAP, proportional-assist ventilation). No study has shown that one of these strategies has any superiority over another. Yet each of these modes has its advocates who believe that the often subtle differences between them may confer some small benefit.

Volume-Cycled Modes. Advantages to assist-control (AC) and intermittent mandatory ventilation (IMV) include their ability to deliver a fixed, assured Vt, the ease with which respiratory system mechanics can be determined, and the general familiarity of the ICU team with their use. These modes should be the first choice in most ICUs. By selecting appropriately low Vt (e.g., 4–8 cc/kg), volutrauma can be avoided. The AC mode has the additional advantage of limiting the work of breathing compared to IMV set at a lower rate, but this difference is likely unimportant in the severely ill, fully sedated patient in whom both modes essentially represent controlled ventilation. Typical settings are listed in Table 7.3.

Pressure-Cycled Modes. Pressure-cycled modes share the advantage of forcing the physician to explicitly choose the inspiratory and expiratory pressures, those parameters most relevant for avoiding ventilator-induced lung injury. Pressure support (PS) also seems more comfortable than volume-cycled ventilation in a subset of patients, perhaps by allowing the patient more control over inspiratory flow and Vt. It is also possible that differences in the flow profile between AC and pressure-control ventilation (PCV) could be exploited to confer benefit (see Figure 7.2). For example, Ppeak can be lowered using PCV at comparable Vt and PEEP, which might reduce the risk of barotrauma. In one study comparing PCV and AC, whereas Ppeak was reduced on PCV by 25%, mean alveolar pressure rose dramatically, an effect that raised the PO_2, may have reduced cardiac output, and has unknown consequences for the risk of barotrauma.[8] In a study comparing volume-cycled and PCV (including inverse ratio ventilation, discussed later), no significant advantages for either method were found.[9] Typical settings for PCV are listed in Table 7.3.

Inverse-Ratio Ventilation. Inverse-ratio ventilation (IRV) describes a group of ventilatory modes (volume-controlled IRV [VC-IRV]; pressure-controlled IRV [PC-IRV])

Table 7.3. Initial ventilator settings

Mode	Assist-control
VI	60 Lpm, square wave
Vt	7 cc/kg
RR	20
FiO2	1.0
PEEP	10 cm H$_2$O

Mode	Pressure–support
IPAP	30 cm H$_2$O
EPAP	10 cm H$_2$O
RR	Set by patient
FiO$_2$	1.0

Mode	PC–IRV
IPAP	30 cm H$_2$O
EPAP	10 cm H$_2$O
RR	16
I:E ratio	2:1
FiO$_2$	1.0

Note: Within minutes of initiating mechanical ventilation, these initial ventilator settings can be tailored to the individual patient, guided mostly by pulse oximetry, and supplemented with occasional blood gas determinations.

in which the inspiratory time exceeds the expiratory time (Te). One can prolong the inspiratory time by selecting a very low inspiratory flow rate, an end-inspiratory plateau, or a decelerating flow profile (using VC-IRV) or by adjusting the inspiratory time or I:E ratio (using PC-IRV), so IRV is not a single mode, but an entire array of ventilatory methods (see Figure 7.3). Compared with AC ventilation at a similar tidal volume, these various forms of IRV have in common a lower peak airway pressure (due to the very low end-inspiratory flow rate), a higher mean alveolar pressure, and a much greater tendency to cause autoPEEP (due to the shortened Te). The purported benefits of IRV relate to the potential for improved gas exchange, reduced barotrauma, or dampened inspiratory shear stresses.

Most studies using IRV demonstrate an improvement in arterial PO$_2$, probably in many patients due to the creation of autoPEEP (which, like PEEP, can decrease shunt). Even when IRV is adjusted to avoid autoPEEP, the PO$_2$ increases, providing evidence for additional mechanisms of improved oxygenation not mediated by autoPEEP (such as the higher mean alveolar pressure or the better mixing of alveolar

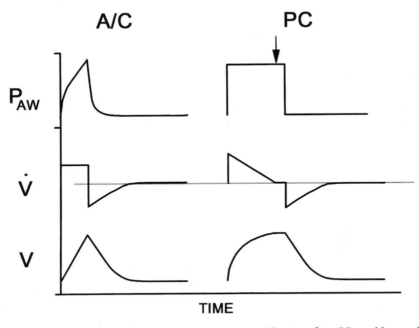

Figure 7.2. Comparison of the airway opening pressure (P_{AW}), airflow (V), and lung volume (V) during assist-control (A/C) and pressure-control (PC) ventilation. Note that if the inspiratory pressure of PC is chosen to equal the plateau pressure during A/C (not shown), the tidal volume is the same for the two modes. Differences include the inspiratory flow profile and the higher mean alveolar pressure (proportional to mean alveolar volume; see lowest tracing) of PC ventilation, which could lead to differences between these modes in gas exchange, hemodynamic impairment, and barotrauma risk. The arrow during PC indicates the point at which the alveolar pressure equals P_{AW}, denoting end-inspiration.

and airway gas).[8] An important caution, however, is that both autoPEEP and higher mean alveolar pressure tend to reduce cardiac output. In one study that compared PC with or without IRV, cardiac output fell with IRV so that systemic oxygen delivery actually worsened.[10] Some investigators have noted a very gradual (over several hours), but progressive tendency for oxygenation to improve following a change to IRV.[11] This phenomenon has led some to suggest that a subset of lung units may be recruitable only through the combined effects of prolonged inspiration and much time. Further studies are needed to shed light on this interesting aspect of IRV.

The impact of IRV on barotrauma risk is hard to predict because the relative contributions of Ppeak, mean alveolar pressure, and PEEP to alveolar disruption are not known. Although the lower Ppeak of IRV may reduce risk, the higher mean alveolar pressure or the frequent occurrence of autoPEEP (often unrecognized) may increase

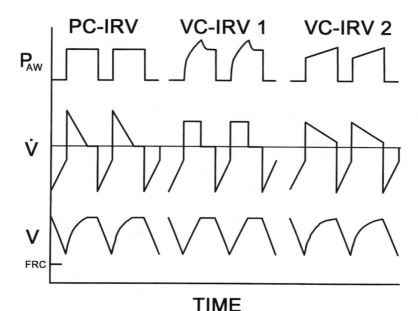

Figure 7.3. Inverse ratio ventilation. Comparison of the airway opening pressure (P_{AW}), airflow (V), and lung volume (V) during three types of inverse ratio ventilation (IRV), including pressure-control IRV (PC-IRV), volume control IRV using an end-inspiratory pause (VC-IRV 1), and volume control using a decelerating inspiratory flow profile (VC-IRV 2). For each mode, note that the end-expiratory lung volume is above functional residual capacity (FRC), implying the presence of autoPEEP.

it. Even the relevance of any of these factors in the causation of pneumothorax is called into question.[12] No clinical studies are available to address the impact of IRV on barotrauma.

The slower inspiratory flow of IRV should apply more gentle shear forces to the alveoli, potentially ameliorating ventilator-induced lung injury, but the relevance of this has not been investigated. In sum, the role of IRV in ARDS is unclear. Although it can often raise the PO_2, a boost in oxygen delivery may not go hand in hand, and even if oxygen delivery is augmented, whether IRV is superior to simply increasing the PEEP is unknown. Further, compared to conventional ventilation, IRV typically requires deeper sedation or therapeutic paralysis with their attendant complications. Typical ventilator settings for PC-IRV are given in Table 7.3.

Investigational Modes. High-frequency ventilation (HFV) involves very high respiratory rates (~ 300/min) and correspondingly low Vt (~ 80 cc). This method is said to take advantage of the reduced lung impedance that results from ventilation near the resonant frequency of the lung. By virtue of its exceedingly short Te, HFV routinely produces high levels of autoPEEP, which may account for its ability to maintain oxygenation and its high incidence of barotrauma (15% in one clinical study[13]). It seems likely that HFV is one way to apply the currently recommended low Vt ventilation, but a way that is unfamiliar to many ICU staff and requires special equipment and monitoring. Whether HFV provides any advantage over conventional ventilation remains to be demonstrated.

Several new modes of ventilation allow some degree of spontaneous ventilation superimposed on pressure-cycled ventilation. Biphasic positive airway pressure (BIPAP) is similar to pressure-control ventilation, but allows spontaneous, unassisted breathing at both the high- and low-pressure levels[14] (see Figure 7.4). The physician can individually adjust the duration and amount of both the upper and lower pressure levels. A related mode is termed *airway pressure-release ventilation* (APRV), which allows spontaneous ventilation at the upper pressure level, but Te is so short (this is a form of IRV) as to make any spontaneous efforts during expiration insignificant. Potential advantages for these modes include a reduced need for sedation and therapeutic paralysis compared to VC-IRV[11] and improved ventilation-perfusion (V/Q) matching,[15] for example due to preservation of ventilation in dependent lung near the diaphragm. This latter point may underlie the interesting time-dependent (over 8–16 hr) improvement in oxygenation seen with APRV.[11] Alternatively, this late gas exchange effect may relate to an ability of the prolonged high airway pressures of IRV to gradually recruit very recalcitrant lung units, as described earlier. In proportional-assist ventilation (PAV), the ventilator adjusts inspiratory pressure in accord with patient demand, allowing the patient to set Vt, I:E ratio, inspiratory flow rate, and respiratory rate. In addition to facilitating ventilator-patient synchrony, PAV may reduce barotrauma by preserving the patient's control of breathing pattern, but any such benefit remains speculative.

Improved patient comfort and reduced sedative needs should not be trivialized, especially in light of recently described complications of therapeutic paralysis. Yet it is unlikely that any of these newer modes of ventilation provides a major breakthrough in ARDS management. Nevertheless, through further clinical investigation it may be possible to tease out subtle benefits of these modes compared to conventional, low Vt ventilation.

A potentially useful adjunctive technique, termed *tracheal gas insufflation* (TGI), involves introducing fresh gas near the carina through a modified endotracheal tube. This added flow washes CO_2-rich gas out of the trachea (and, through turbulence, out of smaller airways as well), reducing anatomic dead space. The PCO_2 reducing effect of TGI is lessened by acute lung injury, but this is partially counterbalanced by the higher PCO_2s used during permissive hypercapnia.[16] In patients with ARDS, TGI with 100% humidified oxygen, delivered throughout the respiratory cycle at a flow of 4 L/minute, successfully lowered PCO_2 from 108 to 84 mmHg.[17] Potential risks of TGI include tracheal erosion, oxygen toxicity related to the unknown FiO_2, and hemodynamic compromise or barotrauma due to the occult presence of autoPEEP.

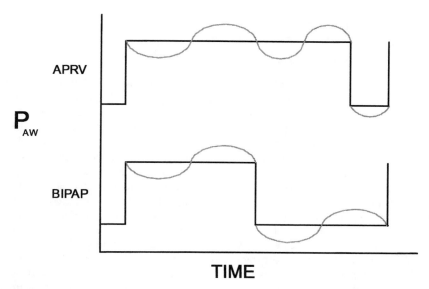

Figure 7.4 Airway pressure release ventilation (APRV) and biphasic positive airway pressure (BIPAP). The solid lines show the two levels of airway opening pressure (P_{AW}). The curving gray lines represent the spontaneous breathing allowed at both pressure levels. Although too little time is spent at the lower pressure during APRV for there to be any significant spontaneous breathing, patients ventilated with BIPAP can breathe freely at both pressures.

Initial Ventilator Settings

The recommended initial ventilator settings are chosen to minimize hypoxemia and circulatory depression (see Table 7.3). In the ensuing minutes these settings can be adjusted optimally as described later. The FiO_2 should be set initially at 1.0 with PEEP of 10 cm H_2O. The assist-control mode of ventilation is often chosen to limit the patient's work of breathing. A tidal volume of 7 cc/kg minimizes pneumothorax and volutrauma risk, and a rate of 20 usually provides adequate ventilation. Alternatively, ventilation can be delivered in a pressure-cycled mode, for example with an inspiratory airway pressure approximately 20 cm H_2O higher than the expiratory pressure (e.g., IPAP 30 cm H_2O, EPAP 10 cm H_2O). Attention should be paid to adjusting inspiratory flow rate and tidal volume (when assist control or IMV are used) or inspiratory pressure (when pressure support is used) to minimize patient effort and distress. Even with appropriately chosen settings, most patients will benefit from sedation and some from therapeutic paralysis (see later). Within minutes of initiating mechanical ventilation, these initial ventilator settings can be tailored to the individual patient, guided mostly by pulse oximetry and supplemented with occasional blood gas determinations. This individualization of ventilator settings, and the rationale underlying them, is described in the sections that follow.

Stabilizing the Patient

If Gas Exchange Is a Problem

In patients with mild ARDS, oxygenation may be maintained with low levels of PEEP and nontoxic concentrations of oxygen, and adequate ventilation can be achieved with ventilator rates less than 24/minute and plateau airway pressures below 30 cm H_2O. More challenging are those patients in whom oxygenation is inadequate despite an FiO_2 of 0.6 and PEEP > 15 cm H_2O or in whom PCO_2 cannot be kept below 45 mmHg without inordinately high respiratory rates or plateau airway pressures.

One of the first priorities following intubation is to adjust ventilatory settings rapidly to minimize any period of potentially injurious oxygen toxicity or alveolar overdistension. This process can typically be achieved in less than 30 minutes, guided by pulse oximetry and airway pressures. In order to attain a pulse oximetry saturation (SpO_2) of greater than 0.9, PEEP should be increased from an initial value of 10 cm H_2O in increments of 2.5 cm H_2O. The PO_2 typically rises within 3 minutes following a change in PEEP, allowing rapid upward titration in the level of PEEP in patients with severe ARDS. It is important to be alert to the occasional patient in whom PEEP does not have the desired effect of increasing oxygenation, so that other strategies for raising PO_2 can be used, as described later. Once the SpO_2 rises above 0.9, the FiO_2 should be promptly reduced. Because the shunt lesion typical of early ARDS is relatively refractory to oxygen, the FiO_2 can often be reduced within minutes from 1.0 to 0.6 with little fall in SpO_2. If oxygenation fails to improve despite FiO_2 of 1.0 and PEEP of 15 cm H_2O, additional measures, described later ("If Hypoxemia Is a Problem"), are needed.

At the same time, ventilator settings should be further individualized to make the patient comfortable and to limit alveolar overdistension, although these two goals are often at odds with one another. Increasing the inspiratory flow rate may reduce the patient's sense of dyspnea, as can changing the mode to PS. In patients with severe ARDS, especially when the PCO_2 approaches or exceeds 40 mmHg, ventilator adjustments will rarely succeed in ameliorating the sense of dyspnea and deep sedation is usually unavoidable. If the plateau airway pressure is greater than 30 cm H_2O (on AC or IMV), the Vt should be progressively reduced. A natural consequence of this approach – and one which should not discourage the physician from proceeding – is that PCO_2 often rises above 45 mmHg (see "When Hypercapnia Is a Problem").

Once the use of PEEP has facilitated a reduction in FiO_2 to 0.6 and the Vt has been lowered until the plateau pressure is no higher than 30 cm H_2O, an arterial blood gas should be obtained to confirm adequacy of oxygenation and to exclude concomitant metabolic acidosis.

If Decreased Venous Return Is a Problem

Positive pressure ventilation and PEEP combine to raise the pleural pressure in patients with ARDS, at times sufficiently to reduce venous return. The degree to which mechanical ventilation causes hypotension or tachycardia is related on the one hand to ventilatory factors (PEEP-induced increment in FRC, chest wall compliance, tidal volume, respiratory rate) and on the other hand to the patient's cardiovascular reflexes and reserve (central vascular volume, autonomic competence, ventricular diastolic function, level of sedation, and others). It follows that lowering the tidal volume or PEEP in a hypotensive patient may restore the circulation. A simple alternative to counter the impact of ventilation and PEEP on venous return, which can be instituted nearly as quickly as ventilatory changes, is to infuse volume (or elevate the legs). Yet volume infusion is likely to exacerbate the lung leak, worsening the shunt and possibly leading to an inferior outcome. Although it would be imprudent to withhold fluids in a hypotensive patient out of fear of compounding edema, once cardiac output has been restored, fluid should be minimized. These issues are more fully discussed in Chapter 6.

If Decreased Capacitance Is a Problem

The magnitude of the plateau airway pressure is determined by the respiratory system compliance (largely due to the lung in patients with ARDS) and the tidal volume (see Chapter 5). Plateau airway pressures greater than 30 cm H_2O indicate overdistension of alveoli and probably lead to amplification of lung injury and an increased incidence of barotrauma. The simplest means to reduce this potentially damaging "volutrauma" is to choose tidal volumes appropriate for the reduced FRC and lung compliance of ARDS, such as 7 cc/kg or lower. A useful guiding principle is to choose the lowest tidal volume that effects adequate CO_2 elimination. The patient whose PCO_2 cannot be held below 45 mmHg while at the same time keeping the plateau pressure below 30 cm H_2O is discussed in "If Hypercapnia Is a Problem."

If Increased Airways Resistance Is a Problem

Airways resistance is often elevated in patients with ARDS, possibly due to damage to conducting airways, airway hyperreactivity related to inflammation, or release of bronchoconstricting mediators. In 10 ARDS patients studied by means which excluded contributions to airway resistance from the endotracheal tube, resistance was elevated in all patients, with the mean value six times normal.[18] Only in occasional ARDS patients, however, is airway resistance increased to a degree that is clinically significant. An exception to this generalization is the use of IRV. As discussed earlier, when the increased airway resistance of ARDS is compounded by the shortened expiratory time of IRV, autoPEEP can usually be detected, often of substantial degree (e.g., > 10 cm H_2O).

A large difference between the peak and plateau airway pressures should prompt an evaluation of the endotracheal tube position and patency. When increased airway resistance can be localized to the patient rather than the endotracheal tube, bronchodilators (e.g., inhaled beta agonist) may be useful. Such patients should be monitored for the presence of autoPEEP and may be at higher risk for barotrauma.

If Hypoxemia Is a Problem

The Use of PEEP

The most common challenge in severe ARDS is providing adequate arterial oxygen saturation with a nontoxic FiO_2 at levels of PEEP unlikely to cause barotrauma. Once the level of PEEP exceeds 15 cm H_2O, many physicians fear catastrophic pneumothorax. Although the link between the level of PEEP and risk of alveolar rupture is far from clear, reaching this level of PEEP should prompt the following questions: (1) is PEEP having the desired effect of improving oxygenation? (2) what else can be done to raise SaO_2, as discussed later? and (3) how can the barotrauma risk be reduced (such as through a lower Vt, or a higher PCO_2)?

PEEP does not always improve oxygenation, especially in patients with unilateral (or predominantly one-sided) lung disease. In such patients postural manuevers, in which the best lung is directed downward, may be rewarding. Because PEEP can even have the effect of overdistending the relatively normal lung and redirecting perfusion through the shunt, PO_2 may improve with reduction of PEEP. In many patients with ARDS, however, levels of PEEP in excess of 20 cm H_2O continue to raise PO_2. In one clinical series, oxygenation increased even as PEEP was pushed to 44 cm H_2O, with no significant depression of cardiac output.[19] Yet when steps are taken to minimize circulating volume, reduce VO_2, and raise oxygen delivery, PEEP in this range is rarely needed.

Once the lung injury moves into a later phase, characterized more by fibrosis than by edema, PEEP is less likely to be helpful and may compound the excessive dead space often seen at this time. Attempts should be made to lower the PEEP if tolerated.

Raising the SvO_2

For a given degree of venous admixture, measures that raise the SvO_2 will improve arterial oxygenation. The SvO_2 can be increased in three fundamental ways – lowering oxygen consumption (VO_2); augmenting oxygen delivery (QO_2); and directly oxygenating the venous blood through IVOX or ECMO (discussed later). Contributors to excessive VO_2 include fever, shivering, agitation, and patient-ventilator dyssynchrony. Oftentimes very simple measures, such as antipyretics, analgesics, or ventilator adjustments, can boost PO_2 importantly. Extreme methods for further reducing VO_2 in the most critical of patients include therapeutic paralysis and intentional cooling. Methods for raising QO_2 are discussed more fully in Chapter 9, but those routinely used in severe ARDS include correction of hypovolemia, transfusion of red blood cells, and infusion of vasoactive drugs.

Prone Position

As early as 1974 it was reported that turning ARDS patients from the supine to the prone position raised PO_2.[20] In a more recent series, when 12 patients were turned prone, PO_2 after 2 hours increased from a mean value of 98 to 146 mmHg, although

4 patients were "nonresponders" (mean PO_2 fell by 20 mmHg).[21] These results have been supported by subsequent studies.[22] "Responders" are often characterized by more severe hypoxemia and hypercapnia and a shorter time since the onset of ARDS.[22] Computed tomographic scanning shows clearing of densities in previously dependent areas when patients are turned prone,[23] and the multiple inert gas elimination technique (MIGET) shows reduced shunt and improved V/Q matching.[21] The duration of the improvement in oxygenation is not known. Although one would predict that after some hours a gravitational gradient of atelectasis would reestablish itself, returning gas exchange to its previous level of derangement, this is not always seen. It may also be possible to prolong the effect of positional maneuvers by simply turning the patient periodically.

This seemingly simple approach is limited in practice by logistic problems (it takes a large fraction of the health care team to turn a critically ill, sedated, cumbersome patient while attending to all of the lines, tubes, and monitors typically in place); the occurrence of poorly understood rhythm disturbances in some patients during turning; the lack of response in roughly one-third of patients; and the availability of simpler methods for improving oxygenation (such as PEEP). Nevertheless, in occasional patients the prone position may allow the reduction of other, more toxic therapies.

Novel Methods for Raising SaO_2

Extracorporeal membrane oxygenation (ECMO) and extracorporeal carbon dioxide removal ($ECCO_2R$) are two similar techniques designed to support the gas exchange properties of the ARDS lung until healing. In both ECMO and $ECCO_2R$, a substantial fraction of the patient's blood flow (one-fourth to one-half of the cardiac output) is passed across a gas-permeable membrane, then returned via either the arterial or venous blood. During ECMO, the extracorporeal circuit is used both to oxygenate the blood and to remove carbon dioxide. $ECCO_2R$ serves predominantly to remove CO_2, allowing the lungs to be rested (e.g., RR 2–4 breaths/minute, Ppeak < 35 cm H_2O). Although both of these techniques can adequately support gas exchange even in the sickest patients, clinical studies in adult patients have been disappointing. In a carefully controlled trial comparing conventional ventilation with PC-IRV plus $ECCO_2R$, overall survival was 38% and did not differ between the two groups.[24] Further, both of these techniques require large investments in training, personnel, and equipment and suffer from a high incidence of complications such as hemorrhage (related to anticoagulation and large-bore cannulas), infection, tubing obstruction, air embolization, and thrombosis. Moreover, the moving force behind $ECCO_2R$, the desire to rest the lung, is more simply achievable with low Vt ventilation and permissive hypercapnia. Unless future clinical trials demonstrate some clinically important benefit, ECMO and $ECCO_2R$ will find no role in the management of adult patients.

Nitric oxide (NO) is a useful adjunctive therapy for severe hypoxemia or physiologically significant pulmonary hypertension in ARDS. This vasodilating gas is introduced into the inspiratory limb of the ventilator and delivered to the lung regions that are still ventilated. Inspired concentrations of 1 to 40 ppm can substantially improve arterial oxygenation in some patients. Often a significant response is observed to inspired concentrations of 1 ppm or less. A dose response relationship is observed in individual patients with maximum effect usually occurring at 10 ppm or less. Rarely further benefit is observed at concentrations as high as 80 ppm. At higher concentrations delivered with high FiO_2 there is the possibility that toxic levels of NO_2 will result. Thus both inhaled NO and NO_2 (NO_X measurement includes additional toxic species) concentrations should be monitored to ensure safe delivery of NO. In addition, methemoglobin concentrations in the blood must be checked intermittently, particularly when inspired concentrations above 10 ppm NO are used. By promoting pulmonary perfusion where ventilation is best, NO raises PO_2. At the same time, pulmonary vascular resistance is lowered, thereby potentially improving cardiac output. In a study of 177 patients with ARDS, NO inhalation of 1.25 to 80 ppm increased PaO_2 by more than 20% in 60% of the patients.[25] This resulted in a reduction in FiO_2 and a reduction in the intensity of mechanical ventilation over the first 4 days of treatment. In this preliminary study[25] and in similar studies,[26] no improvement in mortality has been conclusively shown. Until this is demonstrated in a convincing phase III study, inhaled NO remains investigational.

If Hypercapnia Is a Problem

When the PCO_2 cannot be maintained below 45 mmHg using the guidelines described here (Vt adjusted to keep the plateau pressure < 30 cm H_2O; RR < 30), possible approaches include reducing dead space ventilation, lowering CO_2 production, allowing the PCO_2 to rise above 45 mmHg, or allowing the plateau pressure to rise (raising Vt) (see Table 7.4).

Reducing VCO_2 and Dead Space

Because PCO_2 is directly proportional to CO_2 production, when hypercapnia is a problem, steps should be taken to limit VCO_2. For example, excessive muscle activity can be treated by minimizing painful stimulation, choosing appropriate ventilator settings, and administering judicious sedation. In occasional patients, CO_2 production can be further reduced by deep sedation and therapeutic paralysis, although this intervention carries its own risks. Fever can often be treated with acetaminophen. Cooling blankets are ineffective in lowering VCO_2 in patients who are allowed to shiver, so should not generally be used, except during therapeutic paralysis. Care should be taken to avoid overfeeding because lipogenesis produces a large amount of CO_2. Special, fat-rich, enteral feeding formulas can reduce VCO_2 by lowering the respiratory quotient, but this effect is small and these supplements are expensive. Expired gas analysis using a metabolic cart to determine VO_2, VCO_2, and caloric needs can guide nutrition and prevent overfeeding.

Table 7.4. If hypercapnia is a problem

Inspect the ventilator and tubing for leaks or failure.
Attempt to reduce the level of PEEP (if oxygenation is not a problem).
Exclude autoPEEP.
Rule out hypovolemia.
Treat causes of increased CO_2 production.
Raise the tidal volume as long as the plateau pressure remains below 30 cm H_2O.
Raise the respiratory rate as long as autoPEEP is not present.
Consider deep sedation and paralysis.
Institute permissive hypercapnia.
Consider ECCO2R, if available.

The fraction of tidal ventilation that is dead space (Vd/Vt) is increased as part of the microvascular damage of ARDS. In addition, dead space rises with increasing PEEP or autoPEEP as the alveolar pressure rises above the pulmonary arterial pressure in the nondependent regions of the lungs. In order to reduce dead space, PEEP should be reduced if oxygenation can be maintained with nontoxic fractions of oxygen. If autoPEEP is present, measures to reduce it (e.g., bronchodilators when increased airways resistance is a problem; lowering the respiratory rate when the minute ventilation is very high) may improve alveolar ventilation, lowering PCO_2.

Because the intravascular volume status is reflected in the pulmonary vascular pressures, hypovolemia can exacerbate the dead space–related impact of high alveolar pressures. Hypovolemia should be sought and treated if present. However, because excessive volume adminstration may worsen oxygenation, fluids should not be given indiscriminately.

Permissive Hypercapnia

Historically, physicians have attempted to ventilate patients to a normal PCO_2. In patients with severe lung disease, however, this arbitrary goal has a mechanical cost: the probable amplification of lung injury, as described earlier. Over the past decade, increasing evidence points to the safety and efficacy of allowing the PCO_2 to rise well above 40 mmHg. When patients with severe ARDS are ventilated with volume or pressure limited ventilation as already described, PCO_2 rises typically to 60 to 70 mmHg, but in occasional patients is much higher (in excess of 150 mmHg).[27] The arterial pH falls roughly to 7.2, but at times falls below 7.0. Respiratory acidosis has many physiologic effects, including cellular metabolic dysfunction, depression of myocardial contractility, coronary vasodilation, systemic vasodilation, pulmonary vasoconstriction, enhanced hypoxic pulmonary vasoconstriction, cerebral vasodilation, increased intracranial pressure, renal vasoconstriction, and others. Yet even very high levels of PCO_2 seem remarkably well tolerated by adequately sedated patients. Perhaps this is related to highly efficient and rapidly acting cellular compensatory mechanisms,[28] which tend to defend intracellular pH. Whatever the reasons, some of the dire consequences predicted for hypercapnia, such as arrhythmogenesis, cardiovascular deterioration, or central nervous system injury, have not been clinically apparent. Because respiratory acidosis raises intracranial pressure, permissive hypercapnia should not be used in patients with cerebral edema, trauma, or space-occupying lesions. Some have also speculated that hypercapnia could worsen cardiac ischemia in patients with coronary artery disease through a coronary vasodilation–induced "steal" syndrome, but the significance of this is not known.

The question for the clinician is not whether a normal PCO_2 is desirable, but which is riskier for the patient: a high PCO_2 or alveolar overdistension. Although conclusive evidence from controlled patient trials is still lacking, the preponderance of evidence from animal studies and the limited human data favor the use of permissive hypercapnia. For example, when a group of severe ARDS patients (lung injury score $\geq$ 2.5) were ventilated to keep the Ppeak no higher than 30 to 40 cm H_2O (Vt 4–7 cc/kg), mortality was only 26%, compared to 53% predicted from their APACHE II scores.

How permissive hypercapnic ventilation is best done (magnitude of acidemia, rapidity of changes, use of alkalinizing agents) has not been defined (see Table 7.5). A common approach is to allow the PCO_2 to gradually rise (e.g., 10 mmHg/hr) in order to allow time for cellular compensation. The degree of hypoventilation should be guided by the plateau airway pressure, rather than the absolute level of PCO_2 or pH. Some have advocated the infusion of sodium bicarbonate to raise the blood pH, but this has generally not been done in ARDS patients and no advantage has been shown over simply allowing the pH to fall. Sodium bicarbonate delivers a substantial CO_2 load to a patient already marginally able to excrete what is produced endogenously and further risks volume overload and potassium depletion. Given the questions regarding safety and usefulness, the role of sodium bicarbonate requires validation before it can be advocated clinically. Once the patient begins to improve, ventilation should be increased only gradually, in order to avoid abrupt alkalosis.

Complications

Barotrauma

Pneumothorax is a potentially devastating complication, due in part to the tenuous gas exchange and circulatory state of severe ARDS, and in part to the difficulty of recognizing significant barotrauma in ventilated patients. For example, in one study of 112 pneumothoraces in ventilated patients (not all of whom had ARDS), most

Table 7.5. Permissive hypercapnia

Exclude patients with increased ICP (and possibly with ongoing myocardial ischemia).
Identify and correct increased dead space.
Seek and treat causes of increased CO_2 production.
Assure adequate sedation.
Set the respiratory rate at 20–30 (as long as autoPEEP is not present).
Lower Vt gradually, allowing PCO_2 to rise approximately 10 mmHg/hr.
Continue to reduce Vt until the Pplateau is < 30 cm H_2O.

occurred in anatomic locations generally considered atypical, such as anteromedially (38%), subpulmonic (26%), or posteromedially (11%).[29] Only 22% were seen apicolaterally. Nearly 1 pneumothorax in 3 was missed on the initial reading of the x ray, half of these progressing to tension. In a series of 100 ARDS patients, barotrauma was found to be an independent marker of mortality, but directly contributed to less than 2% of deaths.[30] Perhaps this is explained by the generally low incidence of pneumothorax in ARDS, generally less than 10% (range 0.5% to 41%).

It might seem self-evident that the higher the transpulmonary pressures, the greater the incidence of barotrauma, and such a relationship is seen in animal models, but solid evidence supporting this association in patients is not available. In one study of risk factors for barotrauma, airway pressures were not an independent predictor of pneumothorax, but the number of patients was small.[12] In addition, the incidence of pneumothorax among ARDS patients in this trial (17/41; 42%), nearly all of whom were ventilated with large Vt (10–12 cc/kg) and high plateau airway pressure (exceeding 35 cm H_2O in 35/41 patients), was strikingly higher than in patients managed with a lung protective strategy and permissive hypercapnia (0/53; 0%).[27] Although it may not be fair to compare these two studies, the combined weight of animal studies, uncontrolled human data, and common sense makes a convincing case for a link between transpulmonary pressure and barotrauma risk. If this is true, an additional benefit of the current low Vt, high PCO_2 approach will be a reduction in the rate of pneumothorax.

In the past some have advocated so-called prophylactic chest tubes once an arbitrary value of PEEP is applied, but this approach is hard to justify on several grounds. First, pneumothorax is often loculated and may simply not occur where the chest tube is. Second, bilateral chest tubes probably risk infection and certainly increase patient discomfort. Finally, it is not clear that the absolute value of PEEP is important, as opposed to some other measure of lung overdistension (such as Vt). A prudent approach when PEEP is dialed to the neighborhood of 20 cm of H_2O is to further lower the Vt, seek alternative means to raise the PO_2, such as blood transfusion, therapeutic paralysis, or vasoactive drug infusion (see earlier), notify the entire

Table 7.6. Causes of hypotension in ARDS

Low cardiac output hypotension

  Rhythm disturbance
  Myocardial ischemia
  Hypovolemia, hemorrhage
  Pneumothorax
  Hypoxemia
  PEEP or autoPEEP
  Air or thromboembolism
  Ventilator malfunction
  Inadvertent discontinuation of vasoactive drugs

Low SVR hypotension

  Sepsis
  Multiple systems organ failure
  Vasoactive drugs

ICU team to be especially vigilant for signs of barotrauma, and place chest tube trays at the bedside.

Hypotension

Hypotension commonly complicates the ICU course of patients with ARDS. Some of the causes are listed in Table 7.6. Hypotension is particularly dangerous when due to a fall in cardiac output because the consequent fall in SvO_2 compounds arterial hypoxemia, leading to a rapidly deteriorating cycle of hypoxemia and myocardial dysfunction. A rapid bedside assessment attempts to identify urgent crises while categorizing the hypotension as due to low cardiac output or low systemic vascular resistance (SVR). Attention should be given to the patient, the ventilator, and any drug infusions.

Abrupt Deterioration in Gas Exchange

Abrupt and life-threatening hypoxemia or worsening of acidosis frequently punctuates the ICU course of patients with ARDS. The differential diagnosis for these syndromes is so extensive as to confound the physician at a time when urgent solutions are needed. A pathophysiologic approach, in which causes of hypoxemia are divided into increased shunt (see Table 7.7), decreased oxygen delivery, and increased oxygen consumption aids a rapid bedside analysis. Similarly, causes of worsening respiratory acidosis can be partitioned into increased CO_2 production, rising dead space, and decreased minute ventilation (see Table 7.8).

Table 7.7. Sudden hypoxemia

Increased shunt

> Pneumonia
> Atelectasis
> Pneumothorax
> Severe abdominal distention
> Loss of PEEP (including transient reductions)
> High pressure pulmonary edema, fluid overload
> Airway secretions
> Change in body position
> Malposition of ETT
> Infusion of drug blocking hypoxic vasoconstriction
> Alveolar hemorrhage
> Worsened ARDS
> Pulmonary embolism

Fall in oxygen delivery

> Myocardial dysfunction
> Rhythm disturbance
> Hypovolemia
> Hemorrhage
> Loss of vasoactive drug infusion
> Tension pneumothorax
> Right heart syndromes

Rise in VO_2

> Fever, sepsis, hypermetabolism
> Agitation, respiratory distress
> Shivering

Abrupt Deterioration in Respiratory Mechanics

A final, common crisis in the ventilated ARDS patient is a sudden deterioration in respiratory mechanics, usually signaled by a rise in airway pressures or pressure alarming (when volume-cycled ventilation is used), by new respiratory distress, or by rising PCO_2. When the respiratory mechanics abruptly worsen, the newly elevated peak airway pressure should be divided into its resistive, elastic (lung and chest wall), and PEEP (or autoPEEP) components as described in Chapter 8, in order to focus the diagnostic effort. It is more difficult to recognize deteriorating respiratory system mechanics in patients being ventilated with pressure-cycled modes, but one may see patient distress, falling tidal volumes, or rising PCO_2. It is often useful to return the

Table 7.8. Abrupt worsening of respiratory acidosis

Increased VCO$_2$

> Fever, sepsis, hypermetabolism
> Agitation, respiratory distress
> Shivering

Increased Vd/Vt

> Exclude hypovolemia.
> Seek autoPEEP.
> Try to reduce PEEP.
> Consider pulmonary embolism.

Decreased VE

> Failure of the ventilator
> Change in respiratory mechanics (pressure-cycled modes)
> Leak around the ETT
> ETT obstruction
> Loss of respiratory drive (PS, IMV, BIPAP, APRV)

Table 7.9. Approach to worsened respiratory system mechanics

1. Seek evidence of patient effort as either a cause or symptom of mechanical deterioration: consider reassurance, sedation, analgesia, therapeutic paralysis.
2. Briefly disconnect the ventilator and bag-ventilate, assure patency of the ETT, exclude ventilator malfunction.
3. Determine the components of Ppeak: Pplateau, autoPEEP, Presist
   a. If autoPEEP is up, consider bronchodilators, reducing VE.
   b. If Pplateau is up, exclude pneumothorax, pulmonary edema, atelectasis, right mainstem intubation, distended abdomen.
   c. If Presist is up, examine ETT, consider bronchodilators, seek autoPEEP.

patient to a volume-cycled mode of ventilation in order to determine the peak airway pressure and its components. A bedside approach is given in Table 7.9.

Summary

Mechanical ventilation of ARDS patients is complex, yet taking a rational approach based on understanding of relevant pathophysiology works. Difficult to manage problems or sudden deterioration is approached in the same way. That is, a clinical hypothesis (or list of differential diagnoses) is formulated in pathophysiologic terms. Then the clinical intervention aimed at solving the problem or correcting the sudden deterioration is carefully observed to confirm the clinical hypothesis or, when an unexpected clinical response occurs, to induce the physician to consider other possibilities.

References

1. Marini JJ, Kelsen SG. Re-targeting ventilatory objectives in adult respiratory distress syndrome. Am Rev Respir Dis 1992; 146:2–3.
2. Dreyfuss D, Soler P, Basset G, et al. High inflation pressure pulmonary edema: respective effects of high airway pressure, high tidal volume, and positive end-expiratory pressure. Am Rev Respir Dis 1988; 137:1159–1164.
3. Corbridge TC, Wood LDH, Crawford GP, et al. Adverse effects of large tidal volume and low PEEP in canine acid aspiration. Am Rev Respir Dis 1990; 142:311–315.
4. Tremblay L, Valenza F, Ribeiro SP, Li J, Slutsky AS. Injurious ventilatory strategies increase cytokines and c-fos m-RNA expression in an isolated rat lung model. J Clin Invest 1997; 99:944–952.
5. Slutsky A. Mechanical ventilation. Chest 1993; 104:1833–1859.
6. Roupie E, Dambrosio M, Servillo G, et al. Titration of tidal volume and induced hypercapnia in acute respiratory distress syndrome. Am J Respir Crit Care Med 1995; 152:121–128.
7. Gattinoni L, Pelosi P, Crotti S, et al. Effects of positive end-expiratory pressure on regional distribution of tidal volume and recruitment in adult respiratory distress syndrome. Am J Respir Crit Care Med 1995; 151:1807–1814.
8. Armstrong BW, Macintyre NR. Pressure-controlled, inverse ratio ventilation that avoids air trapping in the adult respiratory distress syndrome. Crit Care Med 1995; 23:279–285.
9. Lessard MR, Guerot E, Lorino H, Lemaire F, Brochard L. Effects of pressure-controlled with different I:E ratios versus volume-controlled ventilation on respiratory mechanics, gas exchange, and hemodynamics in patients with adult respiratory distress syndrome. Anesthesiology 1994; 80:983–991.
10. Mercat A, Graini L, Teboul JL, et al. Cardiorespiratory effects of pressure-controlled ventilation with and without inverse ratio in the adult respiratory distress syndrome. Chest 1993; 104:871–875.
11. Sydow M, Burchardi H, Ephraim E, et al. Long-term effects of two different ventilatory modes on oxygenation in acute lung injury: comparison of airway pressure release ventilation and volume-controlled inverse ratio ventilation. Am J Respir Crit Care Med 1994; 149:1550–1556.
12. Gammon RB, Shin MS, Groves RH, Hardin JM, Hsu C, Buchalter SE. Clinical risk factors for pulmonary barotrauma: a multivariate analysis. Am J Respir Crit Care Med 1995; 152:1235–1240.
13. Gluck E, Heard S, Patel C, et al. Use of ultrahigh frequency ventilation in patients with ARDS. Chest 1993; 103:1413–1420.
14. Hörmann C, Baum M, Putensen C, et al. Biphasic positive airway pressure (BIPAP) – a new mode of ventilatory support. Eur J Anaesthesiol 1993; 11:37–42.
15. Putensen C, Räsänen J, Lopez FA. Ventilation perfusion distributions during mechanical

ventilation with superimposed spontaneous breathing in canine lung injury. Am J Respir Crit Care Med 1994; 150:101–108.

16. Nahum A, Shapiro RS, Ravenscraft SA, Adams AB, Marini JJ. Efficacy of expiratory tracheal gas insufflation in a canine model of lung injury. Am J Respir Crit Care Med 1995; 152:489–495.

17. Belghith M, Fierobe L, Brunet F, Monchi M, Mira J. Is tracheal gas insufflation an alternative to extrapulmonary gas exchangers in severe ARDS? Chest 1995; 107:1416–1419.

18. Wright PE, Bernard GR. The role of airflow resistance in patients with the adult respiratory distress syndrome. Am Rev Respir Dis 1989; 139:1169–1174.

19. Kirby RR, Downs JB, Civetta JM, et al. High level positive end expiratory pressure (PEEP) in acute respiratory insufficiency. Chest 1975; 67:2:156–163.

20. Bryan AC. Comments of a devil's advocate. Am Rev Respir Dis 1974; 110:143S.

21. Pappert D, Rossaint R, Slama K, et al. Influence of positioning on ventilation-perfusion relationships in severe adult respiratory distress syndrome. Chest 1994; 106:1511–1516.

22. Blanch L, Mancebo J, Perez M, Martinez M, Mas A, Betbese AJ, Joseph D, Ballus J, Lucangelo U, Bak E. Short-term effects of prone position in critically ill patients with acute respiratory distress syndrome. Intensive Care Med 1997; 23:1033–1039.

23. Langer M, Mascheroni D, Marcolin R, Gattinoni L. The prone position in ARDS patients: a clinical study. Chest 1988; 94:103–107.

24. Morris AH, Wallace CJ, Menlove RL, et al. Randomized clinical trial of pressure-controlled inverse ratio ventilation and extracorporeal CO_2 removal for adult respiratory distress syndrome. Am J Respir Crit Care Med 1994; 149:295–305.

25. Dellinger RP, Zimmerman JL, Taylor RW, Straube RC, Hauser DL, Criner GJ, Davis K Jr, Hyers TM, Papadakos P. Effects of inhaled nitric oxide in patients with acute respiratory distress syndrome: results of a randomized phase II trial. Inhaled Nitric Oxide in ARDS Study Group. Crit Care Med 1998; 26:15–23.

26. Luhr O, Nathorst-Westfelt U, Lundin S, Wickerts CJ, Stiernstrom H, Berggren L, Aardal S, Johansson LA, Stenqvist O, Rudberg U, Lindh A, Bindslev L, Martling CR, Hornbaek V, Frostell C. A retrospective analysis of nitric oxide inhalation in patients with severe acute lung injury in Sweden and Norway 1991–1994. Acta Anaesthesiol Scand 1997; 41:1238–1246.

27. Hickling KG, Walsh J, Henderson S, et al. Low mortality rate in adult respiratory distress syndrome using low-volume, pressure-limited ventilation with permissive hypercapnia: a prospective study. Crit Care Med 1994; 22:1568–1578.

28. Feihl F, Perret C. Permissive hypercapnia: how permissive should we be? Am J Respir Crit Care Med 1994; 150:1722–1737.

29. Tocino IM, Miller MH, Fairfax WR. Distribution of pneumothorax in the supine and semirecumbent critically ill adult. AJR 1985; 144:901–905.

30. Schnapp LM, Chin DP, Szaflarski N, Matthay MA. Frequency and importance of barotrauma in 100 patients with acute lung injury. Crit Care Med 1995; 23:272–278.

8

Respiratory Muscles and Liberation from Mechanical Ventilation

Rajiv Dhand and Martin J. Tobin

Introduction

Recovery from the acute respiratory distress syndrome (ARDS) may occur within 2 to 3 days in some patients, and early discontinuation of mechanical ventilation and extubation is possible. Unfortunately, most patients with ARDS require prolonged mechanical ventilation, and its discontinuation poses a greater problem. Although precise figures are not available, at least one-third of patients who display difficulties in being weaned from mechanical ventilation are in the recovery phase after acute lung injury.[1,2] Weaning such patients from the ventilator presents a considerable clinical challenge.[3,4] An understanding of the pathophysiologic mechanisms responsible for the inability to resume spontaneous breathing is essential to develop a systematic approach to discontinuation of ventilation.

Pathophysiologic Determinants of Weaning Outcome

The major factors that determine the outcome of a weaning trial are pulmonary gas exchange, respiratory muscle pump failure, and psychological factors.

Pulmonary Gas Exchange

During a weaning trial, hypoxemia may occur as a result of hypoventilation, impaired pulmonary gas exchange, or decreased oxygen (O_2) content of venous blood. In general, severe hypoxemia is uncommon in patients who fail a weaning trial for the simple reason that weaning is not contemplated unless patients display satisfactory oxygenation, such as arterial O_2 tension (PaO_2 > 60 torr with fractional inspired O_2 concentration (FiO_2) of < 0.40 and a positive end-expiratory pressure (PEEP) level of < 10 cm H_2O. Although resumption of spontaneous breathing is associated with worsening of ventilation-perfusion inequality, the degree of impairment does not prevent successful discontinuation of mechanical ventilation.[5] However, correction of hypoxemia is the predominant reason for mechanical ventilation in patients with ARDS, and patients with limited cardiorespiratory reserve may not be able to maintain satisfactory oxygenation following discontinuation of ventilator support even when their baseline PaO_2 values fulfill the criteria mentioned earlier.

Respiratory Muscle Pump Failure

Respiratory muscle dysfunction is the most common cause of weaning failure. This may result from reduced neuromuscular capacity, increased respiratory muscle pump load, or both factors (Table 8.1).

Decreased Neuromuscular Capacity

Respiratory Center Output. Patients failing a weaning trial commonly develop an increase in $PaCO_2$,[6] raising a suspicion of respiratory center depression. However, most patients who fail a weaning trial display an elevated respiratory drive,[6,7] although the level of drive is less than that expected for the degree of chemoreceptor stimulation. This raises the possibility that a relative defect in respiratory center function may exist in some patients. However, abnormalities in respiratory center output are unlikely to be primarily responsible for weaning failure in patients recovering from ARDS.

Phrenic Nerve Function. Approximately 25% to 98% of patients undergoing coronary artery bypass surgery develop an elevated left hemidiaphragm.[4] About 10% of these patients have electrophysiologic evidence of phrenic nerve injury,[8] and thus abnormalities in phrenic nerve function should be suspected if weaning proves difficult in such patients following surgery.[4] However, the incidence of ARDS after coronary artery bypass surgery or cardiopulmonary bypass appears to be very low.[9] ARDS may occur following upper abdominal surgery, such as cholecystectomy. Even without ARDS, many of these patients display a reduction in lung volumes associated with bilateral diaphragmatic elevation and lower lobe atelectasis.[10] These changes are thought to be due to inhibition of diaphragmatic activation secondary to a reflex mediated by mechanical stimulation of the viscera during surgery.[11] The reduction in lung volumes gradually returns to normal over a period of 7 days after surgery.

Respiratory Muscle Dysfunction. Respiratory muscle dysfunction may result from several factors in patients being weaned from mechanical ventilation (Table 8.1), and, of these, hyperinflation is one of the most important. Alterations in the pattern of breathing during weaning may lead to the development of dynamic hyperinflation[6]

Table 8.1. Causes of respiratory muscle pump failure

Decreased neuromuscular capacity

Decreased respiratory center output
Phrenic nerve dysfunction
Decreased respiratory muscle strength and/or endurance
    Hyperinflation
    Malnutrition
    Decreased oxygen supply
    Respiratory acidosis
    Metabolic abnormalities
    Endocrinopathy
    Drug-induced abnormalities
    Disuse muscle atrophy
    Respiratory muscle fatigue

Increased respiratory muscle pump load

Increased ventilatory requirements
    Increased CO_2 production
    Increased dead space ventilation
    Inappropriately increased respiratory drive
Increased work of breathing

(Figure 8.1), which has a number of adverse effects: the respiratory muscles operate at an unfavorable position on their length-tension curve; elastic recoil of the chest wall is directed inward, thereby causing an extra elastic load; and breathing takes place at the upper, less compliant portion of the pressure-volume curve of the lung.[4] These factors cause a decrease in the efficiency of force generation by the respiratory muscles and an increase in the work of breathing.

Malnutrition is common in critically ill patients and is associated with decreases in the ventilatory response to hypoxia, diaphragmatic mass and thickness, and respiratory muscle strength and endurance. The contribution of a decrease in the O_2 *supply* to the respiratory muscles as a cause of failure to wean has been studied. Lemaire and co-workers studied the hemodynamic changes in patients with preexisting heart disease who repeatedly failed weaning attempts. After 10 minutes of spontaneous ventilation, the patients showed evidence of acute left ventricular failure as well as acute ventilatory failure.[12] The transmural pulmonary artery wedge pressure increased from 8 mmHg during mechanical ventilation to 25 mmHg after 10 minutes of spontaneous breathing. Concomitantly, the PCO_2 rose from 42 to 58 mmHg. *Acute respiratory acidosis* decreases the contractility and endurance of the diaphragm.[13] The presence of *metabolic abnormalities,* such as hypophosphatemia, hypokalemia, hypocalcemia, or hypomagnesemia, adversely affects respiratory muscle function. *Endocrine disturbances* such as hypothyroidism and hyperthyroidism may impair respiratory muscle function,

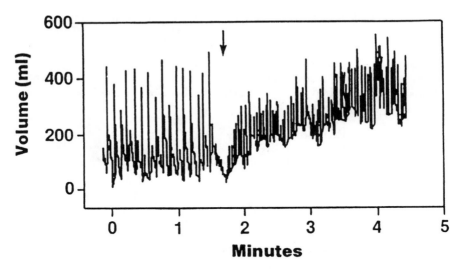

Figure 8.1 In a patient who failed a weaning trial, discontinuation of ventilator support and the onset of spontaneous breathing (arrow) was associated with the development of tachypnea and an increase in end-expiratory lung volume, indicating the development of dynamic hyperinflation. (From Tobin MJ, Perez W, Guenther SM, et al. The pattern of breathing during successful and unsuccessful trials of weaning from mechanical ventilation. Am Rev Respir Dis 1986; 134:1111–1118. Reproduced with permission.)

as may corticosteroid therapy. *Drug-induced disorders* need to be considered, such as the occurrence of prolonged respiratory muscle weakness after discontinuation of neuromuscular blocking agents.[14] Studies of limb immobilization have shown that *skeletal muscle atrophy* develops rapidly and produces a marked decline in muscle mass. The same occurs for the respiratory muscles during controlled mechanical ventilation[15]; whether this process is likely to occur with assisted modes of ventilation is not known. *Respiratory muscle fatigue* has been considered an important cause of failure to wean,[16] although definite proof of its role is not available.[6] Moreover, it has been suggested that the development of rapid shallow breathing and inward motion of the abdomen during inspiration (paradox) signify respiratory muscle fatigue. However, the onset of rapid shallow breathing and abnormal rib cage-abdominal motion occurs immediately upon discontinuation of ventilator support in patients who fail a weaning trial with no further progression during the period of the weaning trial[6,17] (Figure 8.1) – a pattern that is difficult to reconcile with the development of fatigue. In a study conducted in healthy subjects breathing against resistive loads and using an experimental design that permitted the separation of the effect of loading from fatigue, fatigue was shown to be neither necessary nor sufficient to induce abnormal rib cage-abdominal motion.[18] In contrast, respiratory loading was sufficient to induce abnormal motion. These findings do not mean that respiratory muscle fatigue is not a mechanism of weaning failure, but rather that changes in the pattern of breathing cannot be used in its detection. The role of diaphragmatic fatigue as a cause of weaning failure continues to be debated, and efforts to resolve this issue are complicated by the lack of a simple, reliable means to detect respiratory muscle fatigue in patients who are being weaned from mechanical ventilation.

Increased Respiratory Muscle Pump Load

Increased respiratory muscle pump load may result from increased ventilatory requirements or increased work of breathing (Table 8.1).

Increased Ventilatory Requirements. Increased ventilation requirements may result from increased CO_2 production, increased dead space ventilation, and an inappropriately elevated respiratory drive. Overfeeding, lipogenesis, and a high ratio of carbohydrate to fat may result in increased production of CO_2.[19] Although an increase in CO_2 production predisposes to CO_2 retention, it is never the sole cause of hypercapnia. In patients with ARDS, a significant proportion of the ventilation is wasted to regions of dead space.[20] The physiologic dead space, that is, V_D/V_T ratio in healthy subjects, is between 0.33 and 0.45. If CO_2 production is high, an increase in V_D/V_T to 0.6 or above is generally considered to predict an unsuccessful weaning outcome because the associated increase in minute ventilation necessary for satisfactory gas exchange causes marked encroachment on ventilatory reserve; however, exceptions do exist.[21] In addition, patients with increased dead space frequently have decreased lung compliance and increased airway resistance, which cause further increases in the work of breathing. However, the importance of V_D/V_T as a determinant of weaning outcome needs to be studied systematically in a large group of patients. Patients who fail a weaning trial often have a high level of anxiety, which may be associated with increased respiratory drive. Excessive agitation in these patients can lead to an inappropriate increase in work of breathing for the level of minute ventilation.

Increased Work of Breathing. The lungs of patients with ARDS are relatively stiff due to pulmonary edema, consolidation, or fibrosis. Besides the decrease in respiratory system compliance, increases in airway resistance and V_D/V_T also contribute to increase in the work of breathing. Several investigators have examined the relationship between work of breathing and ability to sustain spontaneous breathing. Although respiratory work is greater in weaning failure patients, the threshold values separating weaning success from weaning failure patients differ between the various studies.[4] Furthermore, these threshold values were determined on a post hoc basis, and the value of work measurements as a predictor of weaning outcome has not been examined in a prospective fashion. The O_2 cost of breathing, which reflects respiratory workload, is excessively high in patients who fail to wean from mechanical ventilation. In resting healthy subjects, the O_2 cost of breathing is < 5% of the total body O_2 consumption, whereas it can exceed 50% in patients being weaned from mechanical ventilation.[22]

Such a marked increase in the O_2 cost of breathing markedly decreases the availability of O_2 for delivery to other vulnerable tissue beds and may precipitate myocardial ischemia or other problems. Conflicting results have been reported by investigators who studied the O_2 cost of breathing in patients being weaned from mechanical ventilation. Lewis et al.[22] found that the O_2 cost of breathing was higher in patients who failed a weaning trial, compared to patients who were successfully weaned. However, Kemper and co-workers[23] and Hubmayr et al.[24] found no significant difference in the O_2 cost of breathing in patients who succeeded and those who failed a weaning trial (Figure 8.2).

The workload encountered during spontaneous breathing may determine whether a patient can sustain spontaneous breathing successfully. A systematic evaluation of respiratory mechanics, obtained while the patient was receiving passive ventilation *before* a trial of spontaneous breathing, could not distinguish patients who succeeded from those who failed the subsequent trial of spontaneous breathing.[25] However *during* the trial, patients who failed developed rapid shallow breathing and progressive worsening of pulmonary mechanics compared to those who were weaned successfully.[26] These trials were conducted in patients with chronic obstructive pulmonary disease (COPD). Similar studies need to be conducted in patients with ARDS to determine whether the mechanisms underlying weaning failure in these patients are different from those in patients with COPD.

Psychological Problems

Dependence on mechanical ventilation can be associated with feelings of insecurity, anxiety, fear, and panic.[27] Many patients develop a fear that they will remain dependent on mechanical ventilation and that discontinuation of ventilator support will result in sudden death. Studies are needed to determine the prevalence and nature of psychological disturbances in ventilator-dependent patients and the degree to which they contribute to ventilator dependency.

Predicting Weaning Outcome

The decision to wean depends on the resolution of the underlying condition responsible for ARDS, the patient's clinical status, and the aggressiveness of the physician. The initiation of the weaning process requires careful timing. If delayed unnecessarily, the patient remains at risk of ventilator-associated complications. If performed prematurely, weaning may cause severe cardiorespiratory and psychological decompensation. In addition, development of respiratory muscle fatigue during an unsuccessful weaning trial could lead to structural damage in the muscles.[28] Thus repeated unsuccessful weaning trials should be avoided. However, resting the respiratory muscles by continuing mechanical ventilation may cause muscle atrophy.[15] The optimal time to initiate a weaning trial is a difficult decision as illustrated by the report that

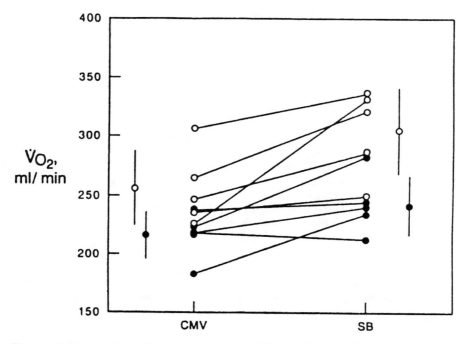

Figure 8.2 Measurements of oxygen consumption (VO_2) during controlled mechanical venti-lation (CMV) and spontaneous breathing (SB) in weaning success (closed circles) and weaning failure (open circles) patients. The increase in VO_2 between CMV and SB, a measure of the oxygen cost of breathing, was not significantly different in the two groups of patients. (From Hubmayr RD, Loosbrock LM, Gillespie DJ, et al. Oxygen uptake during breathing from mechanical ventilation. Chest 1988; 94:1148–1155. Reproduced with permission.)

the judgment of attending physicians was often unreliable in predicting short-term weaning outcome.[2] The positive and negative predictive values were only 0.50 and 0.67, and were mostly biased toward continuation of mechanical ventilation. These findings emphasize the need for objective tests, such as those listed in Table 8.2, to guide the timing of weaning trials.

Gas Exchange

Discontinuation of ventilator support is generally not contemplated in a patient with ARDS who exhibits persistent hypoxemia, for example, PaO_2 of <55 mmHg with an inspired oxygen concentration (FiO_2) of ≥ 0.40. A number of indices derived from arte-rial blood gas (ABG) measurements have been proposed as predictors of weaning out-come. However, none of the ABG criteria listed in Table 8.2 have ever been subjected to prospective investigation. In patients with ARDS who have limited cardiorespiratory

Table 8.2. Variables used to predict weaning success

Gas exchange

PaO_2 of ≥ 60 torr with FiO_2 of ≤ 0.35
Alveolar-arterial PO_2 gradient of < 350 torr
PaO_2/FiO_2 ratio of > 200

Ventilatory pump

Vital capacity of > 10–15 mL/kg body weight
Maximum negative inspiratory pressure < -30 cm H_2O
Minute ventilation < 10 l/min
Maximum voluntary ventilation more than twice resting
    minute ventilation
Frequency to tidal volume ratio (f/V_T) < 105 b/min/L
Abnormal rib cage–abdominal motion
CROP index > 13 ml/breath/min

reserve, successful weaning cannot be predicted on the basis of satisfactory oxygenation alone. Instead, the outcome of a weaning trial is more commonly determined by the ability of the cardiorespiratory system to cope with the increased workload.

Maximum Inspiratory Pressure

Maximum inspiratory pressure (P_Imax), a global assessment of the strength of all the respiratory muscles, is one of the standard measurements employed to predict weaning outcome. In a classic study, Sahn and Lakshminarayan[29] found that a P_Imax value of -30 cm H_2O or less predicted successful weaning, and a P_Imax value higher than -20 cm H_2O predicted weaning failure. However, most subsequent studies have found that these threshold values have poor sensitivity and specificity.[4,26] Improvement in the performance of the test by maintaining occlusion for 20 seconds and attaching a one-way valve to ensure that inspiratory efforts are made at low lung volumes did not improve the predictive value of the test.[30]

Minute Ventilation

A minute ventilation of < 10 L/minute is another index conventionally used to predict a successful weaning outcome.[29] However, most investigators have found it to have a high rate of false negative and false positive results.[30,4]

Rapid Shallow Breathing

Patients who fail a weaning trial develop an immediate increase in respiratory frequency and a decrease in tidal volume upon discontinuation of ventilator support.[6] An increase in respiratory rate to greater than 40 breaths per minute is by itself an excel-lent predictor of weaning failure.[30] However, in one study,[30] measurements of fre-quency (f) and tidal volume (V_T) were combined into an index of rapid shallow breathing – the f/V_T ratio. The f/V_T ratio was measured with a hand-held spirometer over 1 minute of spontaneous breathing after the patient was disconnected from the ventilator circuit. In an initial "training data set" obtained in 36 patients, an f/V_T value of 105 breaths per minute/L was the best discriminator between patients who were successfully weaned and those in whom weaning failed. The predictive power of this value was then assessed in 64 patients who constituted the "prospective-validation data set" (Figure 8.3). The positive and negative predictive values were 0.78 and 0.95, respectively, which were the highest values noted for any of the predictive indices in the study. Other studies that evaluated f/V_T during weaning with gradually decreasing levels of pressure support did not find it to be as discriminatory in predicting weaning failure or success.[31,32] This is not surprising because pressure support ventilation is known to decrease f and increase VT. Epstein[32] studied the value of f/VT as a predic-tor of weaning outcome with the methodology of Yang and Tobin[30] and reported the positive predictive value of f/VT < 100 breaths/minute/L to be 0.83. Only 1 of the 14 patients who required reintubation within 72 hours failed extubation because of their underlying respiratory process; instead, they failed because of problems that f/VT was physiologically or temporally unlikely to predict, such as congestive heart failure, upper airway obstruction, aspiration, encephalopathy, or a new pulmonary abnormality. The negative predictive value – weaning success despite f/VT > 100 breaths/minute/L – in Epstein's study (0.40) was much lower than that originally reported. However, only 10 patients were included in this arm of the study, of whom 6 required > 72 hours of additional weaning before successful extubation. The author acknowledged that the negative predictive value may have been higher if extubation had been attempted at the same time that f/VT was measured.

Rib Cage–Abdominal Motion

The potential importance of abnormal rib cage–abdominal motion as a guide to weaning was first emphasized by Cohen et al.[16] Asynchronous and paradoxic motion of the rib cage and abdomen can be assessed by an index termed *maximum compart-mental amplitude to VT ratio* (MCA/VT), and a high value suggests that weaning is unlikely to be successful.[17] An increase in the breath-to-breath variation of compart-mental contribution in tidal volume, assessed in terms of the standard deviation of the rib cage to tidal volume ratio (RC/VT), also appears to predict weaning failure.[17]

Integrative Indices

Weaning failure is commonly multifactorial in origin, and thus it is not very surprising that an index which assesses a single function is unreliable. Accordingly, an index that integrates a number of physiologic functions should have greater predictive accuracy. Such an index is the CROP index,[30] which incorporates a measure of pulmonary gas

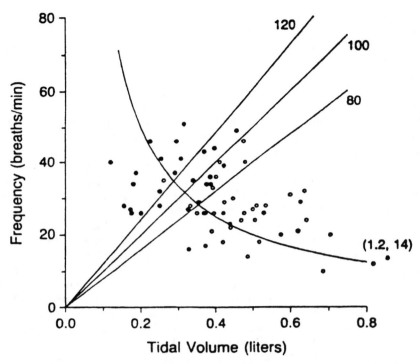

Figure 8.3 Isopleths for the ratio of frequency to tidal volume (f/V_T) representing different degrees of rapid shallow breathing. Patients who fell to the left of the 100 breaths per minute /L isopleth had a 95% likelihood of failing a weaning trial; patients who fell to the right of this isopleth had an 80% likelihood of a successful weaning outcome. The hyperbola represents a minute ventilation of 10 L/minute, a criterion commonly used to predict weaning outcome; it is apparent that this criterion was of little value in discriminating between weaning success (open circles) and weaning failure patients (solid circles). Values for one patient (V, 1.2 L, f 14 breaths/minute) lay outside the graph. (From Yang KL, Tobin MJ. A prospective study of indexes predicting the outcome of trials of weaning from mechanical ventilation. N Engl J Med 1991; 324:1445–1450. Reproduced by permission of the New England Journal of Medicine. Copyright 1991 Massachusetts Medical Society. All rights reserved.)

exchange and an assessment of the demands placed on the respiratory system and the capacity of the respiratory muscles to handle them:

$$\text{CROP index} = \frac{C_{dyn} \times P_I\text{max} \times (PaO_2/P_AO_2)}{\text{Respiratory Rate}}$$

in which C_{dyn} is "dynamic compliance," $P_I max$ is maximal inspiratory pressure, and PaO_2/P_AO_2 is a measure of gas exchange. When prospectively examined, this index had positive and negative predictive values of 0.71 and 0.70, respectively.[30] These values were less than simpler indexes such as f/V_T possibly because the amount of noise or uncertainty of a parameter increases in proportion to the number of terms in the equation.

Another integrative index was developed by Jabour et al.[33] This consists of a measure of ventilatory endurance, pressure-time product (PTI), and an estimate of the efficiency of gas exchange, the minute ventilation needed to bring $PaCO_2$ to 40 mmHg (V_E40):

$$\text{Integrative Index} = PTI \times (V_E40/V_Tsb)$$

where V_Tsb is the tidal volume during spontaneous breathing. The investigators found that this integrative index had a positive predictive value of 0.96 and a negative predictive value of 0.95. However, assessment was performed on a post hoc basis, and they did not examine its accuracy prospectively.

Methods of Weaning

Clinical Approach to Weaning

Before discontinuing mechanical ventilation, particularly in patients with limited cardiorespiratory reserve or unusually high workloads, attention must be directed to several factors. An organized plan of action and a team approach are particularly helpful in weaning problem patients. Adequate control of pain, fever, arrhythmias, and infection is necessary. Correction of fluid and electrolyte imbalance and control of blood glucose levels is helpful. Metabolic alkalosis, which decreases the ventilatory drive, can usually be corrected by chloride and potassium replacements. Although adequate sleep is necessary, medications that cause excessive sedation or impairment of respiratory muscle function may be harmful. The patient should receive adequate nutrition and be prepared psychologically for the weaning process. Promoting verbal communication helps in relieving the patient's fear. A tracheostomy can be advantageous in the patient requiring prolonged mechanical ventilation because it promotes patient comfort, enhances ability to swallow, and improves oral hygiene.[34] In patients with airways obstruction, suctioning of the airways and administration of bronchodilators may facilitate weaning by reducing airway resistance and, thus, the work of breathing.[35,36] Patients with ARDS receiving mechanical ventilation show high airway resistance that is responsive to bronchodilators.[37] Recent studies have shown that bronchodilators can be delivered effectively and conveniently to mechanically ventilated patients with a MDI and spacer in the inspiratory limb of the ventilator circuit.[36] During a weaning trial, the ideal posture for a patient depends on the underlying pathophysiology.[4] Although most patients do better while sitting, some find greater relief from dyspnea in the supine position. A variety of measures have been suggested to help wean problem patients, such as biofeedback and endurance training of the respiratory muscles; however, their application has been limited to a select group of patients, and further studies are needed to document their efficacy in a wider spectrum of mechanically ventilated patients.

Weaning Techniques

Several ventilatory strategies (trials of spontaneous breathing, intermittent mandatory ventilation, and pressure support ventilation) have been prospectively evaluated for their ability to expedite weaning.

To assess a patient's ability to sustain spontaneous ventilation, he or she can be disconnected from the ventilator and receive supplemental O_2 through a T-tube system.[4] The traditional approach has been to employ relatively brief trials of spontaneous breathing (approximately 5 minutes) interposed with resumption of mechanical ventilation, and gradually increase their duration according to a patient's performance. The optimal period of rest between these trials has never been defined, but is commonly 1 to 3 hours. Extubation is performed when the patient is able to sustain spontaneous breathing for 1 to 2 hours without developing respiratory distress. Another approach is to go directly from a high level of ventilator assistance to a spontaneous breathing trial and if the patient does not develop signs of intolerance, extubation is performed without any further weaning. In a study of over 500 patients, Esteban et al.[1] reported that two-thirds of the patients could be extubated after an initial trial of spontaneous breathing. If a patient develops respiratory muscle fatigue during such a trial, the duration of mechanical ventilation required to rest the respiratory muscles has not been defined. Laghi, D'Alfonso, and Tobin[38] demonstrated that diaphragmatic contractility remains significantly depressed for at least 24 hours following the induction of fatigue. Similar studies have not been undertaken in patients who fail a weaning trial, and it is conceivable that the rate of recovery may be even further delayed.

Application of continuous positive airway pressure (CPAP)[39] and flow triggering (Flow-by) have been reported to improve oxygenation and enhance patient comfort during mechanical ventilation[40]; however they cannot be easily employed following extubation.

Intermittent mandatory ventilation (IMV) is the most popular weaning technique in North America.[41,42] When employed for weaning, the IMV rate is usually reduced in steps of 1 to 3 breaths/minute, and an arterial blood gas sample is obtained after about 30 minutes. With application of IMV, patient effort has been thought to be spared in proportion to the number of breaths delivered by the ventilator, but recent evidence suggests that this is not the case. Instead, as the IMV rate is decreased, inspiratory work and pressure-time product increase progressively not only for the spontaneous breaths but also for the assisted breaths.[43] This is largely due to the inability of the respiratory center output to adapt to intermittent support as demon-

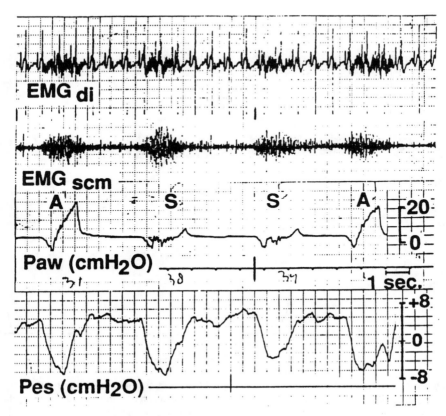

Figure 8.4 Electromyograms of the diaphragm (EMGdi) and of the sternocleidomastoid muscles (EMGscm) in a representative patient receiving synchronized intermittent mandatory ventilation, showing similar intensity and duration of electrical activity in successive assisted (A) and spontaneous (S) cycles. Paw = airway pressure; Pes = esophageal pressure. (From Imsand C, Feihl F, Peffet MD, Fitting JW. Regulation of inspiratory neuromuscular output during synchronized intermittent mechanical ventilation. Anesthesiology 1994; 80:13–22. Reproduced with permission.)

strated in a study employing electromyograms of the diaphragm and sternomastoid muscles[44] (Figure 8.4).

Pressure support ventilation (PSV) augments a spontaneous breath with a fixed amount of positive pressure,[45] and is commonly used to counteract the work of breathing imposed by endotracheal tubes and ventilator circuits. Theoretically, this should help with weaning because a patient who is comfortable at the level of PSV that compensates for imposed work should be able to sustain ventilation following

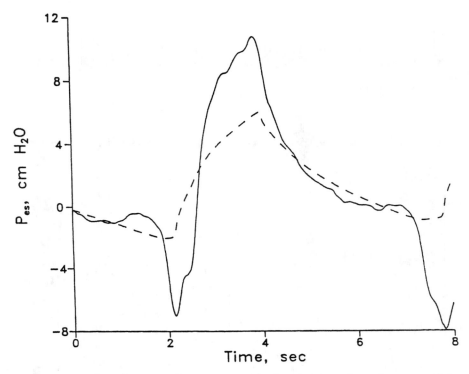

Figure 8.5 Esophageal pressure (Pes, continuous line) and estimated recoil pressure of the chest wall (Pes cw, interrupted line) tracings in a patient receiving pressure support ventilation of 20 cm H_{20}. Pressure tracings have been superimposed so that Pes cw is equal to Pes at the onset of the rapid fall in Pes during late expiration. Times at which Pes tracing are higher than Pes cw represent lower bound expiratory effort. Note the presence of expiratory muscle activation during late inspiration. (From Jubran A, Van de Graaff WB, Tobin MJ. Variability of patient-ventilator interaction with pressure support ventilation in patients with chronic obstructive pulmonary disease. Am J Respir Crit Car Med 1995; 152:129–136. Reproduced with permission.)

extubation. However, the resistance posed by an endotracheal tube varies with the diameter of flow rates, and even when these are constant, resistance will vary as a result of tube deformation and adherent secretions. Indeed, Brochard et al.[46] demonstrated that the level of PSV necessary to eliminate imposed work varied considerable (3–14 cm H_2O) from patient to patient. Likewise, Nathan et al.[47] could not define a level of PSV that predicted respiratory work following extubation. These studies[46,47] indicate that use of PSV to predict a patient's ability to sustain ventilation following extubation is likely to be very misleading. In difficult to wean patients, Stroetz and Hubmayr[2] showed that ventilatory changes following stepwise reductions in PSV did not predict the outcome of weaning trials. Furthermore, ventilator-patient asynchrony may occur during PSV in patients with airway obstruction.[48] At higher levels of PSV, Jubran et al.[48] observed that many patients with airway obstruction revealed evidence of increased expiratory effort during the late inflation phase (Figure 8.5). Thus it may be difficult to predict the decrease in work of breathing with a given level of PSV in any patient, and ventilator-patient asynchrony may occur during PSV, with detrimental effects on the weaning process, in some patients.

Another method of weaning patients is to employ a single daily trial of spontaneous breathing through a T-tube circuit.[1] If spontaneous ventilation can be sustained for 2 hours without undue distress, the patient is extubated. In contrast, if the patient develops signs of respiratory distress on physical examination, the trial is stopped and mechanical ventilation is reinstituted. To allow the respiratory muscles to recover from excessive stress,[38] the patient is rested for about 24 hours with a high level of ventilator assistance such as assist-control ventilation, followed by another trial of spontaneous breathing. This process is repeated until the patient can be extubated successfully.

Relative Efficacy of Weaning Techniques

Two rigorously controlled studies have prospectively compared the efficacy of three different weaning techniques: IMV, PSV, and trials of spontaneous breathing.[49,1] Brochard et al. found that weaning time was significantly shorter with PSV (5.7 ± 3.7 [SD] days) than with IMV (9.9 ± 8.2 days) or trials of spontaneous breathing (8.5 ± 8.3 days). In contrast, using a similar experimental design, Esteban et al.[1] found that a once-daily trial of spontaneous breathing led to extubation about three times more quickly than did IMV, and about twice as quickly as PSV (Figure 8.6). There was no difference in the rate of successful weaning between a once daily trial of spontaneous breathing and intermittent trials of spontaneous breathing (attempted at least twice a day), nor between IMV and PSV. The reason for the different outcomes in the two studies is probably due to the constrained manner in which IMV and trials of spontaneous breathing were employed in the study of Brochard et al.[49] During application of IMV, patients had to tolerate a ventilator rate of ≤ 4 breaths per minute for ≥ 24 hours before extubation[49]; this constitutes a significant ventilatory challenge.[42] In contrast, Esteban et al.[1] extubated patients when they tolerated a ventilator rate of 5 breaths per minute for 2 hours. For the trials of spontaneous breathing in the study of Brochard et al.,[49] physicians could request up to 3 separate trials over a 24-hour period, each lasting 2 hours, before deciding to extubate a patient, whereas in the study of Esteban et al.[1] patients in the once-daily trials of spontaneous breathing were extubated when this was tolerated for 2 hours. The findings in these two studies are complementary; both demonstrate that the pace of weaning depends on the manner in which the technique is applied. When IMV and trials of spontaneous breathing are employed in a constrained manner, weaning is delayed compared with PSV. When a spontaneous breathing trial is employed once a day, weaning is expedited.

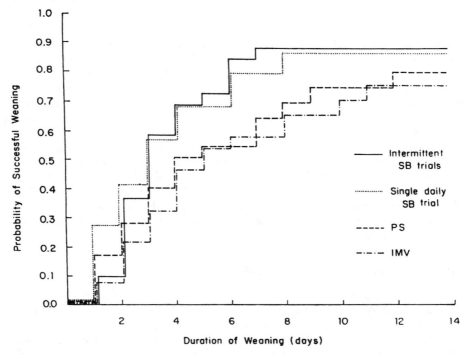

Figure 8.6 Kaplan-Meier curves of the probability of successful weaning with intermittent mandatory ventilation, pressure-support ventilation, intermittent trials of spontaneous breathing, and a once-daily trial of spontaneous breathing. After adjustment for baseline characteristics in a Cox proportional-hazards model, the rate of successful weaning with a once-daily trial of spontaneous breathing was 2.83 times higher than that with intermittent mandatory ventilation ($P < 0.006$) and 2.05 times higher than that with pressure-support ventilation ($P < 0.04$). (From Esteban A, et al. A comparison of four methods of weaning patients from mechanical ventilation. N Engl J Med 1995; 332:345–350. Reproduced by permission of the New England Journal of Medicine. Copyright 1995 Massachusetts Medical Society. All rights reserved.)

A weaning strategy employing the combination of systematic measurement of predictive indices and a once-daily trial of spontaneous breathing was evaluated in a randomized controlled trial in patients receiving mechanical ventilation for acute respiratory failure from multiple causes.[50] The patients were screened each morning; if their PaO_2/FiO_2 ratio was >200, PEEP < 5 cm H_2O, $f/V_T \leq$ 105 breaths/minute/L, cough was satisfactory on suctioning, and no sedative or vasopressor agents were being used, the patients underwent a 2-hour trial of spontaneous breathing the same morning. In the invention group (n = 149), if the patients were able to breathe spontaneously for 2 hours, their physicians were notified of the result and told the patient had a high likelihood of breathing without mechanical ventilation. Patients who were unable to breathe spontaneously for 2 hours underwent daily screening and trials of spontaneous breathing until successful extubation or death. In contrast, patients in the control group (n = 151) were screened daily but did not undergo trials of spontaneous breathing, nor was any feedback provided to their physicians. The patients in the intervention group received mechanical ventilation for a shorter duration (median 4.5 days) compared to those in the control group (6 days; p = 0.003). The rate of complications (p = 0.001), reintubation (p = 0.04), and ICU charges (p = 0.03) were also lower in the intervention compared to the control group.

Summary

A significant proportion of patients recovering from ARDS pose considerable difficulty in weaning from mechanical ventilation. These patients present enormous clinical, economic, and ethical problems. The major determinant of weaning outcome is respiratory muscle function with the adequacy of pulmonary gas exchange and psychological problems playing subsidiary roles. Many of the physiologic indices that have been used to predict weaning outcome are frequently inaccurate, and, of those available, the ratio of frequency to tidal volume appears to be the most reliable. A number of techniques can be used for weaning, and of these a once-daily trial of spontaneous breathing appears to be the most expeditious.

Acknowledgment

Supported in part by a RAG grant from the Department of Veterans Affairs.

References

1. Esteban A, Frutos F, Tobin MJ, et al. A comparison of four methods of weaning patients from mechanical ventilation. N Engl J Med 1995; 332:345–350.
2. Stroetz RW, Hubmayr RD. Tidal volume maintenance during weaning with pressure support. Am J Respir Crit Care Med 1995; 152:1034–1040.
3. Tobin MJ. Mechanical ventilation. New Engl J Med 1973; 330:1056–1061.
4. Tobin MJ, Alex CA. Discontinuation of mechanical ventilation. In Principles and practice of mechanical ventilation, ed. MJ Tobin, McGraw-Hill, New York, 1994, pp. 1177–1206.
5. Torres A, Reyes A, Roca J, Wagner PD, Rodriguez-Roison R. Ventilation-perfusion mismatching in chronic obstructive pulmonary disease during ventilator weaning. Am Rev Respir Dis 1989; 140:1246–1250.

6. Tobin MJ, Perez W, Guenther SM, Semmes BJ, Mador MJ, Allen SJ, Lodato FF, Dantzker DF. The pattern of breathing during successful and unsuccessful trials of weaning from mechanical ventilation. Am Rev Respir Dis 1986; 134:1111–1118.
7. Sassoon CSH, Te TT, Mahutte CK, Light RW. Airway occlusion pressure: an important indicator for successful weaning in patients with chronic obstructive pulmonary disease. Am Rev Respir Dis 1987; 135:107–113.
8. Markand ON, Moorthy SS, Mohamed Y, King R-D, Brown JW. Postoperative phrenic nerve palsy in patients with open-heart surgery. Ann Thorac Surg 1985; 39:68–73.
9. Zapol WM, Frikker MJ, Pontoppidan H, Wilson RS, Lynch KE. The adult respiratory distress syndrome at Massachusetts General Hospital: etiology, progression and survival rates 1978–1988. In Adult respiratory distress syndrome, eds. WM Zapol, F Lemaire. Lung biology in health and disease, vol. 50. Marcel Dekker, New York, 1991, pp. 367–380.
10. Ford GT, Whitelaw WA, Rosenal TW, Cruise PJ, Guenter CA. Diaphragm function after upper abdominal surgery in humans. Am Rev Respir Dis 1983; 127:431–436.
11. Ford GT, Grant DA, Rideout KS, Davison JS, Whitelaw WA. Inhibition of breathing associated with gallbladder stimulation in dogs. J Appl Physiol 1988; 65:72–79.
12. Lemaire F, Teboul JL, Cinotti L, Giotti G, Abrouk F, Steg G, Macquin-Mavier I, Zapol WM. Acute left ventricular dysfunction during unsuccessful weaning from mechanical ventilation. Anesthesiology 1988; 69:171–179.
13. Juan G, Calverley P, Talamo C, Schnader J, Roussos C. Effect of carbon dioxide on diaphragmatic function in human beings. N Engl J Med 1984; 310:874–879.
14. Hansen-Flaschen J, Cowen J, Raps EC. Neuromuscular blockade in the intensive care unit: more than we bargained for. Am Rev Respir Dis 1993; 147:234–236.
15. Anzueto A, Peters JI, Tobin MJ, et al. Effects of prolonged mechanical ventilation on diaphragmatic function in healthy adult baboons. Crit Care Med 1997; 25:1187–1190.
16. Cohen C, Zagelbaum G, Gross D, Roussos C, Macklem PT. Clinical manifestations of inspiratory muscle fatigue. Am J Med 1982; 73:308–316.
17. Tobin MJ, Guenther SM, Perez W, Lodato R-F, Mandor JM, Allen SJ, Dantzker DR-. Konno-Mead analysis of ribcage-abdominal motion during successful and unsuccessful trials of weaning from mechanical ventilation. Am Rev Respir Dis 1987; 135:1320–1328.
18. Tobin MJ, Perez W, Guenther SM, Lodato R-F, Dantzker D.R-. Does ribcage-abdominal paradox signify respiratory muscle fatigue? J Appl Physiol 1987; 63:851–860.
19. Silberman H, Silberman AW. Parenteral nutrition, biochemistry, and respiratory gas exchange. JPEN 1986; 10:151–154.
20. Ralph DD, Thomas Robertson H, Jean Weaver L, Hlastala MP, Canico CJ, Hudson LD. Distribution of ventilation and perfusion during positive endexpiratory pressure in the adult respiratory distress syndrome. Am Rev Respir Dis 1985; 131:54–60.
21. Teres D, Roizen MF, Bushnell LS. Successful weaning from controlled ventilation despite high deadspace-to-tidal volume ratio. Anesthesiology 1973; 39:656–659.
22. Lewis WD, Chwals W, Benotti PN, Lakshman K, O'Donnell C, Blackburn GL, Bistrian BR. Bedside assessment of the work of breathing. Crit Care Med 1988; 16:117–122.
23. Kemper M, Weissman C, Askanazi J, Hyman AI, Kinney JM. Metabolic and respiratory changes during weaning from mechanical ventilation. Chest 1987; 92:979–983.
24. Hubmayr R-D, Loosbrock LM, Gillespie DJ, Rodarte JR. Oxygen uptake during weaning from mechanical ventilation. Chest 1988; 94:1148–1155.

25. Jubran A, Tobin MJ. Passive mechanics of lung and chest wall in patients who failed or succeeded in trials of weaning. Am J Respir Crit Care Med 1997a; 155:916–921.

26. Jubran A, Tobin MJ. Pathophysiologic basic of acute respiratory distress in patients who fail a trial of weaning from mechanical ventilation. Am J Respir Crit Care Med 1997b; 155:906–915.

27. Criner G, Isaac L. Psychological problems in the ventilator-dependent patient. In Principles and practice of mechanical ventilation, ed. MJ Tobin, McGraw-Hill, New York, 1994, pp. 1163–1175.

28. Zhu E, Petrof BJ, Gea J, Comtois N, Grassino AE. Membrane and sarcomere injury in diaphragm following inspiratory resistive loading. Am J Respir Crit Care Med 1997; 155:1110–1116.

29. Sahn SA, Lakshminarayan S. Bedside criteria for discontinuation of mechanical ventilation. Chest 1973; 63:1002–1005.

30. Yang K, Tobin MJ. A prospective study of indexes predicting outcome of trials of weaning from mechanical ventilation. N Engl J Med 1991; 324:1445–1450.

31. Lee KH, Hui KP, Chan TB, Tan WC, Lim TK. Rapid shallow breathing (frequency-tidal volume ratio) did not predict extubation outcome. Chest 1994; 105:540–543.

32. Epstein SK. Etiology of extubation failure and the predictive value of the rapid shallow breathing index. Am J Respir Crit Care Med 1995; 152:545–549.

33. Jabour ER, Rabil DM, Truwit JD, Rochester DF. Evaluation of a new weaning index based on ventilatory endurance and the efficiency of gas exchange. Am Rev Respir Dis 1991; 144:531–537.

34. Heffner JE. Timing of tracheotomy in mechanically ventilated patients. Am Rev Respir Dis 1993; 147:768–771.

35. Mancebo J, Amaro P, Lorino H, Lemaire F, Harf A, & Brochard L. Effects of albuterol inhalation on the work of breathing during weaning from mechanical ventilation. Am Rev Respir Dis 1991; 144:95–100.

36. Dhand R-, Jubran A, Tobin MJ. Bronchodilator delivery by metered-dose inhaler in ventilator-supported patients. Am J Respir Crit Care Med 1995; 151:1827–1833.

37. Wright PE, Carmichael LC, Bernard G.R-. Effect of bronchodilators on lung mechanics in the acute respiratory distress syndrome (ARDS). Chest 1994; 106:1517–1523.

38. Laghi F, D'Alfonso N, Tobin MJ. Pattern of recovery from diaphragmatic fatigue over 24 hours. J Appl Physiol 1995; 79:539–546.

39. Venus B, Jacobs KH, Lim L. Treatment of the adult respiratory distress syndrome with continuous positive airway pressure. Chest 1979; 76:257–261.

40. Sassoon CSH, Lodia R-, Rheeman CH, Kuei JK, Light RW, Kees Mahutte C. Inspiratory muscle work of breathing during flow-by, demand flow, and continuous-flow systems in patients with chronic obstructive pulmonary disease. Am Rev Respir Dis 1992; 145:1219–1222.

41. Venus B, Smith RA, Mathru M. National survey of methods and criteria used for weaning from mechanical ventilation. Crit Care Med 1987; 15:530–533.

42. Sassoon CSH. Intermittent mandatory ventilation. In Principles and practice of mechanical ventilation, ed. MJ Tobin, McGraw-Hill, New York, 1994, pp. 221–237.

43. Marini JJ, Smith TC, Lamb VJ. External work output and force generation during synchronized intermittent mandatory ventilation: effect of machine assistance on breathing effort. Am Rev Respir Dis 1988; 138:1169–1179.

44. Imsand C, Feihl F, Peffet C, Fitting JW. Regulation of inspiratory neuromuscular output during synchronized intermittent mechanical ventilation. *Anesthesiology* 1994; 80:13–22.

45. Brochard L. Pressure support ventilation. In Principles and practice of mechanical ventilation, ed. MJ Tobin, McGraw-Hill, New York, 1994, pp. 239–257.

46. Brochard L, Rua F, Lorino H, Lemaire F, Halt A. Inspiratory pressure support compensates for the additional work of breathing caused by the endotracheal tube. Anesthesiology 1991; 75:739–745.

47. Nathan SD, Ishaaya AM, Koerner SK, Belman MJ. Prediction of minimal pressure support during weaning from mechanical ventilation. Chest 1993; 103:1215–1219.

48. Jubran A, Van de Graaff WB, Tobin MJ. Variability of patient-ventilator interaction with pressure support ventilation in patients with chronic obstructive pulmonary disease. Am J Respir Crit Care Med 1995; 152:129–136.

49. Brochard L, Rauss A, Benito S, Conti G, Mancebo J, Rekik N, Gasparetto A, Lemaire F. Comparison of three methods of gradual withdrawing from ventilatory support during weaning from mechanical ventilation. Am J Respir Crit Care Med 1994; 150:896–903.

50. Ely EW, Baker AM, Dunagan DP, et al. Effect on the duration of mechanical ventilation of identifying patients capable of breathing spontaneously. N Engl J Med 1996; 335:1864–1869.

9

Clinical Assessment and Total Patient Care

James A. Russell, Vinay Dhingra, and Keith R. Walley

Introduction

Attentive assessment and detailed management of all issues related to total patient care are fundamental to care of patients who have ARDS. This chapter provides information regarding clinical assessment and management of common clinical problems and complications that occur in patients who have ARDS. Because this is not a general textbook of critical care medicine, discussion of common investigations, common procedures, and standard treatment are not covered in detail here. Readers are referred to general textbooks of critical care medicine. We do, however, cover issues that relate specifically to managing patients who have ARDS.

Airway Management

Airway assessment and management, fundamental to treating ARDS, are covered briefly in Chapter 7. The major indications for endotracheal intubation of patients at risk for or who have ARDS are for airway protection, prevention of airway obstruction, ventilation (i.e., elimination of CO_2), oxygenation (i.e., to improve abnormal oxygenation), and resuscitation of severe shock (Table 9.1). The most common indication for intubation of patients who have ARDS is to correct inadequate oxygenation despite use of high-flow mask oxygen. Less commonly, patients who have ARDS require intubation because of a depressed level of consciousness that may be secondary to the underlying cause of ARDS (i.e., drug overdose, head trauma), secondary to sedation, or secondary to progressive respiratory failure with

Table 9.1. Indications for intubation of patients with ARDS

Airway protection	For example, decreased level of consciousness
	Inability to clear secretions
	Decreased reflexes protecting upper airway
	Prevention of aspiration of gastric contents
Prevention from airway obstruction	For example, upper airway edema
Ventilation	For example, CO_2 elimination
	Increased work of breathing and decreased ventilatory capability
Oxygenation	For example, to maximize FiO_2
	To add positive pressure ventilation to improve oxygenation
Shock	For example, refractory shock requiring inotropic support

onset of ventilatory failure superimposed on oxygenation failure. Many patients who have ARDS also have shock, which impairs respiratory muscle function and increases the risk of acute deterioration. Therefore, patients in refractory shock may also require intubation for stabilization of cardiovascular and respiratory status. Patients who require air transport or land transport may benefit from earlier intubation prior to transport to decrease the risk of complications during transport.

Airway assessment prior to intubation of the patient in respiratory distress must be done rapidly. During assessment, patients should have high-flow oxygenation at the maximum fraction of inspired oxygen while monitoring ECG and pulse oximetry. Some causes of difficult intubation include short neck, large tongue, obesity, inadequate mouth opening, short mandible, mouth secretions, trauma, cervical instability, and history of previous difficult intubation.[1] Emergent intubation is necessary in patients in full cardiopulmonary arrest, and urgent intubation is necessary in patients who have a declining level of consciousness, inadequate airway protection, and/or refractory hypoxemia.

Assessment of the airway includes assessment of gag reflex, cough reflex, and level of consciousness. In obtunded patients, positioning of the jaw to alleviate airway obstruction by the tongue while administering high-flow oxygen is necessary prior to intubation. In general, use of an oral airway is inappropriate for any sustained period of time in a patient with depressed level of consciousness and hypoxemic respiratory failure. Patients with ARDS who have a depressed level of consciousness usually should be intubated.

Ventilation is difficult to assess clinically and requires measurements of arterial blood gases and interpretation of the pH and PCO_2. Patients with significant respiratory acidosis who have a pH < 7.20 often require intubation and ventilation. However, this is a general guideline. Most often the finding of significant respiratory acidosis that necessitates intubation coincides with clinical findings such as depressed level of consciousness, findings of respiratory muscle fatigue, and signs of significant sympathetic stimulation such as tachycardia, hypertension, and diaphoresis. Patients who have ARDS develop respiratory alkalosis first; ventilatory failure and respiratory acidosis are late findings and usually indicate imminent cardiopulmonary arrest. Ventilatory efforts are assessed by observing respiratory rate, depth of respiratory effort, accessory muscle use, indrawing, and abdominal excursion. Most patients who have progressive ARDS develop tachypnea as a result of decreased lung compliance, stimulation of receptors in the lung secondary to lung inflammation, hypoxemia, and respiratory muscle fatigue. In general, patients cannot maintain respiratory rates greater than 35 to 40 per minute for any significant period of time because of development of respiratory muscle fatigue and failure.

Onset of accessory muscle use reflects relative diaphragmatic weakness. Accessory muscle use is followed by so-called paradoxical respiratory movement indicating more severe diaphragm fatigue. Paradoxical respiratory movement means that during inspiration the chest expands but the abdomen collapses because the fatigued diaphragm moves up in response to the negative intrathoracic pressure generated by the inspiratory effort. During normal inspiration the diaphragm descends and so the abdomen does not collapse.

Significant hypoxemia is now most often assessed by pulse oximetry and by arterial blood gas measurement. Central cyanosis is a very late finding and indicates severe hypoxemia. In addition, many patients who are significantly hypoxemic do not have central cyanosis. In general, patients who are unable to maintain an arterial hemoglobin saturation greater than 85% to 90% on more than 60% to 70% face mask oxygen require additional support including intubation, ventilation, positive airway pressure, and positive end-expiratory pressure to correct arterial hypoxemia.

Mask CPAP

The role of mask CPAP in management of acute hypoxemic respiratory failure due to ARDS is somewhat controversial.

Mask CPAP is reported to be a successful intervention in acute cardiogenic pulmonary edema[2,3] because it improves oxygenation, reduces work of breathing, and decreases left ventricular afterload.[4] Mask CPAP is contraindicated in patients who have significantly decreased level of consciousness and depressed airway protective reflexes, patients who are hemodynamically unstable, patients who do not obtain a good tight seal of the mask (because of anatomy), and patients who have a full stomach. Patients who do not improve with mask CPAP need to be intubated and ventilated. In general, mask CPAP can be used for short periods of time in patients who are awake, responsive, able to protect their airway, and who can withstand the mild discomfort of a tight-fitting mask. Mask CPAP clearly improves oxygenation in cardiogenic pulmonary edema.[2-4] The greater duration of respiratory failure and slower recovery of oxygenation of patients who have ARDS limit the use of mask CPAP in this patient group.

In general, impaired ventilation is evaluated by assessing arterial pH.

Endotracheal Intubation

Endotracheal intubation of the patient who has ARDS is a high-risk intubation that requires skill and experience to be undertaken safely and effectively. Physicians who are relatively unfamiliar with endotracheal intubation should request assistance from qualified personnel such as anesthesiologists and/or intensivists because of the high risk of complications of intubation of these patients.

The equipment needed for intubation is shown in Table 9.2. The technique of intubation is only reviewed briefly here to highlight points relevant to patients who have ARDS. Again, we emphasize that intubation is high risk and should be done or supervised by experienced, skilled operators. First, unless the patient is in full cardiopulmonary arrest or is on the verge of arrest, it is necessary to carefully prepare equipment, drugs, and organize a team approach to intubation to minimize complications of intubation. While preparing for intubation, an intravenous line should be established and reassessed. Intubation equipment should be checked to be sure it is working. The patient should be evaluated to assess difficulty of intubation. While doing these evaluations and preparations, the patient must receive high-flow face mask oxygen while ECG, blood pressure, and pulse oximetry are monitored.

It is prudent to assume that patients requiring urgent intubation who have ARDS have a full stomach and require an intubation procedure that minimizes the risk of aspiration of gastric contents.[5] In patients who have a nasogastric (NG) tube already in place, the NG tube should be placed on suction. In patients who do not have an NG, if a patient is stable and cooperative, then an NG tube can be placed to provide partial gastric emptying.

The technique of intubation by so-called crash induction is reviewed in much more detail in textbooks of anesthesiology and critical care.[5] In general, large-bore rigid tip (Yankauer) suction must be prepared for use during the intubation procedure. The patient must be appropriately sedated and paralyzed to allow cricoid pressure (Sellick maneuver) prior to and during intubation. Firm pressure on cricoid cartilage is applied to collapse the esophagus. Pressure is maintained until the endotracheal tube has clearly been placed in the trachea.

Most commonly, patients have orotracheal intubation by direct laryngoscopy. After preoxygenation, preparation of equipment, and orientation of patient and assistants to the procedure, the patient should be given adequate sedation and paralysis (as discussed later) to allow optimal visualization of the glottis. Usually a number 8.0 or 8.5 endotracheal tube (ETT) is used in adults. A stylette should be inserted to stabilize the endotracheal tube and usually a MacIntosh number 3 or 4 blade is used in adults. The chances of successful intubation are significantly improved by careful positioning into the "modified sniffing" position unless there is high risk of cervical spine instability (i.e., head-injured unconscious patients, patients who have rheumatoid arthritis, etc.). Using a curved or straight blade laryngoscope, the upper airway is visualized followed by the vocal cords, and endotracheal intubation is attempted. The endotracheal tube should be passed through the vocal cords and to a position such that the proximal end of the cuff is just below the vocal cords. Sometimes the

Table 9.2. Intubation equipment

Oxygen
Bag (Ambu bag)
Laryngoscope with working light and blades (Macintosh 3 and 4, Miller 3 blades)
Airway (oral airways sizes 7–10)
Endotracheal tubes (cuff checked, sizes 6.5–8.5 mm) and syringe (10 mL)
Stylet
Suction and Yankauer tip
Mask (small, medium, and large sizes)
Magill forceps (for nasotracheal intubation)

epiglottis cannot be visualized and the tube must be passed blindly. Blind intubation increases the risk of inadvertent esophageal intubation. If attempts are not successful, the tube should be removed and oxygenation should be maintained while repositioning the patient and attempting intubation again.

Once the endotracheal tube is in place, its position should be verified by listening over the stomach to confirm absence of epigastric sounds during each positive pressure inspiration and over the chest to verify bilateral air entry during each inspiration. Patients should be bagged with 100% oxygen and the airway should be fixed in position. If an NG tube is not already in place it should be inserted at this point. An urgent ("stat") chest radiograph should be obtained to confirm position of the endotracheal and NG tubes and and to confirm lack of complications such as gastric distension and pneumothorax.

Adequate preoxygenation is essential before endotracheal intubation of patients who have increased intrapulmonary shunting due to acute hypoxemic respiratory failure. Normally the body has very low stores of oxygen when breathing room air. The functional residual capacity (FRC) of the lungs is the only site of storage of oxygen. Preoxygenation with 100% oxygen increases the total quantity of oxygen by increasing the percentage of oxygen in FRC. The risk of hypoxemia during the apneic phase of intubation is increased in ARDS for several reasons. First, the FRC is dramatically reduced in ARDS and so the available oxygen stores are decreased in these patients. Second, during the preoxygenation period while the patient is breathing spontaneously, oxygen consumption may be significantly increased because of increased respiratory muscle work and oxygen consumption. Third, the increased sympathetic tone and catecholamine state characteristic of these acutely ill patients also directly increases oxygen demand of the heart and other organs. Therefore, this abnormal physiology limits the available oxygen stores in FRC during preoxygenation, which therefore shortens the time that apneic oxygenation is safe. Thus patients who have ARDS are at risk of significant hypoxemia if intubation is difficult, prolonged, or if preoxygenation has been inadequate.

The drugs used to facilitate orotracheal intubation in critically hypoxic patients must be used only with thorough understanding of the pharmacology, pharmacokinetics, and side effects. Furthermore, they should only be used by individuals who have learned the technical skill of intubation or are closely supervised by an appropriate skilled operator. Many patients can be intubated with topical anesthesia alone with minimal or no sedation. Lidocaine spray (4%) is sprayed into the oropharynx and can be followed by lidocaine jelly (2%) on an oral airway. The dose of lidocaine should not exceed 6 mg/kg.

Patients who have acute hypoxemic respiratory failure due to ARDS are high-risk intubation because of the frequent association of hypoxia, rapid worsening of hypoxia if oxygen supply is interrupted, hemodynamic instability from hypovolemia, ventricular dysfunction, peripheral vasodilation, and heightened sympathetic tone. As a result, drugs used to facilitate intubation are much more potent in this population than in the usual elective intubation patient. Furthermore, doses must be adjusted so that respiratory and cardiac arrest are not precipitated by the drugs. Commonly used agents to be used only by experienced operators include intravenous lidocaine, midazolam, diazepam, pentothal, fentanyl, propofol, and ketamine. Drugs such as ephedrine and epinephrine should be readily available to treat severe hypotension after intubation. The use of neuromuscular blocking agents again requires use by a skilled operator who can manage the airway by bag and mask and who can intubate difficult airways. Patients who have ARDS have decreased respiratory compliance, increased oxygen demand, may have retained secretions, and are therefore much more difficult to ventilate and oxygenate using an Ambu bag and mask than are patients without lung disease.

The commonest complications of intubation are esophageal intubation, right mainstem intubation, aspiration of gastric contents, the effects of high airway pressure, and hemodynamic instability (Table 9.3). Intubation of critically ill patients in the ICU is associated with increased risk of serious complications and death.[6] Several physiologic changes can be anticipated before, during, and after intubation. These physiologic changes are induced by the drugs used to facilitate intubation, by the stimulus of largynoscopy, and by the change from negative airway pressure to positive airway pressure ventilation. During largynoscopy, patients frequently develop hypertension and tachycardia from sympathetic stimulation. Following intubation, blood pressure often falls, and hypotension, shock, and even cardiac arrest can occur. The major causes of hypotension after intubation include withdrawal of sympathetic tone from sedation and from correction of hypoxemia, positive airway pressure that decreases venous return and cardiac output, and vasodilating effects of drugs used for sedation. Finally, complications of intubation, such as right mainstem intubation, esophageal intubation, and pneumothorax, should be considered in patients who deteriorate following intubation.

Right mainstem intubation is avoided by placing orotracheal tubes at the appropriate site (20 cm at the lip in females, 23 cm at the lip in males). Right mainstem intubation may only be diagnosed at the time of chest x ray following intubation. Aspiration of gastric contents, a major complication of endotracheal intubation of the critically ill, is avoided by adequate preoxygenation, intubation assuming the stomach is full using crash induction, and techniques for awake intubation such as

Table 9.3. Important acute complications of endotracheal intubation

Mouth/dental injury
Esophageal intubation
Pharyngeal, esophageal, and tracheal tears
Aspiration of gastric contents
Right mainstem intubation
Hypertension
Hypotension
Arrhythmias
Increased intracranial pressure
Laryngeal injury

nosotracheal intubation. The major effects of positive airway pressure include decreased cardiac output, hypotension, pneumothorax, air trapping, and auto-PEEP. Hypotension following endotracheal intubation and positive airway pressure is usually managed by rapid infusion of volume using normal saline or Ringer's lactate. If hypotension is severe and sustained, ephedrine or epinephrine should be given intravenously. If hypotension is sustained despite volume infusion, endotracheal tube position and hypoxia and hypercapnia should be corrected. Occasionally, patients will require vasopressors such as dopamine for a longer period of time, but this is unusual.

Tracheostomy

The timing and role of tracheostomy in the critically ill is controversial.[7,8] Because many patients with ARDS require prolonged ventilation, the issue of tracheostomy comes up frequently. In the patient who clearly requires prolonged ventilation, tracheostomy should be considered because it has several advantages such as patient comfort, better oral hygiene, easier removal and reinstitution of mechanical ventilation, and reduced risk of laryngeal injury. In general, we recommend tracheostomy after several weeks of endotracheal intubation in patients who will require further mechanical ventilation for at least several more weeks. In some patients who are difficult to wean because of hypercapnia, there is some benefit from reducing anatomic dead space by tracheostomy as opposed to endotracheal intubation. This technique is controversial, however, because the net effect is relatively small and probably only benefits patients who have extremely marginal nutrition, muscle strength, and impaired respiratory system mechanics.

Complications of tracheostomy include dislocation of the tracheostomy tube into the pretracheal space, airway and neck hemorrhage, and pneumomediastinum/pneumothorax. Hemorrhage into the neck with hematoma formation causes airway obstruction that may present with deviation of the trachea, increasing airway pressures, and an expanding mass in the neck. This is an emergency that requires urgent evacuation of the hematoma to prevent progressive airway obstruction. Tracheostomy tubes can slip out of the trachea into the pretracheal space, which presents with relatively rapid distress, hypoxia, and increased airway pressure on the ventilator. If an acute tracheostomy becomes displaced it is safer to reintubate the patient orotracheally than to struggle with repositioning of the tracheostomy tube unless the operator has a good understanding of the anatomy and skills necessary to reinsert the tracheostomy tube.

Late complications of tracheostomy include obstruction by mucus and secretions, tracheosphageal fistula, tracheoinnominate fistula, tracheomalacia, and tracheal stenosis.

Respiratory System Support Other Than Ventilation

The major forms of respiratory system support other than ventilation (covered in Chapter 7) include endotracheal suctioning, placement of chest tubes for pleural effusion, hemothorax, and pneumothorax, and respiratory drugs such as bronchodilators.

Most patients on mechanical ventilation, including patients who have ARDS, require regular endotracheal suctioning. This is usually done by respiratory therapists or nurses, but physicians should be aware of the technique and its complications. Unless special suctioning tubes are used that direct the suction catheter into the left mainstem bronchus, most suctioning effectively goes down the right mainstem bronchus. In patients who have head injury, increased intracranial pressure, hemodynamic instability, or myocardial ischemia, suctioning can be associated with transient complications such as increased intracranial pressure, arrhythmias, hypertension, hypotension, and hypoxemia. Intracranial and systemic hypertension secondary to suctioning may be avoided by pretreatment with bolus intravenous lidocaine (75 mg). Hemodynamic complications and arrhythmias may also be avoided by using intravenous lidocaine prior to suctioning. The oropharynx must also be suctioned regularly to remove oropharyngeal secretions. Recent studies have suggested that regular suctioning of oropharyngeal secretions decreases the risk of nosocomial pneumonia in ventilated patients.[9,10] Suctioning requires careful attention to sterile procedure to reduce the risk of cross infection of patients and development of nosocomial pneumonia.

Chest tube placement is most often necessary for simple pneumothorax and tension pneumothorax in mechanically ventilated patients. In general, chest tubes are not recommended for other complications of barotrauma such as pulmonary interstitial emphysema, pneumomediastinum, pneumoperitoneum, or subcutaneous emphysema. These complications require careful search for associated pneumothorax. In general we do not recommend "prophylactic" chest tubes in patients at high risk of barotrauma such as patients who have ARDS who have high airway pressures. Instead, we recommend adjusting ventilation as discussed in Chapter 7 to minimize airway pressure. In patients who require air transport and who already have barotrauma, prophylactic chest tube placement may be appropriate because of the risk of pneumothorax during flight and because of the difficulties of correcting pneumothorax during flight. Chest tubes are also required for patients who have chest trauma for management of hemothorax, pneumothorax, or hemopneumothorax. In patients with chest trauma who have hemothorax or pneumothorax, chest tube placement is necessary to correct the problem and to monitor ongoing air leak and blood loss.

Inhaled bronchodilators are necessary in patients who have airways obstruction due to reversible airway smooth muscle contraction. Wheezing may be caused by airway secretions and airway wall edema, as well as airway smooth muscle contraction. In patients who have wheezing, increased airways resistance, decreased dynamic compliance, or significant auto-PEEP, we recommend a trial of inhaled bronchodilators including beta$_2$-selective agents (e.g., salbutamol, terbutaline, albuterol, metaproterenol) and/or the anticholergineric bronchodilator ipratropium bromide. In patients who have severe wheezing we administer salbutamol hourly and ipratropium every 4 hours by puffer directly into the inspiratory limb of the ventilator tubing.

Most patients who have ARDS do not have significant clinically recognizable airway obstruction. Most wheezing associated with ARDS is probably caused by underlying preexisting chronic obstructive pulmonary disease or asthma with superimposed ARDS.

Cardiovascular Assessment and Care

See details in Chapter 6.

Gastrointestinal Assessment and Care

The major gastrointestinal disorders and issues that require attention in patients who have ARDS are prevention of gastric stress ulceration, and management of nutrition, hepatic dysfunction, upper and lower gastrointestinal hemorrhage, acute pancreatitis, and gut ischemia. Nutrition is discussed next, and the other gastrointestinal disorders are discussed later in this chapter under complications.

Nutritional support is necessary in all critically ill patients at risk of ARDS and who have ARDS. Several studies in other groups of patients (such as abdominal trauma) indicate metabolic and physiologic benefits of nutrition, but it has been difficult to prove that nutrition improves survival.[11-15] Increased catabolism and higher energy needs characterize the metabolic changes of critically ill patients and therefore determine their nutritional requirements. Nutrition is provided to minimize negative nitrogen balance and to meet the increased energy requirements. Determining the protein and energy requirements of the critically ill is a complex and controversial process. Techniques such as indirect calorimetry (to measure oxygen consumption and carbon dioxide production), measurement of urinary nitrogen, and calculation of the nonprotein respiratory quotient are used to prescribe each individual patient's nutrition supplementation requirements. Alternatively, energy requirements may be estimated by calculating average energy expenditure based on weight, height, and age (i.e., Harris-Benedict equation) with a further adjustment of the effects of critical illness. Nutrition may be provided as total parenteral nutrition (TPN) or enteral nutrition.

Enteral nutrition is preferred over total parenteral nutrition because it is safer, cheaper, easier, and may improve outcome compared to TPN. Enteral nutrition maintains gastrointestinal muscosal integrity, decreases the risk of upper GI hemorrhage from stress gastritis and ulceration, and has been associated with decreased morbidity and mortality in critically ill patients. After the period of stabilization and resuscitation (24–48 hours), the harder plastic NG tube used for suction is removed and replaced with a soft polyurethane feeding tube that can be left in the stomach or directed using weighted tips or gastroscopy into the duodenum. Some clinical trials suggest that enteral nutrition may improve outcomes compared to TPN in trauma patients.[12–14] In hypermetabolic patients such as patients who have ARDS, enteral nutrition did not prevent multiple organ failure.[15]

Enteral feeding also has potentially positive effects on immune function in critically ill patients. Recent evidence suggests that glutamine has positive effects on immune function such as gut lymphoid tissue and circulating macrophages. Other ingredients in enteral nutrition that may have positive effects on immune function include arginine nucleotides, omega-3 fatty acids, and polyunsaturated fatty acids.

There is a large choice in enteral feed preparations. These products may be classified as follows: whole protein, semi-elemental, and elemental feeds. There is also standard versus high-energy feeds and fiber-containing feeds. Following nutritional assessment, we generally administer enteral nutrition by continuous infusion using a roller pump. We select a feed with input from a dietary consultant and we consider preexisting nutritional status, energy requirements, and renal function/volume status in selecting the appropriate enteral nutrition.

Enteral nutrition may not be tolerated because of limited absorption or because of diarrhea. Limited absorption is handled by addition of prokinetic agents, by decreasing the rate of infusion, and by changing the type of feed. If absorption still remains incomplete, TPN may be necessary. Diarrhea in patients requiring enteral feeds must be approached with a differential diagnosis because there are other causes of diarrhea in the patient who has ARDS such as antibiotic-associated colitis, infectious colitis, gut ischemia, and malabsorption. Whatever the cause of diarrhea, enteral feeding will usually need to be decreased or discontinued. The enteral feeding algorithm used in our ICU is shown in Figure 9.1.

Total parenteral nutrition (TPN) is provided as a combination of water, electrolytes, vitamins, elements (e.g., zinc, copper, etc.), carbohydrate (as hyperosmolar dextrose solution), protein (as essential and nonessential amino acids), and lipid (often as Intralipid, an emulsion of lipids). Usually, protein (0.6–1.5 g protein/kg) is provided by choosing one of several commercially available solutions. Lipid provides more energy than carbohydrate, which decreases the volume requirements that can be relevant in patients who have ARDS. However, lipid solutions are more expensive than carbohydrate. Hyperosmolar solutions of carbohydrate (e.g., 50% dextrose) necessitate infusion via large central veins.

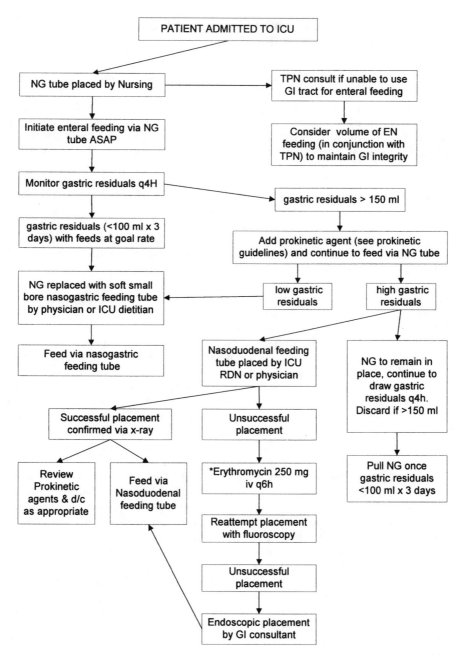

Figure 9.1. Enteral feeding algorithm.

Neurologic Assessment and Care: Pain Control, Sedation, and Neuromuscular Blockers

Most patients who have ARDS require sedation, many require pain control, and only the minority will require neuromuscular blockade.

Pain control and sedation necessitate assessment of pain and sedation needs. Most assessment methods are relatively inexact. Pain can be assessed qualitatively and may be supplemented by pain rating scales. Similarly, level of consciousness may be assessed by the Glasgow Coma Scale, which may be supplemented by the Ramsay sedation scale (Table 9.4).[16]

Following assessment, pain control in patients who have ARDS is usually provided by parenteral narcotics. Narcotics such as morphine also depress respiratory drive, which eases ventilator management and relieves dyspnea. Most patients who have ARDS require relatively prolonged mechanical ventilation, and therefore intravenous morphine (hourly or by infusion) is preferred.[14] Morphine is the drug of choice because of its gradual onset of action (30 minutes), duration of action (2 to 4 hours), and low cost. Morphine's side effects include vasodilation, hypotension, and less often bronchospasm (due to histamine release). Tolerance to intravenous narcotics develops with continued use, and it is not clear whether intermittent bolus or continuous infusion of narcotic leads to more rapid tolerance.[17]

Prolonged use of morphine can cause prolonged sedation because one of its metabolites (morphine-6-flucuronide) is more potent than morphine and it accumulates in patients who have impaired renal function. Other narcotics (such as fentanyl, hydromorphone, meperidine) are used less in patients who have ARDS because of their different pharmacokinetics, pharmacodynamics, and cost. Fentanyl has a more rapid onset of action than morphine, shorter duration of action (at small doses), and fewer hemodynamic side effects than morphine. Therefore, fentanyl may have advantages in the hemodynamically unstable patient.

Surgical and trauma patients who have ARDS may benefit from epidural anesthesia using local anesthetics or intraspinal narcotics.

Sedation in patients who have ARDS is most often achieved by intravenous benzodiazepines, by bolus or continuous infusion. Diazepam, midazolam, and lorazepam are most often used. Diazepam has a long half-life, accumulates in patients who have hepatic or renal dysfunction, and is cheapest. Midazolam is three times more potent than diazepam, has a shorter half-life (1 to 4 hours), and is more expensive than diazepam. Thus midazolam is appropriate for short-term use.[17] Lorazepam has a short half-life, penetrates the brain more slowly than diazepam or midazolam, and its metabolites are inactive.[18] An approach to sedation in critically ill patients used in our ICU is shown in Figure 9.2.

Neuromuscular blocking agents have been used in patients who have refractory hypoxemia to improve oxygenation by decreasing skeletal muscle (especially respiratory muscle) oxygen consumption, by improving thoracic compliance, and by favoring redistribution of blood flow to vital organs.[19]

Neuromuscular blockers are used much less often now in critically ill patients

Table 9.4. The Ramsay Scale of Sedation

Level	Response
1	Anxious and agitated or restless, or both
2	Cooperative, oriented, and tranquil
3	Responding to commands
4	Brisk response to stimuli[a]
5	Sluggish response to stimuli[a]
6	No response to stimuli[a]

[a]Loud voice or glabellar tap.

because of the risk of severe, prolonged muscle weakness associated with nondepolarizing neuromuscular blockers and because of new approaches to management of severe hypoxemia. Succinylcholine (a depolarizing neuromuscular blocker) is still used to facilitate intubation. However, the use of nondepolarizing agents has changed significantly and is very relevant in management of ARDS because in the past, many patients who had severe ARDS and refractory hypoxemia received neuromuscular blockers. In addition to toxicity limiting use of neuromuscular blockers, other techniques to improve refractory hypoxemia such as heavy sedation, prone positioning, nitric oxide, and inverse ratio ventilation are used and diminish the need for neuromuscular blockers.

Prolonged muscle weakness after neuromuscular blocking agents can be caused first by prolonged elevated levels of active drug and active metabolites and second by development of syndromes of neuromuscular pathology. Prolonged paralysis caused by abnormal drug metabolism occurs with vecuronium because one of its metabolites (3-desacetylvecuronium) accumulates and causes prolonged paralysis.[20]

Neuromuscular blocking agents can cause several syndromes of prolonged weakness including myopathy, peripheral neuropathy, and overlap syndromes.[21–23] The original reports described patients who had severe asthma requiring mechanical ventilation who received corticosteroids and steroid muscle relaxants.[21,23] Profound myopathy causes weakness necessitating ventilation for months. Therefore, concomitant use of corticosteroids and steroid muscle relaxants must be avoided.

In our ICU, all critically ill patients who are receiving neuromuscular blockers have monitoring of neuromuscular blockade. This is done at the bedside by critical care nurses trained to interpret train-of-four muscle twitch monitoring.

Neuromuscular blocking agents should be used in patients who have refractory hypoxemia only if measures such as increased sedation, nitric oxide, prone positioning, and pressure control ventilation have been unsuccessful. Muscle relaxation is necessary in patients on pressure control-inverse ratio ventilation. If neuromuscular blocking agents are used, duration of use should be as brief as possible, drug selection must be based on pharmacokinetics, on assessment of hepatic and renal function, and monitoring of neuromuscular blockade may lead to use of lower doses that may decrease complications.

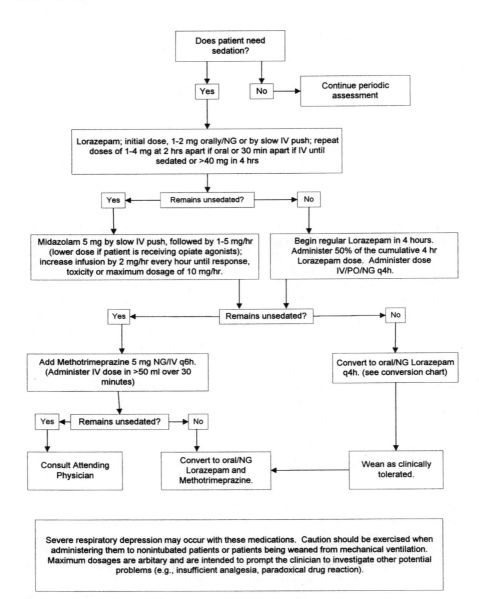

Figure 9.2. Sedation algorithm.

Trauma Assessment and Care

Trauma is a common cause of ARDS and important in management of ARDS for several reasons. First, skillful assessment and management of the early, intermediate, and late phases of trauma may prevent or lessen the severity of ARDS. Second, specific aspects of trauma management overlap with prevention and management of ARDS. For example, early, aggressive resuscitation of shock may prevent lung injury, whereas excessive fluid resuscitation in patients who have increased pulmonary capillary permeability will lead to noncardiogenic pulmonary edema and ARDS. The third important management issue relevant to trauma and ARDS is that ARDS secondary to trauma may have a lower mortality than ARDS secondary to sepsis.

Several types of traumatic injury are associated with increased risk of ARDS. First, multiple trauma complicated by shock is associated with ARDS. Second, multiple transfusions (e.g., more than 10 units in 24 hours) of trauma patients is associated with ARDS. Third, severe head injury can cause intracranial hypertension and neurogenic pulmonary edema, can lead to aspiration of gastric contents because of decreased level of consciousness, and can complicate fluid and ventilator management (e.g., levels of PEEP and $PaCO_2$) of patients who have ARDS. Fourth, multiple long bone fractures are associated with increased risk of ARDS, can be complicated by fat embolism syndrome, and may be an indication for early corticosteroids to prevent fat embolism syndrome. Finally, severe burns can lead to acute lung injury and ARDS because of smoke-inhalation pulmonary injury and because of burn sepsis-induced lung injury. Fluid, airway, and ventilator management of patients who have severe burns intersect with management of ARDS.

Multiple Trauma and ARDS

Effective assessment and management of multiple trauma is fundamental to minimize risk of complications such as ARDS. The epidemiology of trauma shows a trimodal distribution of mortality. The first mode is deaths at the scene caused by lethal injuries such as severe head injury, airway injury, disruption of major vessels, and cardiac tamponade. The second peak of deaths occurs over the next few hours and is caused by potentially treatable life-threatening injuries. Effective management of trauma is characterized by early recognition and skillful correction of treatable life-threatening problems such as airway problems, tension pneumothorax, cardiac tamponade, acute respiratory failure, and hypovolemic shock. The Advanced Trauma Life Support (ATLS) course of the American College of Surgeons is an outstanding educational program that emphasizes the importance of effective immediate management of trauma to prevent early trauma deaths.[24] The third peak of deaths in trauma occurs over days to weeks and is caused by sepsis and multiple system organ failure.

The priorities of emergency management of trauma are similar to the general airway, breathing, and circulation management discussed earlier in this chapter with the following modifications. Airway management must include cervical spine control.

Circulation management includes control of hemorrhage as well as volume resuscitation. Brain resuscitation necessitates early restoration of cerebral perfusion pressure and arterial oxygenation. These priorities are summarized as follows: A (airway with C spine control), B (Breathing), C (Circulation), and D (Neurologic Disability). These priorities take precedence in a sequence called the Primary Survey (ATLS). The second order of priorities are stabilization of fractures and the secondary survey that occurs only after resuscitation and stabilization.

We emphasize several aspects of resuscitation in trauma because early, effective resuscitation is critical to minimize morbidity and mortality of trauma and because intensivists are often called to assist with and even lead resuscitation of trauma victims.

A detailed discussion of airway management in multiple trauma is beyond the scope of this book. Important fundamentals of management are to provide high-flow oxygen by face mask, to alleviate upper airway obstruction by the tongue in unconscious patients by use of nasopharyngeal or oropharyngeal airway, and to intubate if these measures are inadequate. Unconscious patients, patients who have injuries above the clavicles, and patients who have symptoms and signs of cervical spine injury must be intubated with careful attention to control and immobilization of the cervical spine because of the risk of worsening the neurologic spinal injury during the intubation procedure. Therefore, approaches to intubation are blind nasotracheal intubation while providing in-line immobilization and maintaining a neutral neck position; direct orotracheal intubation while maintaining cervical spine immobilization; fiber-optic bronchoscopic intubation (if equipment and skilled personnel are immediately available); and if intubation is unsuccessful, emergency cricothyroidotomy using large-bore needle (14 gauge) or scalpel and placement of 6 French endotracheal or tracheostomy tube. After emergency cricothyroidotomy, a conventional tracheostomy should be done in the operating room.

Resuscitation from hemorrhagic shock requires accurate assessment of the severity of hemorrhagic shock so as to judge the volume necessary for adequate fluid resuscitation. The ATLS course uses four classes of hemorrhagic shock as shown in Table 9.5. Several points deserve emphasis. When there is resting hypotension, there is at least a 1,500 mL blood volume deficit. Second, we strongly agree with the ATLS emphasis on signs of inadequate perfusion (e.g., delayed capillary refill, altered mental status, cool diaphoretic skin) to supplement vital sign assessment. Third, it is recommended that crystalloid (normal saline or Ringer's lactate) be used for initial resuscitation. The volume of crystalloid for resuscitation is three times the estimated blood volume deficit because only one-third of crystalloid is retained in the vascular space. Fourth, peripheral venous access (two large-bore IVs) is preferred over central venous catheterization. Central venous catheterization should be used only if peripheral intravenous cannulation is impossible. Finally, blood transfusion using type-specific blood should be used for severe class IV shock and if patients remain in shock and profoundly hypotensive after 3 to 4 L of crystalloid. If type-specific blood is not available, type O packed red blood cells should be infused.

Patients who have uncontrolled shock despite aggressive resuscitation and correction of pneumothorax should be considered for emergency room thoracotomy. Emer-

Table 9.5. Classification of hemorrhagic shock

Criterion	Class I	Class II	Class III	Class IV
Blood loss (mL)	Up to 750	750–1500	1500–2000	> 2000
Blood loss (% blood volume)	Up to 15	15–30	30–40	> 40
Pulse	< 100	> 100	> 120	> 140
Blood pressure	Normal	Normal	Decreased	Decreased
Pulse pressure	Normal or increased	Decreased	Decreased	Decreased
Capillary refill test	Normal	Positive	Positive	Positive
Respiratory rate	14–20	20–30	30–40	> 35
Urine output (mL/h)	> 30	20–30	5–15	Negligible
CNS-mental status	Slightly anxious	Mildly anxious	Anxious and confused	Confused or lethargic
Fluid replacement (3:1 rule)	Crystalloid	Crystalloid	Crystalloid + blood	Crystalloid + blood

Source: Adapted from Committee on Trauma, American College of Surgeons: Advanced Trauma Life Support Manual. Chicago, American College of Surgeons, 1998.

gency thoracotomy permits correction of cardiac tamponade, control of intrathoracic hemorrhage from major pulmonary vessels, and cross clamping of the aorta to optimize cerebral and coronary perfusion. In the profoundly hypotensive and fully arrested patient, internal cardiac massage can be done.

Head and Spine Injury and ARDS

Severe head injury is associated with increased risk of ARDS and complicates management of ARDS. Severe head injury causes direct (primary) brain injury by causing cerebral contusion, laceration, hemorrhage, and contre-coup contusion. Secondary insults to the brain of head-injured patients exacerbate the primary brain injury, and these include hypoxia, hypoperfusion, cerebral edema, increased intracranial pressure, seizures, and infection. These secondary insults are more severe, more difficult to manage, and more frequent if the head-injured patient develops ARDS.

ARDS can be associated with intracranial hypertension and the development of neurogenic pulmonary edema. Neurogenic pulmonary edema can occur after a variety of severe brain insults such as brain injury and status epilepticus. Neurogenic pulmonary edema develops very rapidly and presents as hypoxemia (or increased A-aDO$_2$), diffuse bilateral pulmonary infiltrates suggestive of pulmonary edema with normal heart size and no pleural effusion, decreased lung compliance, and need for ventilation. If hemodynamic monitoring is done, the pulmonary capillary wedge pressure is normal indicating noncardiogenic pulmonary edema. Thus, clinical presentation is consistent with the diagnosis of ARDS. Noncardiogenic pulmonary edema can be induced in animal models of brain injury and status epilepticus.

The pathophysiology of neurogenic pulmonary edema is sudden, massive sympathetic nervous system discharge at the time of brain injury that dramatically increases pulmonary hydrostatic pressures and causes massive pulmonary edema. Over a short period of time, hydrostatic pressures fall to normal and pulmonary edema persists. Clinically, hemodynamic assessment usually occurs after this primary sympathetic discharge (when pulmonary artery pressures are extremely high) when pulmonary artery and pulmonary capillary wedge pressures have returned to normal. Thus, the pathophysiologic studies suggest that the primary insult is hydrostatic (high-pressure) pulmonary edema that appears noncardiogenic clinically because of the delay to assess hemodynamic status in patients. In addition, the pulmonary endothelium may be injured, which could also account for the later development of noncardiogenic pulmonary edema.[25]

Neurogenic pulmonary edema is usually short lived and often clears in 24 to 48 hours. Management of neurogenic pulmonary edema includes usual airway and ventilatory support, use of diuretics to enhance clearance of pulmonary edema, and prevention of complications because of its short course.

Management of intracranial hypertension is important in severe head injury, but only features relevant to ARDS are discussed here. Increased intracranial pressure (ICP) is associated with poor outcome from head injury and many trauma centers measure and manage ICP to try to decrease morbidity and mortality of head injury. ICP is measured by ventriculostomy and intraventricular catheter or by subdural bolt. The cerebral perfusion pressure is the difference between mean arterial pressure and intracranial pressure. In general, management is aimed to keep cerebral perfusion pressure above 60 mmHg and to keep ICP less than 20 mmHg (normal is < 10 mmHg). Several of the maneuvers used to decrease ICP have effects on management of ARDS. Common interventions to decrease ICP are elevation of the head of the bed to 30 degrees, neutral head position, drainage of CSF from a ventriculostomy catheter, acute hyperventilation, intravenous mannitol, intravenous furosemide, and cooling to 37°C if febrile. Furthermore, intracranial hypertension will often necessitate urgent brain CT scanning to diagnose the cause of intracranial hypertension. Intravenous bolus mannitol (0.25 to 0.5 g/kg of 20% mannitol) transiently increases intravascular volume and osmolality and so can cause or worsen pulmonary edema. This transient effect is followed by an osmotic diuresis. Repeated doses of mannitol can cause hypovolemia, hypotension, and electrolyte imbalance (hyper- and hyponatremia). Osmotic diuresis secondary to mannitol must be followed closely, and replacement fluid (e.g., normal saline) must be given to maintain intravascular volume but to avoid pulmonary edema.

Furosemide also effectively decreases intracranial pressure. Furosemide causes diuresis, decreases CSF production, and decreases brain water content. Furosemide will also have effects on gas exchange in ARDS by decreasing pulmonary edema and by modifying pulmonary vasculature.[26]

Aspiration of gastric contents in the comatose head-injured patient is the other major cause of ARDS complicating head injury. This emphasizes the importance of early endotracheal intubation for prevention of aspiration because treatment of established aspiration is nonspecific support. There is no evidence that early or prophylactic use of antibiotics prevents aspiration pneumonia or decreases the risk or severity of acute lung injury caused by aspiration of gastric contents.

Cervical spine injury complicates airway management and critical care of the patient who develops ARDS after multiple trauma. Control of the cervical spine during intubation has already been emphasized. High cervical spine injury is associated with acute respiratory failure because of abdominal, intercostal, and diaphragm muscle weakness/paralysis. The patient who also has ARDS will develop respiratory distress earlier and more rapidly if there is also respiratory muscle weakness. If the injury is below C5, most patients can breathe spontaneously unless there is coincident lung injury. Injuries above C5 cause phrenic nerve involvement, diaphragm weakness, and increase the risk of acute and chronic respiratory failure. In patients who are initially managed without intubation, there may be deterioration over 3 to 5 days because of development of atelectasis, retained secretions, pneumonia, or pulmonary edema. Intubation and ventilation may then be necessary and may lead to prolonged ventilation with attendant complications such as nosocomial pneumonia.

Chest Trauma and ARDS

Blunt and penetrating chest injuries may be complicated by ARDS because of lung contusion, shock, need for multiple transfusions, and development of nosocomial pneumonia. When ARDS complicates blunt chest injury, the mortality of chest injury increases.

Seven chest injuries are immediately life threatening, may precede development of ARDS, and thus may influence management of ARDS, as follows:

1. Upper airway obstruction.
2. Tension pneumothorax.
3. Open pneumothorax.
4. Massive hemothorax.
5. Cardiac tamponade.
6. Traumatic air embolism.
7. Flail chest.

The recognition and treatment of upper airway obstruction was discussed earlier. Tension pneumothorax, open pneumothorax, and massive hemothorax are managed in the emergency department primarily by large-bore catheter and then chest tube insertion and drainage. Open pneumothorax occurs when a sucking chest wound permits air to enter the pleural space through the chest wall. The open chest wound must be covered with an occlusive dressing (to prevent air entry), taped on three sides and open on the fourth side to allow gas escape. Chest tube and definitive chest wall, and if indicated, lung repair are also necessary.

Massive hemothorax causes shock and acute hypoxemic respiratory failure from ipsilateral lung collapse, and occasionally can even cause shift of the mediastinum because of increased intrapleural pressure. Massive hemothorax is treated by immediate large bore (32F or 36F) chest tube insertion and monitoring of ongoing hemorrhage. In general, if the initial hemorrhage is greater than 2 L or ongoing blood loss exceeds 100 mL/hour, thoracotomy is required to identify and correct the bleeding lesion.

Cardiac tamponade is suggested by ongoing hypotension and jugular venous distension. Because tension pneumothorax can have the same presentation, is commoner, and more easily treated, tension penumothorax must be excluded or corrected to make the diagnosis of cardiac tamponade. Cardiac tamponade is treated by pericardiocentesis or by emergency thoracotomy drainage of the pericardial space and repair of heart injury.

Traumatic air embolism is a difficult diagnosis to make; it is suggested by sudden shock and a focal neurologic deficit in a patient with major chest injury. The diagnosis is confirmed at thoracotomy during which air is vented from cardiac chambers and the lung lesion is repaired.

Flail chest is diagnosed clinically by observing a segment of the chest wall that moves inward during spontaneous ventilation. The flail segment moves inward because there are fractures at two sites of multiple ribs producing a "floating" segment that moves inward when pleural pressure becomes more negative during inspiration. Conversely, a flail segment will not collapse inward when the patient is placed on positive pressure-controlled ventilation. Because of the high force necessary to break multiple ribs at multiple sites, there is often underlying lung contusion that may range from mild to severe.

The treatment of flail chest is primarily the treatment of acute hypoxemic respiratory failure: intubation and positive pressure ventilation to correct hypoxemia, to relieve excessive work of breathing, and to prevent progression to respiratory arrest. The duration of mechanical ventilation is determined by the resolution of lung contusion and lack of complications such as pneumonia, atelectasis, and ARDS. If lung contusion resolves, gas exchange will improve and weaning can occur while attending to the pain caused by the rib fractures.

Some patients who have flail chest may be treated without mechanical ventilation by oxygen by face mask and pain control including systemic narcotics, epidural morphine, or intercostal nerve block.

The seven immediately life-threatening chest injuries require immediate attention. Other important chest injuries that also require attention, some of which may precede the occurrence of ARDS, are lung contusion, aortic rupture, myocardial contusion, esophageal rupture, and diaphragmatic rupture.

Lung contusion is caused by blunt trauma to the lung parenchyma. Lung contusion progresses over the first 24 to 48 hours as hemorrhage and injury edema progress in the area of contusion. Lung contusion is therefore evaluated both on baseline chest radiograph and also on subsequent radiographs. Clinical presentation depends on the extent of lung contusion and severity and extent of other injuries. Severe lung contusion causes acute hypoxemic respiratory failure presenting as dyspnea, tachypnea, diaphoresis, tachycardia, hypertension, and impaired oxygenation. Chest examination may reveal flail chest, rib fractures, crackles, dullness, and rarely wheezes. There may be hemoptysis. The chest radiograph displays focal parenchymal airspace consolidation, and there are often adjacent rib fractures. Management of lung contusion focuses on provision of oxygen and then intubation and ventilation for the usual indications of acute hypoxemic respiratory failure.

Lung contusion is sometimes associated with progression to acute lung injury and full-blown ARDS. Restriction of fluids and careful hemodynamic and fluid management may decrease the risk of progression to ARDS. However, fluids must not be restricted to the extent that shock is not corrected.

Esophageal rupture is a less common injury after blunt or penetrating chest trauma. Esophageal rupture occurs in the setting of upper abdominal blunt trauma in the patient who closes the glottis during injury. The esophageal rupture allows pharyngeal and gastric contents to leak into the mediastinum, which causes mediastinitis and air in the mediastinum on chest radiograph. Esophageal rupture also can cause pneumothorax (especially left-sided), apical cap, and pleural effusion. Insertion of a chest tube for pneumothorax or pleural effusion may drain fluid that has food and particulate matter, raising the suspicion of esophageal rupture. Pleural fluid can be tested for pH (low) and amylase (very high) if suspicion is high and gross examination of fluid shows that it is not clear. The diagnosis of esophageal rupture is usually made by hypaque infusion into the upper esophagus and demonstration of leak into mediastinum or pleural space.

Esophageal rupture can present acutely with severe shock, need for significant volume replacement, and signs of systemic sepsis (systemic inflammatory response syndrome). Resuscitation should be prompt using crystalloid, oxygen, and chest tube insertion for pneumothorax or pleural effusion. Esophageal rupture may be repaired directly if the diagnosis is made acutely (within 12 to 24 hours). However, if the diagnosis is delayed, the morbidity and mortality increase because of complications such as sepsis and ARDS. If diagnosis is delayed, direct esophageal repair may not be possible and instead the patient is managed by esophageal diversion, gastrostomy, mediastinal and pleural drainage, antibiotics, and total parenteral nutrition.

Abdominal Trauma and ARDS

Abdominal trauma can cause ARDS because of severe hemorrhagic shock, the need for massive transfusion, traumatic pancreatitis, and peritonitis secondary to visceral perforation. In patients who have uncontrolled or incompletely controlled shock in the setting of blunt trauma, an abdominal source of hemorrhage must be considered. Exclude tension pneumothorax, massive hemothorax, and cardiac tamponade before concluding that the abdomen is the source of hemorrhage. In patients who are obtunded, emergency department peritoneal lavage is usually necessary to assess the abdomen as a source of hemorrhage. In addition, CT scanning of the abdomen is sometimes helpful for more specific assessment of intra-abdominal injury. However,

CT scanning can only be done if the patient is relatively stable. Peritoneal lavage and CT scanning of the abdomen may also be useful in assessing patients who will have prolonged surgery and in patients who have pelvic and other long bone fractures that could cause shock but an abdominal source of hemorrhage could coexist.

In patients who have abdominal trauma and who require laparotomy, postoperative management to prevent ARDS focuses on early and complete resuscitation from shock using appropriate volume resuscitation and transfusion, maintenance of ventilation and oxygenation with appropriate postoperative ventilation, and early detection and management of septic complications. There is no evidence that prophylactic PEEP prevents the development of ARDS. However, most patients who do not have ARDS who are ventilated benefit from low levels of PEEP (3 to 5 cm H_2O) to prevent atelectasis and to minimize FiO_2 requirements.

Fractures and ARDS

Major fractures and multiple fractures are associated with development of ARDS. Major blood loss, massive transfusion, and fat embolism are the mechanisms of ARDS after major fractures. Early and complete stabilization of fractures allows earlier mobilization of patients and is associated with decreased risk of respiratory complications. Pelvic fractures often cause massive hemorrhage, shock, need for massive transfusion, and thus may precede ARDS. Early external stabilization using external frames can be done in the emergency department and leads to earlier arrest of hemorrhage from pelvic fractures.

Major long bone fractures and pelvic fracture may be complicated by fat embolism syndrome (FES). The clinical presentation of FES is confusion, agitation (neurologic changes), a petechial rash (upper chest, axilla, shoulders commonly), dyspnea, hypoxemia, and diffuse bilateral pulmonary infiltrates developing 2 to 3 days after injury. Other common clinical features are fever, tachycardia, thrombocytopenia, and fat (lipid) in the urine. Fat embolism syndrome may be prevented by early stabilization of fractures and by prophylactic use of corticosteroids.[27]

Burns and ARDS

Extensive burns and smoke inhalation injury are both associated with ARDS. Smoke inhalation injury is a complex lesion that includes carbon monoxide poisoning, upper airway obstruction, and pulmonary parenchymal injury from smoke. Smoke inhalation injury should be suspected in burn victims who have soot in the nose or oropharynx, upper airway edema, carbonaceous sputum, dyspnea, or hypoxemia. Fiber-optic laryngoscopy may be used to assess the upper airway and to facilitate endotracheal intubation. Upper airway burn injury can lead to upper airway obstruction, which calls for early prophylactic intubation in high-risk patients. Patients who have face and neck burns, patients who have extensive burns, and patients who require large-volume fluid resuscitation are at especially high risk and usually require early intubation.

Smoke inhalation can cause lung injury. Progressive hypoxemia, bilateral pulmonary infiltrates, and need for increased ventilation over 24 to 48 hours after burn indicate pulmonary injury. Smoke inhalation, unlike other causes of ARDS, also often causes extensive bronchial secretions, production of thick sputum, wheezing, and decreased dynamic lung compliance. Small airway obstruction is caused by smooth muscle spasm, airway wall edema, and luminal secretions. Thus bronchodilators may be only partially effective in reversing airways obstruction.

Respiratory management of smoke inhalation focuses first on control of the airway; second, correction of hypoxemia from all causes, including carbon monoxide poisoning; and third, control of ventilation. Often fluid management is complicated because of the large fluid resuscitation necessary for the surface burns and because of the need to avoid fluid overload and pulmonary edema. However, correction of shock and maintenance of intravascular volume takes precedence. Mechanical ventilation with PEEP is often necessary for support during the early (24 to 36 hour) resuscitation phase.

Another unique respiratory system complication of burns is circumferential chest burns that can cause progressive constriction as edema accumulates in the burn area. Decreased chest wall compliance leads to increased work of breathing and impaired cough. The primary treatment of circumferential chest burns is bilateral escharotomy of the chest wall burns and mechanical ventilation if necessary.

Sepsis Syndrome and ARDS

Sepsis syndrome and ARDS are closely related for many reasons. First, sepsis syndrome is the commonest precipitating cause of ARDS and septic ARDS has a higher mortality than does ARDS of other etiologies. Second, the clinical features of sepsis syndrome and ARDS overlap, making differentiation sometimes difficult. Third, sepsis syndrome, especially secondary to ventilator-associated nosocomial pneumonia, is a frequent complication of ARDS. Next, ARDS is considered by some as simply the lung's expression of organ dysfunction and organ failure when sepsis causes multiple system organ failure. Furthermore, the pathophysiology of sepsis syndrome and of ARDS is similar. Finally, many of the experimental therapies investigated for sepsis syndrome and ARDS are anti-inflammatory and if successful could have favorable effects on either ARDS or sepsis or both.

Sepsis syndrome is defined as fever (or hypothermia), tachycardia, tachypnea (or need for mechanical ventilation), and at least one new organ system dysfunction that could be secondary to sepsis. Also, there must be a proven or suspected source of infection. The mortality of sepsis syndrome in critically ill patients in the ICU is 30% to 35%, and increasing organ failure is associated with increasing mortality.

Sepsis syndrome is caused by the host's reaction to severe infection and is likely caused by release of pyrogenic, inflammatory mediators. Indeed, only about one-quarter to one-third of patients who have sepsis syndrome have positive blood cultures. In 1992 the term *systemic inflammatory response syndrome (SIRS)* was proposed to emphasize that sepsis syndrome can be caused by noninfectious conditions such as multiple trauma and pancreatitis.[28] The American College of Chest Physicians/Society of Critical Care Medicine defined SIRS, sepsis, severe sepsis, septic shock, and multiple organ dysfunction syndrome (MODS) as shown in Table 9.6 (ACCP/SCCM).

Sepsis syndrome is a common problem in hospitalized patients. About 1% to 2% of hospitalized patients have sepsis syndrome amounting to 400,000 to 500,000 cases per year in the United States. The incidence of sepsis syndrome in hospitalized patients is increasing because of more aggressive chemotherapy, major surgery, organ transplantation, vascular cannulation, increasing age, and increasing prevalence of chronic diseases (e.g., diabetes mellitus). Sepsis syndrome is particularly associated with cancer, chemotherapy, neutropenia, lymphoproliferative disease, multiple trauma, burns, major abdominal surgery, chronic indwelling vascular catheters, and organ failure such as cirrhosis, chronic obstructive pulmonary disease, and renal failure.

The pathophysiology of sepsis syndrome is extremely complex; detailed discussion is beyond the scope of this text. As an overview, many of the inflammatory cascades activated by sepsis syndrome cause acute lung injury and acute respiratory distress syndrome as discussed in Chapter 4. Briefly, gram-positive and gram-negative bacteria trigger a host inflammatory response because of cell wall molecules (techoic acid of gram-positive bacteria) and lipopolysaccharide (LPS) (gram-negative bacteria). The inflammatory response is a complex series of cellular and humoral cascades that have interacting positive and negative feedback loops. The major mediators of sepsis syndrome are neutrophils, platelets, cytokines, coagulation factors, prostaglandins, kinins, and nitric oxide. A common target of these mediators is the endothelium. Endothelial injury increases vascular permeability, which is expressed in the lung as noncardiogenic pulmonary edema. Noncardiogenic pulmonary edema can progress to acute lung injury and ARDS. Vascular injury also leads to thrombosis, microvascular occlusion (by platelets, fibrin, and neutrophils), and tissue ischemia/hypoxia.

Cytokines such as tumor necrosis factor-alpha (TNF) and interleukin-1 (IL-1) are pro-inflammatory. These pro-inflammatory cytokines amplify injury by direct stimulation of other cytokines (e.g., TNF stimulates synthesis and release of IL-1 and IL-6), by stimulation of neutrophils and endothelial cells (up regulation of adhesion molecules), by increased synthesis and release of other humoral mediators (e.g., kinins, prostaglandins, and thromboxanes), by activation of coagulation (and induction of disseminated intravascular coagulation), and by inducing synthesis of nitric oxide (by inducing inducible nitric oxide synthase). Infusion of TNF into humans mimics many features of sepsis syndrome such as fever, tachycardia, tachypnea, myalgia, increased cardiac output, and decreased vascular resistance.

Both extrinsic and intrinsic coagulation pathways are activated in sepsis syndrome, which causes fibrin deposition and microvascular thrombosis, fibrin depletion, generation of fibrin/fibrinogen degradation products, and thrombocytopenia. Sepsis also causes depletion of protein C and protein S, which further accentuates the DIC process.

Vascular endothelial injury is likely widespread in severe sepsis and may be a fun-

Table 9.6. Definitions of sepsis-related syndromes

Syndrome	Definition
Systemic inflammatory response syndrome (SIRS)[a]	Minimum 2 of the following: 1. Temp. $> 38°$ C or $< 36°$ C 2. Resp. rate > 20/min or $PaCO_2 < 32$ torr 3. Heart rate > 90/min 4. Leukocyte count $> 12,000/\mu L$ or $< 4,000/\mu L$ or $> 10\%$ bands
Sepsis	SIRS that has suspected or proven infection
Severe sepsis[b]	Sepsis (as above) plus > 1 organ dysfunction, e.g., ARDS Oliguria Decreased Glasgow Coma score Metabolic acidosis Hypotension/hypoperfusion
Hypotension	Systolic arterial pressure < 90 mmHg or > 40 mmHg drop from usual systolic arterial pressure (without another cause for hypotension)
Septic shock	Sepsis plus hypotension unresponsive to fluid management plus organ dysfunction as per severe sepsis
Multiple-organ dysfunction syndrome	Dysfunction of more than one organ that requires organ support
Refractory septic shock	Septic shock >1 hour and unresponsive to fluid and vasopressor support

[a]American College of Chest Physicians/Society of Critical Care Medicine Consensus Conference Committee. Definition for sepsis and organ failure and guidelines for the use of innovative therapies in sepsis. Crit Care Med 1992; 20:864.
[b]Severe sepsis corresponds to sepsis syndrome.

damental cause of multiple organ dysfunction syndrome. Vascular injury is amplified when neutrophil and endothelial cell adhesion molecules are expressed causing neutrophil retention and binding to endothelium. Neutrophils bind to endothelium and traverse the endothelium to sites of infection to contain the septic process. However, neutrophils bound to endothelium also release toxic oxygen species and enzymes (e.g., elastase), that directly injure the vascular endothelium.

The hypotension of septic shock is probably caused by inappropriate vasodilation because of exuberant expression of vasodilators such as nitric oxide, bradykinin, histamine, prostacyclin (PGI_2), and platelet-activating factor. Hypotension is exacerbated by hypovolemia caused by loss of plasma into interstitium because of increased vascular permeability ("third-spacing") and by low endogenous blood vasopressin levels.

The host responds to these pro-inflammatory stimuli with a range of anti-inflammatory responses. For example, interleukin-1 receptor antagonist (IL-1ra) synthesis and release increases in sepsis and prevents binding of IL-1 to its active receptors. Soluble TNF receptors similarly bind circulating TNF and prevent binding of TNF to tissue-based TNF receptors. Corticosteroids inhibit synthesis of important cytokines such as TNF. Certain cytokines such as IL-10 are anti-inflammatory and prevent organ injury and death in experimental models of sepsis.

Sepsis syndrome is defined clinically so that sepsis syndrome can be diagnosed quickly at the bedside supplemented by routine stat laboratory tests of organ function. The criteria for diagnosis of sepsis syndrome may be supplemented by finding hyperlactatemia, lactic acidosis, thrombocytopenia, and coagulopathy consistent with DIC. Specific dermatologic findings, such as petechiae, purpura (purpura fulminans), splinter hemorrhages, erythema with sole and palm involvement (suggesting toxic shock syndrome), ecthyma gangrenosum (suggesting *Pseudomonas aeruginosa* infection), and pustules (*Staphylococcus aureus* bacteremia) may indicate sepsis and may suggest a specific etiology.

Lung dysfunction is extremely common in critically ill septic patients. Nearly all critically ill septic patients have increased alveolar-arterial oxygen difference (A-aDO$_2$)/decreased PaO$_2$/FiO$_2$ because of ventilation/perfusion mismatch. Increasing lung involvement in sepsis progresses in severity from mildly impaired oxygenation to increasingly severe hypoxemia that is refactory to supplemental oxygen (due to intrapulmonary shunting), decreased lung static compliance, patchy infiltrates progressing to diffuse bilateral pulmonary infiltrates, and increased minute ventilation because of hyperventilation and because of increased physiologic dead space (Vd/Vt).

Early management of sepsis syndrome focuses on cardiopulmonary support, investigations to identify the source of infection, broad spectrum antibiotics pending the results of cultures, drainage of abscesses, and operation to correct surgical problems (e.g., peritonitis). Broad spectrum (gram-positive and gram-negative bacteria) antibiotic coverage is necessary to manage patients who have severe sepsis because the clinical features of gram-positive and gram-negative sepsis are indistinguishable, sepsis can kill rapidly, and early antibiotic treatment is associated with increased survival. Antibiotics must be given intravenously in high doses that produce high blood levels rapidly. The antibiotic regimen selected must consider associated organ dysfunction (especially renal failure), age (neonatal vs. elderly), size of the patient, and immune status (neutropenia, lymphoproliferative disorder, AIDS, previous splenectomy) as well as likely etiology of sepsis. Suggested antibiotic regimens are shown in Table 9.7.

There have been many phase I, phase II, and large multicenter, pivotal phase III randomized controlled trials of new therapies for sepsis that focused on an anti-inflammatory strategy. The common hypothesis underlying these trials was that inhibition of one or more arms of the inflammatory cascade could decrease/prevent organ dysfunction and death. To date, most of the phase III trials have not shown statistically significant benefit to decrease mortality of sepsis syndrome and septic shock. The strategies that have not yet proven effective are corticosteroids, anti-endotoxins, anti-cytokines (anti-TNF, TNF soluble receptor, interleukin-1 receptor antagonist), prostaglandin synthesis inhibition (ibuprofen), and bradykinin antagonists. Clinical trials continue in an attempt to discover an adjunctive therapy that will decrease morbidity (organ dysfunction) and mortality of sepsis syndrome. In the trials of new agents reported so far, none has been found to be effective in preventing or reversing acute respiratory failure/

Table 9.7. Suggested antibiotic regimens for management of severe sepsis and septic shock

Clinical scenario	Antibiotic regimen
Immune competent host. No clear cause	1. Ampicillin (2 g IV Q6h) + tobramycin (1.5 mg/kg IV Q8h or 3–5 mg/kg IV OD)[a] + metronidazole (500 mg IV Q6h) 2. Imipenem (1 g IV Q6h) 3. Ceftriaxone (2 g IV Q12h) 4. Ciprofloxacin (400 mg IV Q12h) + metronidazole (500 mg IV Q8h) + gentamicin (1.5 mg/kg IV Q8h)
Immune-compromised. No clear cause	1. Piperacillin (3 g IV Q4h) (or ticarcillin, ceftazidime) + tobramycin (1.5 mg/kg IV Q8h) 2. Imipenem (1 g IV Q6h) 3. Ceftazidime (2 g IV Q8h) + vancomycin (500 mg IV Q6h) *If beta-lactam allergic:* 4. Ciprofloxacin (400 mg IV Q12h) + tobramycin (1.5 mg/kg IV Q8h) 5. Imipenem (1 g IV Q6h) + gentamicin (1.5 mg/kg IV Q8h)
Intravenous drug user	1. Vancomycin (500 mg IV Q6h) + tobramycin (1.5 mg/kg IV Q8h) 2. Cloxacillin (2 g IV Q4h) (or nafcillin) + tobramycin[b]
Lung – community-acquired	1. Cefotaxime (2 g IV Q6h) (or ceftriaxone 2 g IV Q24h or cefuroxime 1.5 g IV Q8h) + erythromycin (1 g IV Q6h)
Lung–nosocomial	1. Ceftazidime (2 g IV Q6h) + gentamicin (1.5 mg/kg IV Q8h) 2. Cefotaxime (2 g IV Q6h) + tobramycin (1.5 mg/kg IV Q8h) 3. Ciprofloxacin (400 mg IV Q12h) + cefotaxime (2 g IV Q6h)
Abdomen	1. Ampicillin (2 g IV Q6h) + metronidazole (500 mg IV Q8h) + gentamicin (1.5 mg/kg IV Q8h) 2. Ceftriaxone (2 g IV Q24h) + clindamycin (600 mg IV Q8h) 3. Imipenem (1 g IV Q6h) + gentamicin (1.5 mg/kg IV Q8h)[c]
Brain (meningitis)	1. Cefotaxime (2 g IV Q6h) (or ceftriaxone 2 g IV Q12h) + ampicillin (2 g IV Q4h) 2. Chloramphenicol (1 g IV Q6h) + cotrimoxazole (5 mg/kg TMP + 25 mg/kg SMX IV Q6h).
Brain (abscess)	1. Metronidazole (750 mg IV Q8h) + ceftriaxone (2 g IV Q12h) 2. Chloramphenicol (1 g IV Q6h)

[a]Aminoglycosides should be initiated using a loading dose of 3 mg/kg followed by 1.5 mg/kg Q8h if renal function is normal. Once daily aminoglycoside dosing (3 mg/kg) can be an alternative, although there is less evidence of efficacy in critically ill versus in non-critically ill patients.
[b]Many cities have methicillin-resistant *Staphylococcus aureus* and thus cloxacillin or nafcillin are not appropriate initial therapy until sensitivity is known.
[c]Imipenem alone may not be sufficient in critically ill patients with abdominal sepsis. Imipenem alone may be adequate for abdominal sepsis if the condition is not critical.

ARDS associated with sepsis syndrome. Therefore, at present we do not recommend these adjunctive therapies to try to prevent ARDS or to decrease mortality of sepsis syndrome because to date none have been shown to be clearly effective.

In addition to causing ARDS, sepsis syndrome can occur as a complication of ARDS. When a patient who has ARDS develops sepsis syndrome, a broad differential diagnostic approach must be taken because the source of sepsis may be occult, difficult to prove, and therefore difficult to resolve. The commonest cause of sepsis syndrome complicating ARDS is ventilator-associated nosocomial pneumonia (see Chapter 11). The other common causes of nosocomial sepsis in the ICU are line sepsis, wound infection, and urinary tract infection. However, consider other etiologies such as central nervous system infection (brain abscess, meningitis secondary to bacteremia, open head injury), sinusitis (increased risk because of nasogastric/nasotracheal tubes and ineffective/infrequent swallowing), purulent parotitis, endovascular infection (primary bacteremia, endocarditis), abdominal infection (peritonitis, abdominal abscess, bowel infarction, pancreatic abscess, biliary tract obstruction/sepsis), and genitourinary infection (cystitis, less commonly pyelonephritis, renal abscess, perinephric abscess). In surgical patients, wound infections must be considered as well as specific septic complications of surgery (e.g., mediastinitis after open heart surgery).

Common Complications of ARDS and Its Therapy

ARDS can be associated with many pulmonary and extrapulmonary complications.[29,30] Knowledge of the more common complications will enable prevention, early recognition, and treatment of these conditions (Table 9.8).

Respiratory Complications

Barotrauma and nosocomial pneumonia are the two most common respiratory complications of ARDS. The incidence of pneumothorax with respiratory failure is 1% to 4% but may be over 30% in patients with ARDS.[31,32] Patients with ARDS are at significantly higher risk for barotrauma than many other ventilated patients for two reasons. First, the inflamed lungs of ARDS are more likely to be disrupted by positive airway pressure. Second, patients who have severe ARDS often require higher than usual airway pressures such as higher PEEP, higher peak airway pressure, and higher mean airway pressure. It is not clear whether different forms of airway pressure (e.g., PEEP vs. mean airway pressure) have different risks of barotrauma. Barotrauma is caused by alveolar rupture and subsequent dissection of air along peribronchovascular sheaths.

Pneumothorax can significantly alter the clinical course of patients who have ARDS. Tension pneumothorax usually presents as catastrophic respiratory and hemodynamic compromise.[30] Tension pneumothorax should be considered whenever there is sudden, unexpected respiratory or cardiovascular deterioration in ventilated patients who have ARDS. Cardiovascular presentations of tension pneumothorax include diaphoresis, hypotension, tachycardia, arrhythmias, and pulmonary hyper-

Table 9.8 Prevention and treatment of multiple system organ failure in ARDS

Organ system	Preventive management	Treatment
Respiratory	Treat shock/infection.	Treat shock.
	Minimize toxic FiO_2 (< 60%).	Minimize toxic FiO_2 (< 60%).
	Treat infection.	Treat infection.
	Minimize airway pressure.	
	Institute permissive hypercapnia	Institute permissive hypercapnia
Cardiovascular	Treat shock.	Treat shock.
		Give vasopressor support
Renal	Treat shock/infection.	Treat shock/infection.
	Avoid nephrotoxic drugs.	Avoid nephrotoxic drugs.
	Low-dose dopamine[a]	
	Not mannitol	
	Not furosemide	
Hepatic	Treat shock/infection.	
	Avoid hepatotoxic drugs.	
Coagulation	Treat shock/infection.	Blood replacement therapy.
	Vitamin K	
Gut	Treat shock/infection.	Treat shock/infection.
	Enteral nutrition[a]	Total parenteral nutrition
	Glutamine[a]	
Brain	Treat shock/infection.	Treat shock/infection.

[a]Controversial with studies showing benefit and other studies showing no effect.

tension. Respiratory presentations of tension pneumothorax include decreased oxygenation, increased airway pressure in volume-controlled ventilation, decreased tidal volume in pressure-controlled ventilation, decreased air entry, tracheal shift, and increased resonance on percussion. In a near arrest or full arrest situation, the clinical findings should lead to a presumed diagnosis of tension pneumothorax and therapy should be initiated without obtaining a stat chest radiograph. Therapy should include inspection and attempts to clear any blocked in situ chest tube(s), followed by placement of a 16 gauge intravenous catheter in the second intercostal space, midclavicular line on the affected side. Definitive treatment of tension pneumothorax is placement of a chest tube on the affected side.

Simple pneumothorax may present as an increase in airway pressure during volume-controlled ventilation or decreased tidal volume during pressure-controlled ventilation. Simple pneumothorax is often not suspected clinically but rather is diagnosed by chest radiography. Definitive treatment is placement of a chest tube on the affected side.

Nosocomial pneumonia is discussed in detail in Chapter 11. Clinical studies of mechanically ventilated patients report a risk of nosocomial pneumonia of 1% to 3% per day and crude incidence rates of 7% to 54%.[33] Autopsy examination of lungs from patients with ARDS may reveal pneumonia in up to 75% of cases.[34] The presence of diffuse pulmonary infiltrates with ARDS makes the diagnosis of pneumonia difficult.[35] Clinical features of infection include new fever and left shift in WBC combined with the clinical findings of consolidation, a new and persistent infiltrate on chest radiograph, and purulent sputum with positive culture. These findings are sensitive but not specific for the diagnosis of nosocomial pneumonia in ARDS.[33-36]

Pneumonia is the most common infectious complication of ARDS and can increase mortality.[34,35] The commonest organisms that cause nosocomial pneumonia are enteric gram-negative bacilli such as *Pseudomonas, Acinetobacter, Serratia, E. coli,* and *Klebsiella* as well as S. *aureus*.[33] Standard initial therapy for nosocomial pneumonia includes empiric coverage for the organisms just listed. Subsequently, antibiotics are selected that are active against any organisms identified on culture.

Cardiovascular Complications

Cardiovascular complications of ARDS may be secondary to the underlying disease that leads to ARDS (e.g., sepsis), secondary to ARDS itself, or secondary to therapeutic interventions such as positive pressure ventilation, PEEP, intravenous hemodynamic monitoring, and medications. Hypotension, hypertension, and arrythmias occur frequently in ARDS.[29]

A pathophysiologic approach to hypotension as a complication of ARDS leads to accurate diagnosis and more effective treatment. Because blood pressure is the product of cardiac output and vascular resistance, hypotension may be secondary to a decrease in either cardiac output or vascular resistance or both. Cardiac output is most often diminished in ARDS because of decreased intravascular volume. Decreased intravascular volume may be due to loss of volume (e.g., hemorrhage, diarrhea), decrease in venous return (e.g., positive airway pressure, PEEP), or third space loss of fluids (e.g., sepsis, trauma, pancreatitis). Cardiac output may also be decreased because of systolic or diastolic ventricular dysfunction. Systolic dysfunction may be caused by myocardial infarction or myocardial depression associated with sepsis.[37] Right ventricular diastolic dysfunction decreases ventricular filling. Left ventricular diastolic dysfunction also impairs left ventricular filling and may be caused by leftward shift of the intraventricular septum, sepsis, myocardial edema, or myocardial ischemia or infarction. Finally, obstruction to blood flow (e.g., pulmonary embolism) may decrease cardiac output and cause shock.

Hypotension may also be due to decreased vascular resistance, which is most often caused by sepsis, vasoactive medications, anaphylaxis, and adrenal insufficiency.[29,30] Management of hypotension and shock is discussed in Chapter 6.

Hypertension is less common than hypotension in ARDS. The differential diagnosis of hypertension in patients who have ARDS includes increased sympathetic and adrenal tone secondary to airway problems, hypoxemia, hypercapnia, pain, and inadequate pain relief/sedation. Hypertension may also be due to volume expansion in the patient with preexisting hypertension who is aggressively resuscitated and in the patient who has renal insufficiency.

Arrhythmias in ARDS are caused by hypoxemia, acid-base abnormalities, fluid volume shifts, electrolyte disturbances, and underlying cardiac disease. There is a direct correlation between degree of hypoxemia and incidence of PVCs.[38] Arrhythmias may also be caused by drugs such as inotropes, vasopressors, histamine (H_2) blockers, and gastrointestinal motility agents, and by central venous and pulmonary artery catheters.[30,39,40]

In assessing a patient with arrythmias and ARDS, an ABC approach must be taken to ensure adequate oxygen saturation and tissue perfusion. Any patient with a hemodynamically significant arrhythmia who has a decrease in oxygenation indicated by pulse oximetry should be taken off the ventilator and manually bagged with 100% oxygen during this unstable period. In the hemodynamically stable patient a focused cardiorespiratory examination along with an ECG and laboratory workup should be performed to identify and treat reversible causes.

Gastrointestinal Complications

The common gastrointestinal complications of ARDS are gastric stasis, bowel ileus, failure to tolerate enteral feeding, upper gastrointestinal hemorrhage, acute pancreatitis, gut ischemia, and pneumoperitoneum.

Gastric stasis and ileus are common in critically ill patients who have ARDS and may be caused by shock, hypoxemia, drugs that inhibit gastrointestinal motility (e.g., narcotics, antipsychotics, and other drugs with anticholinergic side effects), electrolyte disturbances (e.g., hypokalemia), and recent abdominal surgery or trauma. Gastric stasis and ileus often present as failure to absorb enteral feeding. Management of gastric stasis and ileus includes search for an underlying cause, withdrawal of drugs that interfere with gastrointestinal motility, and use of prokinetic agents (e.g., metoclopramide).

Upper gastrointestinal hemorrhage is often secondary to the stress of critical illness. Patients ventilated for greater than 48 hours and patients who have coagulopathy are at increased risk for upper gastrointestinal hemorrhage.[30] Approximately 10% to 30% of critically ill, ventilated patients develop upper gastrointestinal hemorrhage.[29] Patients with ARDS may be at even higher risk with incidence of upper gastrointestinal hemorrhage of up to 85%.[41] The causes of upper gastrointestinal hemorrhage include esophagitis, gastritis, peptic ulcer, and stress-induced gastric ulceration.[29]

The prevention and management of gastric stress ulcer prophylaxis is controversial. In a recent meta-analysis of gastrointestinal hemorrhage in the intensive care unit,[42] significant decrease in overt, clinically relevant bleeding was found with H_2 receptor antagonists compared to placebo. When compared to antacids, there was a weak trend in favor of H_2 antagonists for prevention of clinically relevant bleeding. H_2 receptor antagonists, however, were associated with a greater incidence of nosocomial pneumonia when compared to placebo. Enteral feeding is at least as effective as drug prophylaxis in the prevention of stress ulceration.[43] A randomized controlled trial of ranitidine versus sucralfate found no difference in the rate of upper gastrointestinal hemorrhage or nosocomial pneumonia.[42]

The clinical practice guideline for stress ulcer prophylaxis used in our ICU increases appropriateness and decreases costs of care.[44] The guideline is shown in Figure 9.3.

Acute pancreatitis may precede ARDS and can complicate conditions associated with ARDS such as abdominal trauma, abdominal aortic aneurysm rupture, cardio-pulmonary bypass, cardiac transplant, major surgery, and alcoholism. The common-est causes of acute pancreatitis are alcoholism and gallstone disease. In the critically ill, many patients have had shock as a preexisting insult that precedes development of acute pancreatitis.[45,46] Serum enzymes (amylase, lipase), abdominal ultrasound, and computed tomography are used to diagnose pancreatitis, to evaluate progress, and to evaluate complications such as pancreatic necrosis, pancreatic pseudocyst, pancreatic abscess, and peripancreatic necrosis and hemorrhage. Respiratory compli-cations are common in severe pancreatitis and include atelectasis, pleural effusion, noncardiogenic pulmonary edema, and full-blown ARDS. Patients who have severe pancreatitis complicated by acute respiratory failure usually require prolonged venti-lation until there is resolution of the pancreatitis and its severe abdominal complica-tions. Furthermore, ARDS will usually not improve unless these underlying condi-tions improve.

The management of severe, acute pancreatitis is controversial. Mainstays of man-agement are correction of underlying cause (e.g., shock), general resuscitation (ABCs), nothing by mouth (NPO), NG tube drainage of gastric secretions, total par-enteral nutrition, and treatment of complications. Controversial management issues include management of pancreatic necrosis, pancreatic debridement procedures, antibiotics, percutaneous drainage of fluid collections for suspected abscess, and par-tial pancreatectomy. Patients who develop pancreatic abscess or pancreatic pseudocyst will often require drainage and, if unsuccessful, surgical debridement and drainage.[45]

Gut ischemia is a potential complication of ARDS because many patients who have ARDS also have risk factors for gut ischemia. Atherosclerotic heart disease, recent myocardial infarction, hypotension, shock, arrhythmias, and age over 50 years are the common risk factors for gut ischemia. Acute abdominal pain, ileus, abdomi-nal distension, emesis (or increased NG tube returns), and low-grade fever in a patient who has risk factors should trigger the clinician to consider gut ischemia. The diagnosis is difficult because laboratory findings, such as leukocytosis, hyperamy-lasemia, and lactic acidosis, are quite nonspecific in the critically ill. Plain abdominal radiographs may reveal ileus, ascites, separation of small bowel loops (by bowel wall edema), small bowel dilatation, and thickening of valvulae conniventes (thumb printing). More definitive investigations include arteriography and contrast-enhanced computerized tomography. Early diagnosis and treatment are associated with better survival than delayed diagnosis so patients should be evaluated rapidly and early surgical consultation is recommended.[47] Therapy for gut ischemia includes correction of shock in low cardiac output states, minimization of vasoconstrictors, intra-arterial papaverine, and often urgent laparotomy for embolectomy, gut resec-tion, and grafting. Newer approaches include thrombolysis[48] and angioplasty.[49]

Pneumoperitoneum can be a complication of barotrauma or may indicate rupture

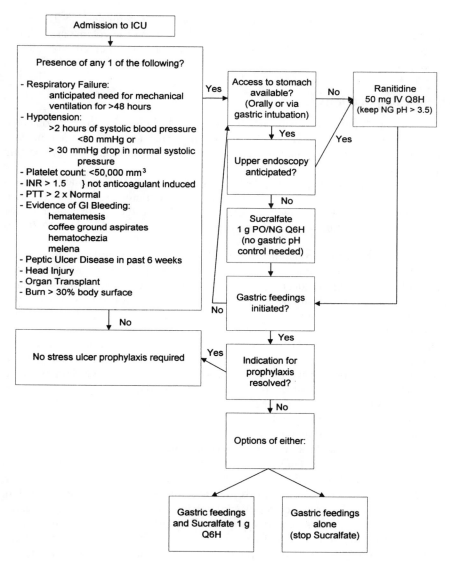

Figure 9.3. Clinical practice guideline for stress ulcer prophylaxis.

of a hollow viscus. Dissection of air from pulmonary barotrauma along fascial planes results in pneumoperitoneum. The presence of extra alveolar air on chest radiograph can be helpful in differentiating potential etiologies. A review of 28 cases of pneumoperitoneum found in all but one case the presence of extra alveolar air, suggesting pulmonary barotrauma was the most likely cause of pneumoperitoneum.[50] Treatment of pneumoperitoneum secondary to barotrauma depends on the volume and clinical effects of the air.[51] Most often pneumoperitoneum is merely observed and resolves spontaneously.

Renal Complications

Renal failure complicates up to 40% of cases of ARDS and is an ominous sign because of the associated high mortality.[52] Underlying risk factors for acute renal failure include increased age, diabetes, preexisting renal dysfunction, and preexisting hypertension.

Acute renal failure complicating ARDS may be secondary to the underlying cause of ARDS (e.g., sepsis, hemorrhagic shock from multiple trauma, severe pancreatitis), secondary to shock associated with ARDS, or secondary to therapy (e.g., vasopressor drugs, nephrotoxic drugs, PEEP). Acute renal failure in patients who have ARDS is often multifactorial.

Patients with respiratory failure who require mechanical ventilation have alterations in renal hemodynamics and tubular function that increase the risk of acute renal failure.[53,54] Oliguria, decreased sodium excretion, and increased antidiuretic hormone (ADH) complicate mechanical ventilation with PEEP. Persistently positive fluid balance in patients with ARDS may worsen already compromised gas exchange and is associated with a worse prognosis.[55,56]

The major contributing factors responsible for acute renal failure in ARDS are shock (hypovolemic, septic, cardiogenic) and nephrotoxins.[53] Hypovolemic shock is most often caused by positive pressure ventilation, PEEP, aggressive diuresis, blood loss, and volume redistribution (e.g., sepsis, peritonitis, burns, pancreatitis). In patients who have sepsis syndrome, acute renal failure almost always follows an episode of overt septic shock and much less often occurs as a complication of sepsis syndrome (SIRS) without septic shock.

The commonest nephrotoxins that patients who have ARDS receive are radiographic dye for CT scanning, nephrotoxic antibiotics, pigments (hemoglobin, myoglobin), nonsteroidal anti-inflammatory agents, and vasopressors. Many drugs used in the ICU can cause interstitial nephritis such as semisynthetic penicillins (ampicillin, methicillin), cephalosporins, ciprofloxacin, cotrimoxazole, sulfonamides, thiazides, furosemide, diphenylhydantoin, and warfarin. The risk of acute renal failure after injection of radiographic dye is increased in patients who are diabetic, volume depleted, or who have preexisting renal dysfunction. Fortunately, acute renal failure secondary to aminoglycosides is much less common because the use of aminoglycosides has decreased dramatically. Other less toxic drugs (e.g., third-generation cephalosporins, carbapenems, quinolones) that are highly bacteriocidal for aerobic gram-negative bacilli have replaced aminoglycosides in most critically ill adults. Alpha adrenergic vasopressors that decrease renal blood flow such as epinephrine, norepinephrine, and high-dose dopamine (> 10 μg/kg/minute) may worsen renal function and may induce acute renal failure.

Table 9.9. Continuous renal replacement therapy in the critically ill

	CHARACTERISTICS			
Type of Therapy	Blood flow (mL/min)	Fluid removal (ultrafiltration)	Ultrafiltrate rate (L/d)	Solute removal
CAVH[1]	50–100[a]	Yes	0–17	Little
CAVHD[2]	50–100[a]	Yes		Yes
CAVHDF[3]	50–100[a]	Yes		Yes
CVVH[4]	50–200	Yes	12–48	Little
CVVHD[5]	50–200	Yes		Yes
CVVHDF[6]	50–200	Yes		Yes

[a]Blood flow depends on patient's arteriovenous pressure gradient.
[1]CAVH: Continuous arteriovenous hemofiltration.
[2]CAVHD: Continuous arteriovenous hemodialysis.
[3]CAVHDF: Continuous arteriovenous hemodiafiltration.
[4]CVVDH: Continuous venovenous hemofiltration.
[5]CVVHD: Continuous venovenous hemodialysis.
[6]CVVDHF: Continuous venovenous hemodiafiltration.

Other causes of acute renal failure are less common causes in ARDS but should be considered in the differential diagnosis. Glomerulonephritis, vasculitis, micro-angiopathy, Goodpasture's syndrome, renal obstruction (embolism, dissection), renal vein thrombosis, papillary necrosis, tubular obstruction by crystals, and renal tract obstruction should be considered.

Renal support of patients who have acute renal failure is discussed in detail in critical care texts. The commonest indications for dialysis in the patient who has ARDS and acute renal failure are volume overload, hyperkalemia, and progressive uremia. The major forms of renal support for the critically ill are peritoneal dialysis, intermittent hemodialysis, and continuous renal replacement. The choice of therapy depends on hemodynamic stability of the patient and availability of appropriate physician and technical expertise. Although intermittent hemodialysis is the gold standard, an increasing proportion of critically ill patients who have acute renal failure are treated by continuous renal replacement therapy.

Intermittent hemodialysis provides very efficient fluid removal (ultrafiltration) and solute removal (clearance) but necessitates vascular access and has important complications such as hypotension, arrhythmias, and bleeding. In the hemodynamically unstable patient, intermittent hemodialysis is often impossible, and continuous renal replacement therapy is necessary.

Continuous renal replacement therapy is commonly used to support patients with ARDS who are hemodynamically unstable, septic, or have multiple system organ failure (Table 9.9). Continuous arteriovenous therapies require both arterial and venous access and usually significant anticoagulation. CAVH allows fluid removal but not much solute removal. Blood flow is determined by the arteriovenous pressure gradient and thus blood flow is low, filtration is less efficient, and hemofilters often clot in hypotensive patients. CAVHD and CAVHDF allow both efficient fluid and efficient solute removal because dialysate fluid flows countercurrent to blood flow in the hemofilter.

Continuous venovenous therapy has emerged in recent years and is the technique of choice now in many ICUs because arterial cannulation is not needed. A double lumen venous dialysis catheter is connected to a blood pump that drives blood flow through the hemofilter.

The complications of continuous renal replacement therapy are caused by anticoagulation, vascular access, fluid and electrolyte shifts, and technical problems with equipment. Because continuous venovenous therapy utilizes a blood pump, there must be alarms for disconnection (for detection of air emboli), air traps, and pressure alarms. Both hemofiltration and hemodiafiltration remove middle molecules such as antibiotics, cytokines, and amino acids. Thus, drug levels and doses must be monitored and adjusted appropriately. Studies suggest that continuous renal replacement therapy improves outcome in comparison to intermittent hemodialysis, but none are prospective randomized controlled trials and thus none are definitive. Furthermore, although continuous renal replacement therapy removes cytokines, it is not clear whether this changes outcome.

Dermatological Complications

Rashes in patients who have ARDS are not uncommon, and the commonest cause of rash is drug reactions. Drug reactions may be maculopapular, erythematous, vesicular, or have other forms.[57] Minor drug eruptions may be a sign of more significant systemic reactions to drug. Severe drug eruptions such as Stevens-Johnson syndrome are very rare but may be life threatening.[57]

Other dermatologic complications of ARDS include petechiae, purpura, and ecchymoses due to underlying disease and/or hematologic conditions. Petechial rashes are related to abnormalities in the platelet number and function or vascular disease (e.g., meningococcemia, vasculitis, septic emboli). Purpura may indicate underlying hematologic conditions such as post-transfusion purpura, thrombotic, thrombocytopenic purpura (TTP), or thrombocytopenia as a result of sepsis, DIC, or drugs.

Neurologic Complications

Neurologic dysfunction with respiratory failure is not uncommon and is usually multifactorial. The major central nervous system complications of ARDS are obtundation, coma, and seizures. The major peripheral nervous system complications of ARDS are myopathy and neuropathy.

Coma in critically ill patients may be caused by primary CNS disease or injury or by systemic insults. The major primary CNS causes of coma in the critically ill are intracranial hemorrhage, trauma, cerebral infarct, meningitis, encephalitis, status epilepticus, brain tumor, brain abscess, and hydrocephalus. Cerebral infarction may be due to ischemia from a decrease in cerebral perfusion, cerebral emboli, or cerebral hemorrhage secondary to coagulopathy.[29] Secondary systemic causes of coma include medications, hypoxemia, hypotension, sepsis, drug toxicity (i.e., drug overdose), acid-base disturbances, and electrolyte imbalance.[29]

The peripheral nervous system complications of ARDS, myopathy and neuropathy, present as muscle weakness. The major myopathic complication of concern in patients who have ARDS is the myopathy and prolonged weakness that occurs secondary to use of neuromuscular blocking agents. Patients who have ARDS are at increased risk because neuromuscular blockers may be used to improve oxygenation and because the risk is increased with certain drugs such as pancuronium, if there is associated renal dysfunction. Furthermore, concomitant use of corticosteroids and neuromuscular blocking agents increases the risk of prolonged and severe myopathy. This problem is best managed by prevention, that is, avoidance of use of neuromuscular blockers.

There is growing recognition of critical illness polyneuropathy, which may occur in ARDS.[58] Usually patients have multiple organ failure and/or sepsis and develop critical illness polyneuropathy as a later complication. The clinical features of critical illness polyneuropathy are flaccid quadriparesis, hypotonia, hyporeflexia, muscle atrophy, respiratory muscle weakness, and distal sensory loss.

The diagnosis of critical illness polyneuropathy is suspected clinically and confirmed by neurophysiologic testing. Often the first clue to the diagnosis is difficulty with weaning from mechanical ventilation despite adequate recovery of the underlying cardiopulmonary pathology.[59] Recovery is slow, may be incomplete, and treatment is nonspecific (i.e., treatment of the underlying disease). To date, there is no known prevention or treatment for critical illness polyneuropathy.

Hematologic Complications

The two most common hematologic abnormalities in ARDS are anemia and thrombocytopenia. Anemia is usually multifactorial secondary to blood loss from hemorrhage, phlebotomy, hemolysis, and decreased red blood cell production.

Thrombocytopenia and coagulation disorders are common in ARDS and can cause hemorrhage, oozing from venipuncture and arterial sites, petechiae, purpura, and ecchymoses. Thrombocytopenia occurs in 50% to 70% of patients who have ARDS and is associated with increased mortality.[60,61] Platelet consumption and sequestration are the dominant causes of thrombocytopenia.[60] Platelet sequestration occurs in the lungs, liver, and spleen. Platelet destruction occurs secondary to drugs, underlying disease (e.g., sepsis), post-transfusion purpura, and disseminated intravascular coagulation (DIC). DIC occurs in up to 25% of patients with ARDS.

Coagulopathy secondary to coagulation factor depletion is also common in ARDS. The commonest causes of coagulopathy are depletion of vitamin K–dependent factors II, VII, IX, and X as a result of malnutrition, malabsorption of feeds, and broad spectrum antibiotics. DIC and hepatic dysfunction also cause coagulation factor depletion. Administration of intravenous vitamin K and correction of coagulopathy both diagnoses and corrects the vitamin K–dependent coagulation factor deficiency. Failure to correct coagulopathy after administration of vitamin K suggests most commonly severe liver disease, accelerated coagulation factor consumption (e.g., DIC), or coagulation factor antibodies.

Blood transfusion is important because blood transfusion may be indicated to increase oxygen delivery. Blood transfusion also is important in ARDS because blood transfusion can cause ARDS (leukoagglutinin reaction), and blood transfusion has acute and chronic complications. Blood transfusion is controversial in the critically ill because there have been few randomized controlled trials. As a result, blood transfusion practice is highly variable. Clinicians often use a transfusion trigger based on experience and based on the results of consensus guidelines.[62,63] Several randomized controlled trials in patients with sickle-cell disease,[64] trauma,[65] and cardiovascular surgery[66] found little difference in mortality whether using conservative or liberal transfusion practices.

Blood transfusion has been shown to increase global oxygen delivery in patients who have ARDS.[67,68] Although some studies found that blood transfusion increased calculated oxygen consumption, oxygen consumption determined by analysis of expired gases did not change.[67,68] Therefore, it is not clear that acute transfusion can diagnose tissue hypoxia or reverse tissue hypoxia.

The safe level of hemoglobin in patients who have ARDS is not known. Anemia is tolerated by increasing cardiac output to maintain oxygen delivery, by increasing tissue oxygen extraction to maintain oxygen consumption, and by shifting the oxyhemoglobin dissociation curve to optimize unloading of oxygen to tissues. Thus anemia is potentially less well tolerated in critically ill patients who have limitations in the ability to increase cardiac output (e.g., acute MI, congestive heart failure) and/or who have impaired ability to regulate peripheral vascular tone and blood flow distribution (e.g., sepsis, vasoactive drugs).

Although blood transfusion clearly increases global oxygen delivery, it is not as clear that tissue oxygen delivery is actually increased. Blood transfusion may not increase microvascular oxygen delivery because of altered blood viscosity and because of the impaired red blood cell deformability of stored blood. Blood transfusion increases viscosity, which alters blood flow distribution in the microvasculature. Stored blood develops the storage lesion. The storage lesion is characterized by changes in red blood cells such that they become more spherical in shape and less deformable, which may impair their transit through the microvasculature.

The indications for red blood cell transfusion must be determined carefully for each patient. Patients who have heart disease and are critically ill tolerate anemia less well.[69] Patients who have ARDS whose oxygen delivery is limited by arterial hypoxemia may also tolerate anemia less well. The question of what is the appropriate transfusion trigger in the critically ill was addressed in a pilot randomized controlled trial.[70] The results of a large multicenter trial of transfusion in critical care (TRICC) will yield important information to guide clinicians in judging an appropriate transfusion trigger. In general, we recommend a transfusion trigger of about 80 g/L in the critically ill and about 100 g/L in critically patients who have myocardial ischemia or who have refactory arterial hypoxemia (i.e., SaO_2 less than 88% despite maximal care).

Deep venous thrombosis (DVT) and pulmonary embolism are complications of ARDS that are potentially preventable. Unless there are contraindications (e.g., head injury, severe coagulopathy, thrombocytopenia, prior heparin-induced thrombocytopenia), subcutaneous heparin (e.g., 5,000 units every 8 to 12 hours) should be given to all immobilized patients who have ARDS to prevent DVT and pulmonary embolism. Patients who have contraindications to heparin (e.g., neurosurgical patients) or who cannot tolerate heparin can be managed with lower extremity, intermittent pneumatic compression cuffs to prevent DVT. Other alternative approaches to prophylaxis of thromboembolism include low molecular weight heparin, antiembolism stockings, aspirin, warfarin, and vena caval interruption.

The diagnosis of deep venous thrombosis and of pulmonary thromboembolism (PTE) is often difficult and is even more challenging in patients who have ARDS. The reasons that diagnosis is difficult in ARDS is that patients are often sedated or obtunded so symptoms cannot be elicited. The presence of low-grade fever, tachycardia, tachypnea, and increased minute ventilation are extremely common in ARDS,[71] and there are many reasons for worsening hypoxemia in patients who have ARDS. Decision analysis and evidence-based decision-making algorithms have been derived and validated in noncritically ill patients; however, they have not been rigorously evaluated in critically ill patients.

Deep venous thrombosis is usually considered when there is asymmetrical edema or when there are signs and changes in clinical status suggestive of pulmonary thromboembolism. Clues to consider PTE include tachypnea (incidence 80%–90%), tachycardia (50%–60%), fever (40%–50%), and shock (5%). Shock appears as "cardiogenic" shock with hypotension, tachycardia, cool diaphoretic skin, peripheral and sometimes central cyanosis, and increased JVP; however, the chest is remarkably clear. Less commonly, examination reveals an increased pulmonary component of the second heart sound, increased JVP or CVP (from right ventricular failure), or pleural friction rub. Subtle presentations that should raise suspicion of pulmonary embolism in critically ill patients include increased minute ventilation to maintain $PaCO_2$ (because of increased physiologic dead space) or increased $PaCO_2$ in the paralyzed patient who has a fixed minute ventilation, increased difficulty with oxygenation (because of increased shunt), sudden episode(s) of respiratory distress, and unexplained failure to wean from mechanical ventilation.

The radiographic features of pulmonary thromboembolism (basal atelectasis, pleural effusion, elevated hemidiaphragm) may be impossible to discern in a patient who has diffuse, bilateral pulmonary infiltrates because of ARDS. Electrocardiographic changes suggestive of PTE include right ventricular strain, incomplete or complete right bundle branch block, right axis deviation, P pulmonale, and $S_1Q_3T_3$ pattern.

Patients who are hemodynamically monitored may have clues to the diagnosis of pulmonary thromboembolism from changes in hemodynamics. Pulmonary thromboembolism increases mean pulmonary artery (PA) and right atrial pressures, decreases cardiac output, decreases mixed venous oxygen saturation, and widens the PA diastolic-wedge pressure gradient.[72] Unfortunately, severe ARDS may also cause many or all of these hemodynamic changes.

Portable bedside echocardiography is being used increasingly and we believe is fundamental to the evaluation of patients who have cardiogenic shock. The echocardiographic features of pulmonary embolism can include poor contraction and dilation of the right ventricle, shift of the ventricular septum to the left, paradoxical movement of the ventricular septum, and decreased left ventricular volume (because of underfilling). Again, the diagnosis of pulmonry embolism is difficult in patients who have ARDS because significant ARDS can cause many of these echocardiographic findings.

The approach to diagnosis of DVT and pulmonary embolism in patients who have ARDS is different than the approach to diagnosis in less critically ill patients. Ventilation-perfusion lung scan in the patient who has ARDS has limited utility because ventilation scanning is usually not done and because perfusion abnormalities are common in ARDS. Furthermore, one multicenter study highlighted the limitations of V/Q scanning and emphasized the need to classify patients clinically as low, moderate, or high risk for PTE.[73] The diagnosis of PTE can usually be excluded in patients who have low clinical probability and a low probability V/Q scan. Conversely, high probability V/Q scan in patients who have moderate or high clinical suspicion of PTE should be treated for pulmonary thromboembolism. However, the vast majority of critically ill patients, especially patients who have ARDS, will have intermediate probability V/Q scans and will require additional investigation.

Additional investigations to consider to establish the diagnosis of PTE include noninvasive leg studies (e.g., venous doppler, impedance plethysmography, and B mode ultrasound), helical chest CT scanning, and pulmonary angiography. Studies have validated the sensitivity and specificity of the noninvasive leg studies, but these validation studies are not focused on critically ill patients. However, in patients who have intermediate (i.e., nondiagnostic) perfusion scans, confirmation of the diagnosis of DVT by noninvasive leg studies leads to the decision to anticoagulate and obviates the need for pulmonary angiography. Therefore, noninvasive leg studies are useful in the investigation of patients who have ARDS in whom pulmonary thromboembolism is suspected.

Pulmonary angiography is the gold standard for the diagnosis of pulmonary embolism. However, pulmonary angiography is more expensive, has increased risks, and is logistically more difficult than other noninvasive tests. Therefore, pulmonary angiography is usually reserved for use in patients who have had other less invasive tests but who do not yet have the diagnosis of PTE established or excluded. In ARDS, pulmonary angiography needs to be seriously considered in patients who have nondiagnostic perfusion scans (e.g., low and intermediate probability) and/or nondiagnostic leg studies.

The safety of pulmonary angiography has increased in recent years. The overall mortality is 0.2%. The risk of death is increased in patients who have moderate or severe pulmonary hypertension. The risks of pulmonary angiography may be reduced by use of non-ionic, low-osmolality contrast agents.

The cornerstone of treatment of deep venous thrombosis and pulmonary thromboembolism is systemic anticoagulation. Patients who present with shock need careful consideration of more aggressive therapy such as thrombolytic therapy, pulmonary embolectomy, or inerior vena caval interruption procedures.

Shock secondary to pulmonary thromboembolism is managed by fundamentals of airway, breathing, and circulatory support to achieve cardiopulmonary stabilization to then permit appropriate diagnostic procedures to proceed. Cardiogenic shock secondary to PTE is treated by optimal oxygenation, support of ventilation, and often will require vasopressor support. Physiologic studies suggest that aggressive fluid resuscitation may not be appropriate because fluid resuscitation can cause further right ventricular dilation and increases right ventricular end-diastolic pressure (RVEDP). Because systemic arterial pressure is reduced and RVEDP is increased, the pressure gradient for coronary perfusion of the right ventricle is decreased. Therefore, drugs such as norepinephrine are recommended to increase systemic arterial pressure, to enhance the coronary perfusion pressure, and to thereby enhance right ventricular contractility.

Thrombolytic therapy should be considered early in treatment of patients who have shock secondary to pulmonary thromboembolism because thrombolytic agents more rapidly lyse clot, more rapidly lower pulmonary artery pressure, and therefore more rapidly resolve shock. Controlled trials of patients who have shock secondary to PTE are lacking. Trials of thrombolysis in PTE showed more rapid clot lysis and earlier hemodynamic improvement compared to heparin; however, at 1 week there were no differences between heparin and thrombolytic-treated patients.[74-77] One study found that streptokinase and heparin decreased mortality compared to heparin in patients who had shock and massive pulmonary embolism. If thrombolytic agents are used, invasive procedures must be minimized to decrease the risk of hemorrhage. Streptokinase may be the drug of choice because of its efficacy, lower cost (compared to alteplase and urokinase), and comparable risk profile. After streptokinase, systemic heparinization is necessary.

Surgical pulmonary embolectomy is used infrequently in management of massive pulmonary embolism because of the efficacy and relative safety of thrombolysis followed by heparin. Surgical pulmonary embolectomy is used in patients who have contraindication to thrombolysis. Recent experience shows improving results compared to older studies of embolectomy.

Catheterization techniques have been developed to permit removal of pulmonary artery clot using a suction device on a catheter.[78]

In patients who are not in shock who have pulmonary embolism, systemic heparinization is standard therapy. Heparin should be given by bolus followed by continuous intravenous infusion to maintain activated partial thromboplastin time greater than 1.5 times control. Heparin should be started if there is strong clinical suspicion of pulmonary embolism while arranging investigations. Heparin can be stopped if pulmonary embolism is excluded or continued if the diagnosis is confirmed.

Nomogram-based dosing of heparin in the ICU is more effective than empiric dosing because nomogram-based dosing shortens the time to achieve therapeutic anticoagulation and also decreases the amount of time at subtherapeutic doses.[79,80] The heparin infusion nomogram used in our ICU is shown in Figure 9.4.

The major complications of systemic heparinization are bleeding (major 3%–4%, all bleeding 10%), heparin-induced thrombocytopenia (HIT), and hypersensitivity. Bleeding secondary to heparin is treated by stopping heparin, if bleeding is minor, and protamine, if bleeding is major or life threatening.

ARDS can occur as a complication of severe hematologic conditions (such as hematologic malignancy) and bone marrow transplantation. In general, ARDS complicating these conditions has a very poor prognosis. Patients who have acute leukemia are at high risk for pneumonia that may progress to ARDS. Leukemic patients who have fever and pulmonary infiltrates require aggressive investigation and broad spectrum antibiotics. Investigation should include sputum (gram stain, acid-fast bacillus, fungal and bacterial cultures), blood, and urine culture; bronchoscopy (with protected specimen brushings and washings) at 12 to 24 hours; CT-guided needle biopsy (if not ventilated), and open lung biopsy requires careful consideration. The pathology of ARDS is discussed in Chapter 3. The role of open lung biopsy is controversial because if broad spectrum antibiotics and antifungal agents are used empirically, it is not common to find at open lung biopsy another treatable cause of diffuse pulmonary infiltrates and respiratory failure in the immunocompromised leukemic patient. Broad spectrum antibiotic regimens include ceftazidime (+/– vancomycin), ciprofloxacin and vancomycin, piperacillin and aminoglycoside, and imipenem (+/– vancomycin).

Many leukemic patients receive granulocyte colony-stimulating factor (G-CSF) or granulocyte-macrophage colony-stimulating factor (GM-CSF) to increase leukocyte count when leukocyte counts are extremely low during the nadir of chemotherapy. Use of G-CSF or GM-CSF may be complicated in the critically ill patient by worsening hypoxemia perhaps because of leukocyte trapping in the pulmonary circulation.

Patients who have leukemia and very high leukocyte counts may also develop fever, tachypnea, hypoxia, and pulmonary infiltrates because of the hyperleukocytosis syndrome. The larger, less deformable immature cells of the leukemic patient lodge in capillaries (leukostasis) and can cause cardiovascular (arrhythmias), neurologic (seizures, coma), and pulmonary (hypoxia, pulmonary infiltrates) complications. The hyperleukocytosis syndrome with these complications is managed by leukapheresis, irradiation (cranial or thoracic, respectively), and systemic chemotherapy.

Patients who have hyperleukocytosis can also develop severe pseudohypoxemia that is caused by consumption of oxygen in blood in the arterial blood gas syringe by the metabolically active leukemic cells. This is avoided by transporting the arterial blood gas syringe on ice and by rapid testing.

Published literature has demonstrated that a nomogram for adjusting the rate of heparin infusion that is based upon the patient's weight is more successful at achieving and maintaining desired degrees of anticoagulation than other available methods. To attempt to improve the success with anticoagulation from heparin, the following nomogram is recommended. Physician's may order heparin dosages to be adjusted based on the nomogram:

INTRAVENOUS HEPARIN ADJUSTMENT NOMOGRAM -ACCORDING TO PTT

For Heparin Concentration 50 u/ml (25,000 u in 500 ml D5W)

The rate of infusion should be rounded to the nearest multiple of 50 units (1 ml) per hour infusion rate.

INITIAL BOLUS = 80 units/kg, followed by 18 units/kg/hr infusion

Adjust Heparin rate according to the following PTT results:

PTT (sec)	BOLUS DOSE IV	STOP INFUSION	RATE CHANGE
<35	80 units/kg	0	Increase by 4 units/kg/hr
35-45	40 units/kg	0	Increase by 3 units/kg/hr
45-60	40 units/kg	0	Increase by 2 units/kg/hr
60-85 (Therapeutic)	0	0	0 (no change)
85-110	0	0	Decrease by 2 units/kg/hr
>110	0	60 min	Decrease by 4 units/kg/hr

Draw PTT every 6-8 hours until within the therapeutic range (60-85 seconds). Once therapeutic range is reached, draw PTT daily while patient is on Heparin.

HEPARIN INFUSION RATE CHANGES BASED ON ABOVE NOMOGRAM

Change the rate of infusion (ml/hr) of heparin according to the weight of the patient based on the following chart. The hospital pharmacy prepares heparin in a concentration of 50 units/ml ie. 25000 units in 500 ml D5W.

	40	50	60	70	80	90	100	110	Wt (Kg)
Increase by 4 units/kg/hr	+3	+4	+5	+6	+6	+7	+8	+9	ml/hr
Increase by 3 units/kg/hr	+2	+3	+4	+4	+5	+5	+6	+7	ml/hr
Increase by 2 units/kg/hr	+2	+2	+2	+3	+3	+4	+4	+4	ml/hr
Decrease by 2 units/kg/hr	-2	-2	-2	-3	-3	-4	-4	-4	ml/hr
Decrease by 4 units/kg/hr	-3	-4	-5	-6	-6	-7	-8	-9	ml/hr

Figure 9.4. Intravenous heparin adjustment nomogram.

Endocrine and Metabolic Complications

The commonest metabolic complications of ARDS are hyperglycemia, hypoglycemia (less common), hyper- and hyponatremia, hypokalemia, hypocalcemia, hypomagnesemia, and hypophosphatemia. Hyperglycemia is secondary to increased glycogenolysis and gluconeogenesis caused by high levels of stress hormones epinephrine, norepi-nephrine, and corticosteroids. Hyperglycemia is more severe in patients who have underlying diabetes. Hyperglycemia is best managed by continuous infusion of insulin using a sliding scale for dosage adjustment. The insulin infusion protocol (unpub-lished) used in our ICU is shown in Figure 9.5.

Hypoglycemia is most often secondary to excessive exogenous insulin, emphasiz-ing the need to monitor blood glucose closely in patients on insulin infusions. Hypo-glycemia may also be caused by lack of countercoagulatory hormones and so may be a clue to occult adrenal insufficiency in the critically ill. Other important causes of hypoglycemia include hepatic insufficiency, inadequate glucose intake, malnutrition, and drugs such as beta blockers, sulfonylureas, and salicylates.

Hyponatremia is commonly multifactorial and may be depletional (secondary to nasogastric losses, diuresis, diarrhea, and other fluid losses), dilutional (secondary to hypotonic fluid replacement in patients who have high ADH levels secondary to stress, mechanical ventilation, and hypovolemia), and rarely factitious (due to hyperglycemia).

Acute hyponatremia can develop rapidly in the postoperative surgical patient because of increased levels of ADH (secondary to narcotics, pain) and infusion of hypotonic fluids (e.g., D5W).[81] In obstetrical cases, acute severe hyponatremia can develop secondary to infusion of oxytocin in D5W. Diuretics such as furosemide and thiazides can lead to mild or moderate and rarely severe hyponatremia.[82] Hypona-tremia leads to cerebral edema, which can present as agitation, delirium, seizures, confusion, and coma. For unclear reasons females are more susceptible to serious cerebral edema and major clinical complications of hyponatremia including status epilepticus, respiratory arrest, and death.[83]

Hyponatremia is best treated by prevention. Preventive measures include careful and regular assessment of volume status, intake, output, and measurement of sodium and by infusion of isotonic (as opposed to hypotonic) fluids. Severe acute hypona-tremia is managed by resuscitation of volume deficit using normal saline, followed by infusion of hypertonic saline. Complications of treatment of hyponatremia include excessively rapid correction of hyponatremia and development of central pontine myelinolysis. Correction of severe hyponatremia is controversial with some recom-mending rapid correction[84] and other suggesting slower correction because rapid cor-rection may cause central pontine myelinolysis.[85]

Hypernatremia is less common and may occur in patients receiving large solute loads, who have large fluid losses (e.g., diarrhea, osmotic, diuresis) and/or have inad-equate free water replacement (e.g., head injury, coma, sedation, and inability to express thirst needs). Patients who have head injury may have acute partial or com-plete diabetes insipidus that presents in the ICU as polyuria and hypernatremia.

Hypokalemia is relatively common in patients who have ARDS and is usually due to inadequate intake and excessive potassium losses secondary to diuresis, vomiting, diarrhea, or magnesium depletion with or without hypomagnesemia. Hypokalemia may also be due to intracellular shifts of potassium by insulin and beta adrenergic agents. Hypokalemia is most often prevented by providing adequate KCl in IV fluids, enteral feeds, and total parenteral nutrition fluids.

GOAL: The goal is to maintain serum glucose between 7 and 11.5 mmol/L

MONITORING: Check glucose q1h (either capillary or blood) until stable (3 values in desired range). Checks can be reduced to q2h x 4 hours → q4h if blood glucose remains in desired range. Restart Q1H checking if any change in insulin infusion rate occurs.
If glucose is changing rapidly (even if in the desired range) or if in a critical range (<3.5 or >20mmol/L Q30 minute checks may be needed. However, blood blucose will not change significantly in <30 minutes with any change in insulin

Initiating Insulin Infusion

Glucose	11.5-14mmol/L	14.1-17mmol/L	17.1-20mmol/L	20.1-24mmol/L	>24mmol/L
	Give 3 units insulin IV push and start @ 2 units/hr	Give 6 units insulin IV push and start @ 2 units/hr	Give 8 units insulin IV push and start @ 2 units/hr	Give 10 units insulin IV push and start @ 2 units/hr	Cal MD for orders

Ongoing Insulin Infusion:
Below Desired Range (7.11.5mmol/L

Glucose Level	Infusion Rate of 1-3 units/hr	Infusion Rate of 4-6 units/hr	Infusion Rate of 7-9 units/hr	Infusion Rate of 10-12 units/hr	Infusion Rate of 13-16 units/hr	Infusion Rate of >16 units/hr
<3.5 mmol/L	D/C infusion and give 1 amp D50 IVP					
3.5-4.5mmol/L	D/C Infusion: Re-check B/S in 1 hour. If >7, re-start but decrease rate by 1 unit/hr.		D/C Infusion: Re-check B/S in 1 hour. If >7, re-start but decrease rate by 2 units/hr.		D/C Infusion: Re-check B/S in 1 hour, If>7, re-start but decrease rate by 3 unit/hr.	
4.6-5.5mmol/L	D/C Infusion: Re-check B/S in 1 hour, if>7, re-start but decrease rate by 1 unit/hr.	Decrease Infusion by 50%				
5-6-7mmol/L	Decrease Infusion by 1 unit/hr	Decrease Infusion by 2 units/hr	Decrease Infusion by 3 units/hr	Decrease Infusion by 4 units/hr	Decrease Infusion by 4 units/hr	Decrease Infusion by 6 units/hr

In Desired Range (7-11.5mmol/L)

7-11.5mmol.:	NO CHANGES/DON'T TAMPER WITH SUCCESS! If Blood sugar continues to decrease within the desired range over 3 consecutive hours, decrease rate by 1 unit/hr.	NO CHANGE/DON'T TAMPER WITH SUCCESS! If Blood sugar continues to decrease within the desired range over 3 consecutive hours, decrease rate by 2 unit/hr.

Above Desired Range (7-11.5mmol/L)

Glucose Level	Infusion Rate of 1-5 units/hr	Infusion Rate of 6-10 units/hr	Infusion Rate of 11-16 units/hr	Infusion Rate of >16 units/hr
11.5-14mmol/L	Give 2 units insulin IVP and increase Infusion by 1 uits/hr	Give 3 units insulin IVP and increase Infusion by 2 units/hr	Give 3 units insulin IVP and increase Infusion by 3 units/hr	Call Physician for New Order
14.1-17mmol/L	Give 3 units insulin IVP and increase Infusion by 1 unit/hr	Give 5 units insulin IVP and increase Infusion by 2 units/hr	Give 5 units insulin IVP and increase Infusion by 3 units/hr	Call Physician for New Order
17.1-20mmol/L	give 8 units insulin IVP and increase Infusion by 1 unit/hr	Give 8 units insulin IVP and increse Infusion by 2 units/hr	Give 8 units insulin IVP and increase Infusion by 3 units/hr	Call Physician for New Order
20.1-24mmol/L	give 10 units insulin IVP and increase Infusion by 1 unit/hr	Give 10 units insulin IVP and increase Infusion by 2 units/hr	Give 10 units insulin IVP and increase Infusion by 3 units/hr	Call Physician for New Order
>24mmol/L	Call Physician for New Order			

Figure 9.5. Insulin infusion protocol – regular human insulin only.

Magnesium deficiency and hypomagnesemia are both extremely common in critically ill patients who have ARDS. Magnesium deficiency is often multifactorial in etiology including inadequate intake, underlying malnutrition, alcoholism, and diuretic use, diarrhea, and vomiting. Magnesium deficiency is often exacerbated in the ICU by ongoing diuretic use, inadequate magnesium repletion, and other ongoing magnesium losses. Magnesium depletion may be severe without overt hypomagnesemia because magnesium, like potassium, is primarily an intracellular cation. Magnesium infusion is necessary in many ICU patients.

The commonest endocrine complications of ARDS are acute adrenal insufficiency and euthyroid sick syndrome.

Acute adrenocortical insufficiency may actually be the acute presentation of chronic, unrecognized adrenocortical insufficiency (primary or secondary). Recent reports suggest that true acute adrenocortical insufficiency may also develop during the course of critical illness.[86,87] Adrenocortical insufficiency may be suspected in patients who have ARDS if there are clues such as hypoglycemia, hyponatremia, hyperkalemia, and, most importantly, hypotension, especially if relatively resistant to inotropic support. If acute adrenocortical insufficiency is suspected clinically, patients should receive intravenous corticosteroids (e.g., dexamethasone 4 mg IV stat and every 4 to 6 hours thereafter to avoid interference with cortisol levels) and have a rapid ACTH stimulation test.[86,87] When the diagnosis is confirmed, dexamethasone can be replaced by intravenous hydrocortisone.

Although true hypo- and hyperthyroidism are rare in the critically ill patient who has ARDS, abnormal thyroid hormone levels are common. Most critically ill patients have euthyroid sick syndrome, which is characterized by low T3, often low T4, and normal or low TSH levels.[88] Furthermore, in postoperative patients who have low T4 and low or normal TSH, mortality is high.[89] It is therefore difficult to determine whether thyroxine should be given to critically ill patients. Several studies show no improvement in mortality when patients who did not have clear preexisting thyroid disease and who had low T4 and TSH were given 1-thyroxine.[90]

References

1. Ferck CM. Predicting difficult intubation. Anaesthesia 1991; 46:1005.
2. Bersten AD, Holt AW, Vedig AE, et al. Treatment of severe cardiogenic pulmonary edema with continuous positive airway pressure delivery by face mask. N Engl J Med 1991; 325:1825.
3. Katz JA, Marks JD. Inspiratory work with and without continuous positive airway pressure in patients with acute respiratory failure. Anesthesiology 1985; 63:598.
4. Buda AJ, Pinsky MJ, Ingels NB et al. Effect of intrathoracic pressure on left ventricular performance. N Engl J Med 1979; 301:453.
5. Sellick BA. Cricoid pressure to control regurgitation of stomach contents during induction of anesthesia. Lancet 1961; 2:404.
6. Schwartz DE, Matthay MA, Cohen NH. Death and other complications of emergency airway management in critically ill adults. Anesthesiology 1995; 82:367.
7. Marsh HM, Gillespie DJ, Baumgartner AE. Timing of tracheostomy in the critically ill patient. Chest 1989; 96:190.
8. Heffner JE. Medical indications for tracheostomy. Chest 1989; 96:186.

9. Cook DJ, Hebert PC, Heyland DK, Brun-Buisson C, Marshall JC, Russell JA, Sprung CL. How to use an article on therapy or prevention: pneumonia prevention using subglottic secretion drainage: I. Are the results of the study valid? Crit Care Med 1997; 25:1502.

10. Valles J, Artigas A, Rello J, et al. Continuous aspiration of subglottic secretions in preventing ventilator associated pneumonia. Ann Int Med 1995; 12:179.

11. Moore EE, Jones TN. Benefits of immediate jejunostomy feeding after major abdominal trauma – a prospective randomized study. J Trauma 1986; 26:874–881.

12. Admas S, Dellinger EP, Wertz MJ, et al. Enteral vs. parenteral nutrition support following laparotomy for trauma: a randomized prospective trial. J Trauma 1986; 29:882–891.

13. Moore FA, Moore EE, Jones TN, et al. TEN vs. TPN following major abdominal trauma-reduced septic morbidity. J Trauma 1989; 29:916–923.

14. Kidsk KA, Croce MA, Fabian TC, et al. Enteral vs parenteral feeding. Effects of septic morbidity after chest and penetrating abdominal trauma. Ann Surg 1992; 215:503–511.

15. Cerra FB, McPerhson JP, Lonstantinides FN, et al. Enteral nutrition does not prevent multiple organ failure syndrome (MOFS) after sepsis. Surgery 1998; 104:727–733.

16. Ramsay MAE, Savege TM, Simpson BRJ, Goodwin R. Controlled sedation with alphax-alone-alphadolone. Br Med J 1974; 2:656.

17. Hansen-Flaschen J, Brazinsky S, Basile C, Lanken P. Use of sedating drugs and neuromuscular blocking agents in patients requiring mechanical ventilation for respiratory failure. JAMA 1991; 266:2870.

18. Shapiro B, Warren J, Egol A, et al. Practice parameters for intravenous analgesia and sedation for adult patients in the intensive care unit: an executive summary. Crit Care Med 1995; 23:1596.

19. Marik P, Kaufman D. The effect of neuromuscular paralysis on systemic and splanchnic oxygen utilization in mechanical ventilated patients. Chest 1996; 109:1038.

20. Segredo V, Caldwell J, Matthay M. Persistent paralysis in critically ill patients after long-term administration of vecuronium. N Engl J Med 1992; 327:524.

21. Griffin D, Fairman N, Coursin D, et al. Acute myopathy during treatment of status asthmaticus with corticosteroids and steroidal muscle relaxants. Chest 1992; 102:510.

22. Kupfer Y, Namba T, Kaldawi E, Tessler S. Prolonged weakness after long-term infusion of vecuronium bromide. Ann Intern Med 1992; 117:484.

23. Leatherman JW, Fluegel WL, David WS, Davies SF, Iber C. Muscle weakness in mechanically ventilated patients with severe asthma. Am J Resp Crit Care Med 1996; 153:1686.

24. Committee on Trauma, American College of Surgeons. Advanced trauma life support manual. American College of Surgeons, Chicago, 1998.

25. Colice GL, Matthay MA, Bass E, Matthay RA. Neurogenic pulmonary edema. Am Rev Respir Dis 1984; 130:941.

26. Ali J, Wood LDH. Pulmonary vascular effects of furosemide on gas exchange in pulmonary edema. J Appl Physiol 1984; 57:160.

27. Kallenbach J, Lewis M, Zaltzman M, et al. Low dose corticosteroid prophylaxis against fat embolism. J Trauma 1987; 27:1173.

28. American College of Chest Physicians/Society of Critical Care Medicine Consensus Conference Committee. Definitions for sepsis and organ failure and guidelines for the use of innovative therapies in sepsis. Crit Care Med 1992; 20:864.

29. Pingleton SK. Complications of acute respiratory failure. Med Clin North Am 1983; 67(3):725–746.

30. Pingleton SK. Complications associated with the adult respiratory distress syndrome. Clin Chest Med 1982; 3(1):143–155.
31. Cullent DJ, Caldera DL. The incidence of ventilatory-induced pulmonary barotrauma in critically ill patients. Anesthesiology 1979; 50:185.
32. De Latorre FJ, Tomasa A, Klamburg J, et al. Incidence of pneumothorax and pneumo-mediastinum in patients with aspiration penumonia requiring ventilatory support. Chest 1997; 72(2):141–144.
33. George DL. Epidemiology of nosocomial pneumonia in intensive care unit patients. Clin Chest Med 1995; 16(1):29–44.
34. Dever LL, Johanson WG. Pneumonia complicating adult respiratory distress syndrome. Clin Chest Med 1995; 16(1):147–153.
35. Niederman MS, Fein AM. Sepsis syndorme, the adult respiratory distress syndrome, and nosocomial pneumonia: a common clinical sequence. Clin Chest Med 1990; 11(4): 633–656.
36. Sutherland KR, Steinberg KP, Maunder RJ, et al. Pulmonary infection during the acute respiratory distress syndrome. Am J Respir Crit Care Med 1995; 152:550–556.
37. Parrillo JE, Burch C, Shelhamer JH, et al. A circulating myocardial depressant substance in humans with septic shock. J Clin Invest 1985; 76:1539–1553.
38. Sideris DA, Katsadoros DP, Valiano G, Assioura A. Type of cardiac dysrhythmias in respiratory failure. Am Heart J 1975; 89(1):32–36.
39. Abernathy WS. Complete heart block caused by the Swan-Ganz catheter. Chest 1974; 65(3):349.
40. Cairns JA, Holder D. Ventricular fibrillation due to passage of a Swan-Ganz catheter. Am J Cardiol 1975; 35:589.
41. Harris SK, Bone RC, Ruth WE. Gastrointestinal hemorrhage in patients in a respiratory intensive care unit. Chest 1977; 72(3):301–304.
42. Cook DJ, Reeve BK, Guyatt GH, et al. Stress ulcer prophylaxis in critically ill patients resolving discordant meta-analyses. JAMA 1996; 275(4):308–314.
43. Pingleton SK, Hadzima SK. Enteral alimentation and gastrointestinal bleeding in mechanically ventilated patients. Crit Care Med 1983; 11(1):13–16.
44. Pitimana-aree S, Forrest D, Brown G, et al. Implementation of a clinical practice guideline for stress ulcer prophylaxis increases appropriateness and decreases cost of care. Int Care Med 1998; 24:217–223.
45. McFadden DW, Reber MA. Indications for surgery in severe acute pancreatitis. Int J Pancreatol 1994; 15:83.
46. Warshaw AL, O'Hara PJ. Susceptibility of the pancreas to ischemic injury in shock. Ann Surg 1978; 188:197.
47. Deehan DJ, Heys SD, Brittenden J, et al. Mesenteric ischemia: prognostic factors and influence of delay upon outcome. J R Coll Surg Edinb 1995; 40:112.
48. Rivitz SM, Geller SC, Hahn C, et al. Treatment of acute mesenteric venous thrombosis with transjugular intramesenteric urokinase infusion. J Vasc Intervent Radiol 1995; 6:219.
49. Matsumoto AH, Tegfmeyer CJ, Fitzcharles FK, et al. Percutaneous transluminal angioplasty of visceral arterial stenosis: results and long-term clinical followup. J Vasc Intervent Radiol 1995; 6:165.
50. Hillman KM. Pneumoperitoneum: a review. Crit Care Med 1982; 10(7):476–481.

51. Stein AL, Lane E. A new treatment modality for pneumoperitoneum associated with mechanical ventilation. Chest 1982; 81(4):519–520.
52. Mancebo J, Artigas A. A clinical study of the adult respiratory distress syndrome. Crit Care Med 1987; 15(3):243–246.
53. Kraman S, Khan F, Patel S, Seriff N. Renal failure in the respiratory intensive care unit. Crit Care Med 1979; 7(6):263–266.
54. Kilburn KH, Dowell AR, Durham NC. Renal failure in respiratory failure. Arch Intern Med 1971; 127:754–762.
55. Humphrey H, Hall J, Sznajder I, et al. Improved survival in ARDS patients associated with reduction in pulmonary capillary wedge pressure. Chest 1990; 97:1176.
56. Mitchell JP, Schuller D, Calandra FS, et al. Improved outcome based on fluid management in critically ill patients requiring pulmonary artery catheterization action. Am J Resp Crit Care Med 1992; 145:990.
57. Manders SM. Serious and life-threatening drug eruptions. Am Fam Physician 1995; 51(8):1865–1872.
58. Zochodne DW, Bolton CF, Wells GA, et al. Critical illness polyneuropathy. A complication of sepsis and multiple organ failure. Brain 1987; 110:819.
59. Coronel B, Mercatello A, Courtrier JC, et al. Polyneuropathy: potential cause of difficult weaning. Crit Care Med 1990; 18:486.
60. Bone RC, Francis FB, Pierce AK. Intravascular coagulation associated with the adult respiratory distress syndrome. Am J Med 1976; 61(5):585–589.
61. Schneider RC, Zapol WM, Carvalho AC. Platelet consumption and sequestration in severe acute respiratory failure. Am Rev Respir Dis 1980; 122:445–451.
62. American College of Physicians. Practice strategies for elective red blood cell transfusion. Ann Intern Med 1992; 116:403.
63. Consensus Conference. Perioperative red blood cell transfusion. JAMA 1988; 260:2700.
64. Vichinsky EP, Haberkern CM, Neumayr L, et al. A comparison of conservative and aggressive transfusion regimens in the perioperative management of sickle cell disease. N Engl J Med 1995; 333:206.
65. Fortune JB, Feustel PJ, Saifi J, et al. Influence of hematocrit on cardiopulmonary function after acute hemorrhage. J Trauma 1987; 27:243.
66. Johnson RG, Thurer RL, Kruskall MS, et al. Comparison of two transfusion strategies after elective operations for myocardial revascularization. J Th Cardio Surg 1992; 104:307.
67. Ronco JJ, Phang PT, Walley KR, et al. Oxygen consumption is independent of oxygen delivery in severe adult respiratory distress syndrome. Am Rev Resp Dis 1991; 143:1267.
68. Marik PE, Sibbald WJ. Effect of stored-blood transfusion on oxygen delivery in patients with sepsis. JAMA 1993; 269:3024.
69. Hebert PC, Wells G, Tweeddale M, et al. Does transfusion practice affect mortality in critically ill patients? Am J Resp Crit Care Med 1997; 155:A20 (abstract).
70. Hebert P, Wells G, Marshall J, et al. Transfusion requirements in critical care. A pilot study. JAMA 1995; 273:1439.
71. Ronco JJ, Belzberg A, Phang PT, et al. No differences in hemodynamics, ventricular function and oxygen delivery in septic and nonseptic patients with the adult respiratory distress syndrome. Crit Care Med 1994; 22:777.

72. Cozzi PJ, Hall JB, Schmidt GA. Pulmonary artery diastolic occlusion pressure gradient is increased in acute pulmonary embolism. Crit Care Med 1995; 23:1481–1485.
73. PIOPED Investigators. Value of the ventilation/perfusion scan in acute pulmonary embolism: results of the Prospective Investigation of Pulmonary Embolism Diagnosis (PIOPED). JAMA 1990; 263:2753–2759.
74. Urokinase Pulmonary Embolism Trial Study Group: Urokinase pulmonary embolism trial. Phase 1 results. JAMA 1970; 214:2163–2172.
75. Dalla-Volta S, Palla A, Santolicandro A, et al. PAIMS 2: Alteplase combined with heparin in the treatment of acute pulmonary embolism. Plasminogen activator Italian multicenter study 2. J Am Coll Cardiol 1992; 20:520–526.
76. Goldhaber SZ, Haire WD, Feldstein ML, et al. Alteplase versus heparin in acute pulmonary embolism: randomized trial assessing right ventricular function and pulmonary perfusion. Lancet 1993; 341:507–511.
77. Jerjes-Sanchez C, Raminoz-Rivera A, Garcia M, et al. Streptokinase and heparin versus heparin alone in massive pulmonary embolism: a randomized, controlled trial. J Thromb Thrombolysis 1995; 2:227–229.
78. Timsit J, Reynaud P, Meyer G, et al. Pulmonary embolectomy by catheter device in massive pulmonary embolism. Chest 1991; 100:655–658.
79. Brown G, Dodek P. An evaluation of empiric vs. nomogram-based dosing of heparin in an intensive care unit. Crit Care Med 1997; 25:1534–1538.
80. Raskhke RA, Reilly BM, Guidry JR, et al. The weight-based heparin dose nomogram compared with a "standard care" nomogram. Am Intera Med 1993; 119:874.
81. Chung HM, Kluge R, Schrier RW, Anderson RJ. Postoperative hyponatremia: a prospective study. Arch Int Med 1986; 146:333–336.
82. Friedman E, Shadel M, Halkin H, Farfer Z. Thiazide-induced hyponatremia. Ann Intern Med 1989; 110:24.
83. Arieff AI. Hyponatremia, convulsions, respiratory arrest and permanent brain damage after elective surgery in healthy women. N Eng J Med 1986; 314:1529.
84. Ayns JC, Krothapalli RK, Arieff AI. Treatment of symptomatic hyponatremia and its relation to brain damage. N Engl J Med 1987; 317:1190.
85. Sterns RH. Severe symptomatic hyponatremia. Treatment and outcome. Ann Intern Med 1987; 107:656.
86. Sovi A, Pepper GM, Wyrwinski PM, et al. Adrenal insufficiency occurring during septic shock: incidence, outcome and relationship to peripheral cytokine levels. Am J Med 1995; 98:266.
87. Baldwin WA, Allo M. Occult hypoadrenalism in critically ill patients. Arch Surg 1993; 128:673.
88. Wartofsky L, Burman KD. Alterations in thyroid function in patients with systemic illness: the "euthyroid sick syndrome." Endocr Rev 1982; 3:164.
89. Barre AE, Gunther B, Hartl W, et al. Altered hormonal activity in severely ill patients after injury or sepsis. Arch Surg 1984; 119:1125.
90. Arem R, Karlsson F, Deppe S. Intravenous levothyroxine therapy does not affect survival in severely ill intensive care unit patients. Thyroidol Clin Exp 1995; 7:79.

10

ARDS: Innovative Therapy

Gordon R. Bernard

Introduction

The search for new therapeutic approaches in ARDS has multiple motivations. First, and foremost, is the persistently high mortality associated with current clinical management which ranges from 35% to 80%. Second, a plethora of mediators have been described, as discussed elsewhere in this text, that may be responsible for or significantly contribute to ARDS. Recently a wide variety of seemingly innocuous agents have been identified and purified that have been shown in vitro or in animal models to be able to block the effects of many of the putative mediators of the syndrome. What follows is a discussion of the pharmacologic agents that have received the most attention for their potential to reduce the incidence, severity, or duration of ARDS.

Surfactant Replacement

When washed clean of surfactant, the alveolar surface of the lung develops a marked increase in surface tension, which causes the lung to become very noncompliant and collapse at low transpulmonary pressure. Surfactant is a naturally occurring complex of phospholipids, neutral lipids, and several specific proteins that is secreted by type II pneumocytes. The clinical model of pure surfactant deficiency is infant respiratory distress syndrome, IRDS. This process is similar to ARDS, but little or no evidence indicates that surfactant abnormalities are fundamentally pathogenetic in ARDS (as they are in IRDS).

The pressure-volume behavior of the diseased lungs with ARDS has been clearly

James A. Russell and Keith R. Walley, eds. *Acute Respiratory Distress Syndrome*. Printed in the United States of America. Copyright © 1999. Cambridge University Press. All rights reserved.

associated with surfactant depletion/dysfunction.[1,2] The surfactant lavaged from ARDS patients functions poorly and is of abnormal composition.[3,4] Native surfactant is impaired by inflammatory substances released by activated granulocytes[5] and is inactivated simply by mixing with pulmonary edema fluid.[6,7] This effect seems to be due to soluble proteins such as fibrin monomers or albumin that accumulate in the alveoli as the normal sieving function of the pulmonary endothelium is lost during acute lung injury.

Surfactant replacement therapy is now part of the everyday clinical management of IRDS after results of several clinical trials established the therapy as beneficial in the neonate. In ARDS there is preclinical evidence of efficacy from surfactant administration to animal models such as acid or bile aspiration, postviral lung injury, hyperoxic injury, vagotomy-induced or lung lavage–induced pulmonary edema. Small, uncontrolled trials of surfactant in human ARDS resulted in transient improvements in lung physiology, and the therapy seems to have been well tolerated.[8-10] Data from a large multicenter, randomized, controlled, prospective trial of inhaled synthetic surfactant have not revealed a survival benefit from the therapy.[11] Whether the dose used was adequate is one potential concern. Routine use of surfactant in ARDS cannot be recommended at this time due to lack of proven efficacy in clinical trials.[11,12]

Nitric Oxide

Nitric oxide (NO) has complex biologic effects but is primarily recognized for its effects as an endothelium-derived relaxing factor/vasodilator intimately involved in regulation of vascular tone. Administration of NO by continuous inhalation reduces vascular pressures in pulmonary hypertension, a regularly observed clinical accompaniment to ARDS. Because high pulmonary vascular pressures and resistance may contribute to the pathophysiology of ARDS, the use of inhaled NO as a pulmonary vasodilator provides an interesting tool to study the effects of reversing these clinical signs. Unlike PGE_1, NO lowers pulmonary pressures without causing systemic hypotension.[13] Its effects when inhaled are local and result in a relatively selective increase in perfusion of well-ventilated lung zones, and thus improve ventilation-perfusion matching. A trial of NO in 10 ARDS patients who served as their own controls showed that inhaled NO at 18 and 36 ppm significantly reduced PAP, reduced intrapulmonary shunting, improved arterial oxygen tension, and allowed the reduction of FiO_2 by around 15%.[14] Importantly, systemic blood pressure was unaffected. Tachyphylaxis to NO was not noted, and the NO doses used were the range of doses given to patients with primary pulmonary hypertension. Results of a recent phase II multicenter study of inhaled NO in ARDS patients demonstrated physiologic effect without evidence of survival benefit.[15] One possible explanation for these results is that death occurs due to multisystem organ failure rather than due to hypoxemia alone.

Another study[16] in a very small number of patients has shown that much lower doses of NO in the 0.060 to 0.230 ppm range can produce significant effects and would presumably have fewer side effects. In fact, these doses of NO are not far different from the observed atmospheric levels of NO, especially in large cities during peak traffic. It is interesting to speculate that mechanical ventilation may exacerbate pulmonary vascular dysfunction due to NO deprivation because wall oxygen and air are free of NO in many, if not most, hospitals.[16]

Another subject of wide discussion has been whether NO might be pathophysiologically involved in other processes including septic shock.[17,18] Endotoxin or cytokines can cause vasodilation and hypotension apparently through a NO mechanism.[19] NO synthase (NOS) inhibitors can increase blood pressure in animal and human septic shock,[20,21] but increased mortality has also been noted in animal studies.[22,23,24] Active study is continuing in this area.

Corticosteroids in the Early Stages of ARDS

Corticosteroids have long been attractive as a group of agents with significant, but well understood, toxicity and the ability to inhibit the production of a wide variety of potent inflammatory mediators, regardless of the source. Drugs in this category have been able to reduce morbidity and mortality in animal models of sepsis and lung injury but generally only if administered prior to the experimental insult.

An early partially prospective trial in the mid-1970s, although not specifically addressing ARDS, implied a survival benefit from corticosteroid therapy in septic patients. However, since that time, data from a number of large, carefully controlled, randomized, prospective trials with corticosteroids have not supported these early results and have failed to demonstrate improvement in survival or in organ function in patients with ARDS (Figures 10.1, 10.2, 10.3) or sepsis.[25–28] Unfortunately, these drugs also do not appear to reduce progression to ARDS among septic patients who are at great risk of developing ARDS.[29] Early administration of steroids may be of benefit in some ARDS-like disorders (*Pneumocystis carinii* pneumonia or prophylactic use in patients at risk for fat embolism syndrome), but their widespread use in ARDS and sepsis cannot be objectively supported.

Corticosteroids in the Late (Fibroproliferative) Stage of ARDS

Although corticosteroids have demonstrated no utility in early but established ARDS (i.e., the first 24 to 72 hours), there has been growing interest in the use of corticosteroids in the so-called late stage of ARDS. After 1 to 2 weeks of persistent ARDS, a subset of patients seems to undergo a fibroproliferative process that can progress to degrees of obliterative scarring of the lungs or cyst formation. It is not exactly clear just how many ARDS patients progress to this stage, but at least three

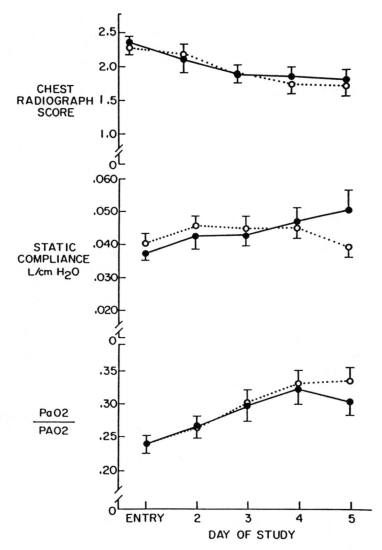

Figure 10.1. Comparison of patients treated with methylprednisolone (___) (n = 50) or placebo (. . . .) (n = 49), according to chest radiograph score (0 denotes normality, 1 mild, 2 moderate, and 3 severe pulmonary edema), effective total thoracic static lung compliance (static compliance), and ratio of arterial to alveolar partial oxygen pressures (PaO_2/PAO_2). There were no significant differences between the methylprednisolone and placebo groups at the time of entry or during the five days immediately following entry (P > 0.05). (Reprinted with permission from Bernard et al. NEJM 1987; 317:1565–1570.)

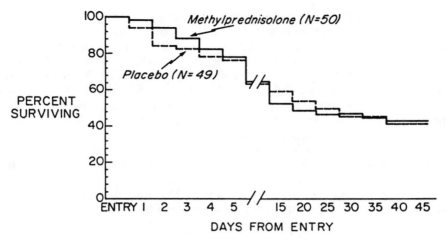

Figure 10.2. Comparison of the survival of patients with ARDS over the first 45 days after entry into the study, according to treatment with methylprednisolone or placebo. There were no significant differences in survival at any time during the 45-day follow-up period (P = 0.77). (Reprinted with permission from Bernard et al. NEJM 1987; 317:1565–1570.)

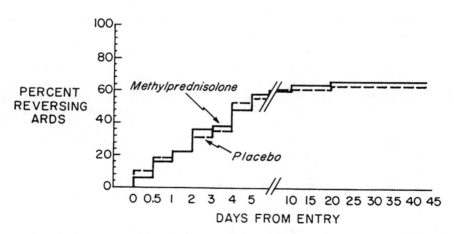

Figure 10.3. Comparison of the percentage of patients in whom ARDS was reversed through reversal of the arterial blood gas criteria alone after treatment with either methylprednisolone (n = 50) or placebo (n = 49). There were no significant differences in the reversal rates between the two groups at any point during the 45-day follow-up period (P = 0.74). (Reprinted with permission from Bernard et al. NEJM 1987; 317:1565–1570.)

uncontrolled studies have examined the use of corticosteroid "rescue" in ARDS patients with persistent respiratory failure and pulmonary fibrosis (e.g.,[30]); these have reported improvement in lung function. In the absence of a prospective, randomized, controlled trial, the true value of this therapy, if any, is difficult to assess. Treatment in the published studies begins generally after some 2 weeks of ARDS. Note that this is a time after which the survival curve in ARDS is fairly flat. Even if a survival bene-fit were not demonstrated by such a study, one could speculate that late corticos-teroid treatment might attenuate the persistent lung abnormalities such as obstruc-tion, restriction, and reduced diffusion capacity that are observed in a subset of ARDS survivors. The severity of pulmonary dysfunction during ARDS (for example, degree of pulmonary hypertension or reduction in lung compliance) may predict abnormal lung function after recovery, but the amount of fibrosis, inflammation, and airspace organization in open lung biopsies from ARDS patients does not appear to correlate with lung function measured 1 year or more after ARDS.[31]

Anti-endotoxin Immunotherapy

Endotoxin infusion in animals can produce physiologic changes similar to sepsis syn-drome and acute lung injury. Various components of endotoxin are humorally immunogenic, and inactivation of endotoxin in vivo by passive immunotherapy has now been extensively investigated. The O-side chain and a toxic core region com-posed of lipid A of gram-negative bacteria are antigenic, but the structure of lipid A is conserved across species and thus cross protection by one antibody against many gram-negative strains is possible in principle.

More than a decade ago, a randomized, controlled trial was published showing that mortality in patients with gram-negative bacteremia was reduced by a human antiserum raised against the J5 strain of *Escherichia coli*.[32] Encouraged by these find-ings, investigators developed two monoclonal anticore IgM antibodies. These were designated HA-1A (a human antibody) and E5 (a murine antibody). Both HA-1A and E5 were used in large, multicenter, randomized, controlled, prospective trials in suspected gram-negative sepsis.[33,34] Each appeared to reduce mortality within a spe-cific subset of patients (those with demonstrable gram-negative bacteremia in the case of HA-1A, those without refractory shock for E5).

For several reasons the conclusions of these studies, that these agents would be use-ful in the treatment of human sepsis, have been called into question.[35,36] First, the util-ity of the two antibodies was questioned on immunologic grounds – it was (and remains) controversial as to whether and under what conditions either product can bind, neutralize, or accelerate the clearance of endotoxin. (In our laboratories, preincu-bation of *E. coli* endotoxin with E5 did not blunt the pulmonary injury induced when the endotoxin was given intravenously to sheep.[37]) Second, the studies were criticized on various methodologic grounds. The E5 trial had shown significant benefit in a rela-tively small subset of the enrolled patients defined retrospectively. In the HA-1A study, imbalances may have occurred in the randomization process, and the primary mortality end point had been extended during the trial from 14 days to 28 days. A follow-up randomized clinical trial of E5 failed to substantiate the benefit seen in the earlier study.[38] A third E5 trial is reportedly in progress. A follow-up randomized clinical trial of HA-1A was terminated due to increased mortality among patients receiving the antibody. In summary, the broad question of the relative benefits of anti-endotoxin therapy remains an open one. The large-scale clinical trials with monoclonal antibodies have failed to demonstrate a role for these specific drugs. Other endotoxin binding or blocking agents with potent neutralizing ability are under investigation.

Cyclooxygenase Inhibitors

As described earlier, animal models of endotoxemia show substantial pulmonary deterioration as one of the physiologic manifestations. Also demonstrable is the massive production of cyclooxygenase-derived eicosanoids as measured in the general circulation and, in much higher concentrations, in lung lymph (interstitial fluid).[39] Eicosanoids such as the cyclooxygenase product thromboxane A_2 (TxA_2), a vasoconstrictor and platelet pro-aggregant, appear to be key mediators. Cyclooxygenase inhibitors such as ibuprofen can attenuate lung injury and reduce pulmonary hypertension and lung lymph flow in sheep even when given after the onset of experimental sepsis.[40] Ibuprofen can also reduce the ARDS-like effect of exogenous tumor necrosis factor in sheep (see section on anticytokine agents later).[41]

Other important cyclooxygenase products include the vasodilators prostaglandin E_2 and prostacyclin ($PG-I_2$), which can attenuate the ovine pulmonary response to endotoxin. Prostaglandin E_2 may also have anti-inflammatory properties. The relative effects of these products versus thromboxane, for example, are not known. An initial phase II randomized, blinded, prospective, pilot study in 30 patients with sepsis showed that ibuprofen was nontoxic, reduced excretion of TxA_2 and prostacyclin degradation products, and reduced fever, tachycardia, and peak airway pressure.[42] The data suggested that shock may have been reversed more rapidly in the treated subjects. A recent multicenter, randomized clinical trial confirmed the observed physiologic effects of the cyclooxygenase inhibitor ibuprofen.[43] In addition, ibuprofen resulted in decreased oxygen consumption and lactic acidosis. However, this trial convincingly demonstrated that ibuprofen does not prevent the development of shock or the development of ARDS and does not improve survival.[43]

Anticytokine Agents

Small mediator proteins produced by a variety of immune cells, principally macrophages and monocytes, termed *cytokines,* are being actively investigated in order to determine their role in sepsis. The best examples of pro-inflammatory cytokines are tumor necrosis factor (TNF) and interleukin-1 (IL-1). These compounds seem to have important functions in host defense in their normally low concentrations, but can be released in large amounts in sepsis. In fact, there is a stereotypical cascading release of these cytokines after endotoxemia with TNF levels increasing 1 to 2 hours after endotoxin, followed by IL-1 and IL-6 a few hours later. TNF seems to be the trigger because data show that blocking TNF levels reduces the subsequent levels of IL-1 and IL-6. Furthermore, when exogenous TNF is infused intravenously, a physiologic response reminiscent of sepsis and ARDS occurs in a wide variety of animal species. IL-1 seems less potent but appears to act synergistically with TNF, and administration of the naturally occurring acute phase reactant termed IL-1 receptor antagonist (IL-1ra) increases survival in experimental sepsis. Large and prolonged elevations of circulating TNF and IL-6 are associated with high mortality in human sepsis; however, the cause-and-effect relationship of IL-6 to morbidity is unclear.[44-46] Sepsis is also associated with release into the circulation of soluble receptors that bind TNF, and administration of exogenous receptors has been observed to improve survival after endotoxemia in animals.

The proximity of cytokine release into the circulation and the severe pathophysiologic responses of sepsis has, as with endotoxin, prompted the development of the hypothesis that neutralization of these cytokines with specific antibodies or interfering with their attachment to cell surface receptors may be of some clinical benefit. However, the potential also exists for such therapy to have adverse effects.

Anti-TNF antibodies, soluble TNF receptors, and exogenous IL-1ra have been the subjects of human trials in sepsis.[47] Initial phase II studies of all of these agents demonstrated safety and suggested significant clinical benefit. Trends toward improved mortality were suggested in several of these studies.[47] However, in subsequent larger trials no benefit in survival has been clearly demonstrated. It is clear that TNF and other cytokines involved in the inflammatory response of ARDS and sepsis play both detrimental and beneficial roles. When these pro-inflammatory cytokines are expressed in high levels in the blood, they initiate and propagate a systemic inflammatory response, contributing substantially to the development of multiple organ failure. In contrast, when expressed locally at the site of infection or other injury, these pro-inflammatory cytokines are essential for the inflammatory response to successfully clear infections and heal injuries. Thus blocking cytokines may impair host defenses or may deprive the organism of low-level exposure to cytokines that induces tolerance to subsequent septic or cytokine-induced insult. Anticytokine therapies are a double-edged sword.

Recombinant IL-1ra appeared to confer an overall survival benefit in an open-label phase II trial,[48] and the effect was more easily demonstrated in patients with particularly high levels of circulating IL-6. This overall benefit was not confirmed in a subsequent large, double-blind multicenter phase III trial.[49] In the second trial, improved survival could be identified but only in a retrospectively defined group of more severely ill patients. A follow-up trial designed to investigate this possible effect prospectively has been halted after interim analysis demonstrated that a survival benefit would be very unlikely upon trial completion.

In spite of the remarkable new understanding of the role of cytokines in sepsis, large trials have yet to prove a consistent benefit from antagonizing the effects of these molecules in sepsis. The potential of these drugs to treat established ARDS is even less clear, and no such studies have been performed to date.

Antioxidants

Very highly reactive metabolites of oxygen usually referred to as free radicals are produced under normal biologic conditions and in significant quantities by activated neutrophils and other inflammatory cells. This process, called respiratory burst, is part of normal host defense against infection. After stimulation by endotoxin or inflammatory mediators such as TNF or interleukins, respiratory burst produces the superoxide radical ($\cdot O_2^-$), which, by a variety of reactions, can result in the generation of the very toxic hydroxyl radical ($\cdot OH$). The superoxide radical $\cdot O_2^-$ can also be transformed by the enzyme superoxide dismutase (SOD) into hydrogen peroxide (H_2O_2), which, in turn, can either oxidize chloride ions to form the antimicrobial substance hypochlorous acid or form OH. Elaborate antioxidant mechanisms involving enzymes (SOD, catalase), sulfhydryl-bearing peptides and proteins (most notably, glutathione), and small molecular weight scavengers (vitamin C, vitamin E, beta-carotene) normally contain these reactions and limit activity to the site of bacterial phagocytosis. However, the oxidant load from the output of the numerous oxidant pathways may overwhelm these defenses and damage surrounding tissues. Evidence that this process is actively occurring in ARDS has been demonstrated by measurement of H_2O_2 concentrations in the exhaled breath of such patients. Studies in this area have shown substantially higher than normal H_2O_2 concentrations in condensates of exhaled breath, supporting the hypothesis of ongoing oxidant stress.[50]

Experimental studies using SOD as rescue therapy for oxidant stress, either alone or in combination with other antioxidants, has had effects ranging from beneficial to harmful. There may be a biochemical explanation for these diverse findings. It is possible that SOD may actually accelerate the production of the deleterious species, $\cdot OH$ or H_2O_2. This process would be especially likely to occur if catalase concentrations in the microenvironment are low and the peroxide is allowed to accumulate. There are fewer data available regarding the utility of catalase, but some studies have shown protective effects in animals. Its utility in clinical situations remains to be tested.

Glutathione is a ubiquitous tripeptide whose cysteine moiety provides reducing potential via its sulfhydryl group.[51] It is interesting to speculate on the role of glutathione in the lung epithelial lining fluid because levels there are the highest in any extracellular fluid of the body. Low levels of glutathione have been noted in epithelial lining fluid, as well as in red blood cells, in patients with ARDS. Although the exact mechanism responsible for this reduction is unknown, speculation centers around increased GSH catabolism due to oxidant stress and reduced cysteine substrate available for regeneration of GSH. Augmentation of glutathione can be accomplished by administration of glutathione itself, or a glutathione derivative (cysteine or cysteine analogue). Glutathione in plasma does not enter cells readily in intact form; it must be dismantled into its constitutive amino acids for incorporation into cells. Cysteine, if administered as the free amino acid, is toxic if given in large amounts. The cysteine analogue oxothiazolidine carboxylate (OTC, Procysteine), is cell permeable, metabolized intracellularly into cysteine via the intermediate S-carboxy-L-cysteine, and non-toxic even in large quantities in humans. This agent may be very useful as a GSH repleting agent.[52]

Use of N-acetylcysteine (NAC) to increase hepatic glutathione stores as part of the treatment of human acetaminophen toxicity has lent credence to the notion that such therapy might be useful in ARDS. NAC has been shown to reduce endotoxin- and hyperoxia-induced lung injury in animals. One study in ARDS patients[52] showed that NAC and OTC increased red cell glutathione from approximately 50% of normal to within the normal range over several days of treatment. These agents also improved static lung compliance and chest x-ray appearance. These agents reduced the number of days of acute lung injury and increased cardiac index, but, in this small study, there was no difference in mortality.[52] NAC has also been observed in preliminary reports to reduce TNF levels in ARDS patients.

Platelet-Activating Factor Antagonists

Platelet-activating factor (PAF), as the name implies, promotes platelet activation but has now been recognized to also activate granulocytes, cause leakiness of blood vessels, and induce bronchoconstriction. PAF is a lipid derived from the membrane phospholipids of a variety of cells. Intravenous infusions of PAF in sheep cause physiologic abnormalities similar to those caused by intravenous endotoxin.[53] Receptor antagonists isolated from animal material or produced synthetically have been employed in studies to determine the effects on the inflammatory response. In animal models of sepsis, improvements in pulmonary abnormalities and survival have been demonstrated.[54,55] A large prospective trial of a PAF antagonist (BN 52021) has recently been completed in a population of patients with sepsis. There was a suggestion of benefit for those patients with documented gram-negative infection as opposed to gram-positive or other infections, and the treated patients appeared to have more rapid resolution of multisystem organ failure.[56]

Eicosanoids

Prostaglandin E_1 (PGE_1) is a synthetic lipid mediator similar to endogenously produced PGE_2. Both compounds have similar vascular and anti-inflammatory actions. PGE_1 improves gas exchange, pulmonary hypertension, and lung edema accumulation in animal models of acute lung injury. In clinical ARDS, PGE_1 actually lowers pulmonary arterial pressures but, in some cases, also lowers arterial oxygen tension.[57,58] In addition, PGE_1 frequently produces a fall in vascular resistance, an increase in cardiac output, and an increase in oxygen delivery. Although these features are not always desirable in ARDS, they suggest the drug may have clinical utility under certain circumstances.

Large-scale trials have been conducted in humans using PGE_1 as interventional therapy. The first prospective trial was in surgical ARDS patients, and the results suggested a survival benefit at 30 days that was no longer significant at 75 days.[59] A more recent prospective multicenter trial in a mix of medical and surgical ARDS patients revealed no survival benefit.[60]

As might have been predicted from the preclinical animal data, side effects included hypotension, fever, and arrhythmias. There were also the anticipated effects on cardiac index and oxygen delivery.[61] These data are not strong enough to support a recommendation for routine use of the drug in ARDS.

To avoid some of these side effects, one clinical trial has tested the use of prostaglandin E_1 encapsulated in artificial liposomes in 17 patients with ARDS compared to 8 patients given placebo.[62] Drug-related adverse events were reported twice as frequently in the liposomal PGE_1 group compared to placebo. Liposomal PGE_1 resulted in improved PaO_2/FiO_2 and lung compliance and earlier liberation from mechanical ventilation. At 28 days 1 of 17 patients in the liposomal PGE_1 group died; 2 of 8 patients in the placebo group died.[62]

Inhaled prostacyclin I_2 has been used as a selective pulmonary vasodilator in ARDS patients.[63-65] Inhaled PGI_2 results in improved PaO_2/FiO_2 ratios and improves pulmonary shunt, similar to inhaled NO. Like inhaled NO, improved gas exchange during PGI_2 inhalation appears to be due to selective pulmonary vasodilation and redistribution of blood flow from shunt areas to well-ventilated regions.[63-65]

Ketoconazole is a thromboxane synthetase inhibitor that decreases thromboxane A_2 concentrations in ARDS patients.[66] Leukotriene B_4 and thromboxane A_2 production by alveolar macrophages are decreased by ketoconazole.[67] An early report suggested that ketoconazole may prevent the development of ARDS in critically ill surgical patients (6% in ketoconazole group compared to 31% in placebo group) and decrease mortality.[68] A subsequent randomized prospective clinical trial of ketoconazole was conducted in septic patients at risk of developing ARDS.[69] ARDS occurred in 15% of the patients randomized to receive ketoconazole compared to 64% of the patients randomized to receive placebo. This reduction was statistically significant as was the reduction in mortality, although there was no significant difference in ventilator or ICU days.[69]

Pentoxifylline

The phosphodiesterase (PDE) inhibitor pentoxifylline, a methylxanthine derivative, has been in clinical use in humans for several years as a promoter of improved perfusion in chronic peripheral vascular disease. This agent also is an adenosine receptor antagonist and possesses anti-inflammatory properties. It reduces the responsiveness of granulocytes to stimulation by endotoxin and cytokines and granulocyte oxidative burst. Mouse survival in septic shock was increased when the drug was given even 4 hours after the initial insult,[70] although some studies show less impressive effects.[71]

Pentoxifylline does not block the fever or the hyperdynamic cardiovascular responses in human volunteers given experimental endotoxin infusion.[72,73] A small study in ARDS patients has been performed in which substantial doses of pentoxifylline administered over a short period seemed to be safe.[73,74] No immediate physiologic benefits were apparent, and use of pentoxifylline in ARDS is not recommended at this time.

Antiproteases

Inflammatory cells release proteolytic enzymes when stimulated. These enzymes are capable of digesting elastin, collagen, and other structural and humoral proteins essential to homeostasis. The levels and activity of proteases, especially serine proteases, such as neutrophil elastase, have been described in bronchoalveolar lavage fluid (BALF) from ARDS patients.[75–80] Actual proteolytic activity, however, was not usually elevated. This is presumably due to the wide variety of antiproteases present in the alveolar milieu. BALF elastase activity and the urinary elastin fragment, desmosine, are associated with the development of ARDS among high-risk patients.[78,81]

The enhancement of antiprotease activity in ARDS is an attractive intervention to contemplate as a potential treatment for ARDS. Animal studies have shown that exogenous antiproteases can blunt lung injury, and exogenous alpha-1-antiprotease (alpha$_1$AP) is well tolerated by patients in its current use for hereditary alpha$_1$AP deficiency. Increasing endogenous alpha$_1$AP levels via gene therapy, a therapy which is under current study, may also eventually be shown to be useful. A limitation of the use of alpha$_1$AP is that it is a large molecule and thus it may not gain access to the microenvironment between activated inflammatory cells and adjacent structures. Small molecules with otherwise similar properties exist, and at least one of these has been observed to reduce endotoxin-induced lung injury in sheep.[82] Clinical trials of small molecular weight antielastases are now being initiated.

Summary

Despite an explosion in the level of understanding of molecular and cellular processes in the pathogenesis and perpetuation of acute lung injury, no therapy has been proven beneficial in patients with ARDS. However, all is not lost because the research efforts expended thus far have produced a better understanding of the clinical illness along with better means to study it in all of its complexity and heterogeneity.[83–90] Many of the agents listed have not had the opportunity to be tested in large-scale trials where these latter aspects of ARDS can be dealt with. Some of the previously studied drugs not useful in all patients may yet prove useful in carefully selected subsets of patients. Of course, this limits their utility. Perhaps effective therapy will require combinations of pathway-specific agents, which will be very complex to study, or entirely new approaches to drug and oxygen delivery.[91] For now, it seems most prudent for clinicians to await further trials of new agents while continuing to strive for safer and more effective supportive care of ARDS victims.

Supported by NIH Grant HL43167, "Cardiopulmonary Effects of Ibuprofen in Human Sepsis"; NIH Grant HL19153, "Specialized Center of Research in Acute Lung Injury"; and the Bernard Werthan, Sr., Fund for Pulmonary Research.

References

1. Petty TL, Reiss OK, Paul GW, Silvers GW, Elkins ND. Characteristics of pulmonary surfactant in adult respiratory distress syndrome associated with trauma and shock. Am Rev Respir Dis 1977; 115:531–536.
2. Petty TL, Silvers GW, Paul GW, Stanford RE. Abnormalities in lung elastic properties and surfactant function in adult respiratory distress syndrome. Chest 1979; 75:571–574.
3. Hallman M, Spragg R, Harrell JH, Moser KM, Gluck L. Evidence of lung surfactant abnormality in respiratory failure. Study of bronchoalveolar lavage phospholipids, surface activity, phospholipase activity, and plasma myoinositol. J Clin Invest 1982; 70:673–683.
4. Gregory TJ, Longmore WJ, Moxley MA, et al. Surfactant chemical composition and biophysical activity in acute respiratory distress syndrome. J Clin Invest 1991; 88:1976–1981.
5. Ryan SF, Ghassibi Y, Liau DF. Effects of activated polymorphonuclear leukocytes upon pulmonary surfactant in vitro. Am J Respir Cell Mol Biol 1991; 4:33–41.
6. Seeger W, Stohr G, Wolf HR, Neuhof H. Alteration of surfactant function due to protein leakage: special interaction with fibrin monomer. J Appl Physiol 1985; 58:326–338.
7. Kobayashi T, Nitta K, Ganzuka M, Inui S, Grossmann G, Robertson B. Inactivation of exogenous surfactant by pulmonary edema fluid. Pediatr Res 1991; 29:353–356.
8. Spragg RG, Gilliard N, Richman P, et al. Acute effects of a single dose of porcine surfactant on patients with the adult respiratory distress syndrome. Chest 1994; 105:195–202.
9. Heikinheimo M, Hynynen M, Rautiainen P, Andersson S, Hallman M, Kukkonen S. Successful treatment of ARDS with two doses of synthetic surfactant. Chest 1994; 105:1263–1264.
10. Weg JG, Balk RA, Tharratt RS, Jenkinson SG, Shah JB, Zaccardelli D, Horton J, Pattishall EN. Safety and potential efficacy of an aerosolized surfactant in human sepsis-induced adult respiratory distress syndrome. JAMA. 1994; 272:1433–1438.
11. Anzueto A, Baughman RP, Guntupalli KK, Weg JG, Wiedemann HP, Raventos AA, Lemaire F, Long W, Zaccardelli DS, Pattishall EN. Aerosolized surfactant in adults with sepsis-induced acute respiratory distress syndrome. Exosurf Acute Respiratory Distress Syndrome Sepsis Study Group. N Engl J Med 1996; 334:1417–1421.
12. Gregory GA, Phibbs RH. Surfactant replacement for respiratory failure: lessons from the neonate. Anesth Analg 1993; 76:465–466.

13. Frostell CG, Blomqvist H, Hedenstierna G, Lundberg J, Zapol WM. Inhaled nitric oxide selectively reverses human hypoxic pulmonary vasoconstriction without causing systemic vasodilation. Anesthesiology 1993; 78:427–435.
14. Rossaint R, Falke KJ, Lopez F, Slama K, Pison U, Zapol WM. Inhaled nitric oxide for the adult respiratory distress syndrome. N Engl J Med 1993; 328:399–405.
15. Dellinger RP, Zimmerman JL, Taylor RW, Straube RC, Hauser DL, Criner GJ, Davis K Jr, Hyers TM, Papadakos P. Effects of inhaled nitric oxide in patients with acute respiratory distress syndrome: results of a randomized phase II trial. Inhaled Nitric Oxide in ARDS Study Group. Crit Care Med 1998; 26:15–23.
16. Gerlach H, Pappert D, Lewandowski K, Rossaint R, Falke KJ. Long-term inhalation with evaluated low doses of nitric oxide for selective improvement of oxygenation in patients with adult respiratory distress syndrome. Intensive Care Med 1993; 19:443–449.
17. Wink DA, Hanbauer I, Krishna MC, DeGraff W, Gamson J, Mitchell JB. Nitric oxide protects against cellular damage and cytotoxicity from reactive oxygen species. Proc Natl Acad Sci USA 1993; 90:9813–9817.
18. Kilbourn RG, Griffith OW. Overproduction of nitric oxide in cytokine-mediated and septic shock. J Natl Cancer Inst 1992; 84:827–831.
19. Evans T, Carpenter A, Kinderman H, Cohen J. Evidence of increased nitric oxide production in patients with the sepsis syndrome. Circ Shock 1993; 41:77–81.
20. Kilbourn RG, Jubran A, Gross SS, et al. Reversal of endotoxin-mediated shock by NG-methyl-L-arginine, an inhibitor of nitric oxide synthesis. Biochem Biophys Res Commun 1990; 172:1132–1138.
21. Petros A, Lamb G, Leone A, Moncada S, Bennett D, Vallance P. Effects of a nitric oxide synthase inhibitor in humans with septic shock. Cardiovasc Res 1994; 28:34–39.
22. Minnard EA, Shou J, Naama H, Cech A, Gallagher H, Daly JM. Inhibition of nitric oxide synthesis is detrimental during endotoxemia. Arch Surg 1994; 129:142–147; discussion 147–148.
23. Pastor C, Teisseire B, Vicaut E, Payen D. Effects of L-arginine and L-nitro-arginine treatment on blood pressure and cardiac output in a rabbit endotoxin shock model. Crit Care Med 1994; 22:465–469.
24. Nava E, Palmer RM, Moncada S. The role of nitric oxide in endotoxic shock: effects of NG-monomethyl-L-arginine. J Cardiovasc Pharmacol 1992; 20 Suppl 12:S132–S134.
25. Bernard GR, Luce JM, Sprung CL, et al. High-dose corticosteroids in patients with the adult respiratory distress syndrome. N Engl J Med 1987; 317:1565–1570.
26. Sprung CL, Caralis PV, Marcial EH, et al. The effects of high-dose corticosteroids in patients with septic shock. A prospective, controlled study. N Engl J Med 1984; 311:1137–1143.
27. Anonymous. Effect of high-dose glucocorticoid therapy on mortality in patients with clinical signs of systemic sepsis. The Veterans Administration Systemic Sepsis Cooperative Study Group. N Engl J Med 1987; 317:659–665.
28. Bone RC, Fisher CJ Jr, Clemmer TP, Slotman GJ, Metz CA, Balk RA. A controlled clinical trial of high-dose methylprednisolone in the treatment of severe sepsis and septic shock. N Engl J Med 1987; 317:653–658.
29. Luce JM, Montgomery AB, Marks JD, Turner J, Metz CA, Murray JF. Ineffectiveness of high-dose methylprednisolone in preventing parenchymal lung injury and improving mortality in patients with septic shock. Am Rev Respir Dis 1988; 138:62–68.
30. Meduri GU, Chinn AJ, Leeper KV, et al. Corticosteroid rescue treatment of progressive

fibroproliferation in late ARDS: patterns of response and predictors of outcome. Chest 1994; 105:1516–1527.

31. Suchyta MR, Elliott CG, Colby T, Rasmusson BY, Morris AH, Jensen RL. Open lung biopsy does not correlate with pulmonary function after the adult respiratory distress syndrome. Chest 1991; 99:1232–1237.

32. Ziegler EJ, McCutchan JA, Fierer J, et al. Treatment of gram-negative bacteremia and shock with human antiserum to a mutant Escherichia coli. N Engl J Med 1982; 307:1225–1230.

33. Ziegler EJ, Fisher CJ Jr, Sprung CL, et al. Treatment of gram-negative bacteremia and septic shock with HA-1A human monoclonal antibody against endotoxin. A randomized, double-blind, placebo-controlled trial. The HA-1A Sepsis Study Group. N Engl J Med 1991; 324:429–436.

34. Greenman RL, Schein RM, Martin MA, et al. A controlled clinical trial of E5 murine monoclonal IgM antibody to endotoxin in the treatment of gram-negative sepsis. The XOMA Sepsis Study Group. JAMA 1991; 266(8):1097–1102.

35. Natanson C, Hoffman WD, Suffredini AF, Eichacker PQ, Danner RL. Selected treatment strategies for septic shock based on proposed mechanisms of pathogenesis. Ann Intern Med 1994; 120:771–783.

36. Glauser MP, Heumann D, Baumgartner JD, Cohen J. Pathogenesis and potential strategies for prevention and treatment of septic shock: an update. Clin Infect Dis 1994; 18 Suppl 2:S205–S216.

37. Wheeler AP, Hardie WD, Bernard G. Studies of an antiendotoxin antibody in preventing the physiologic changes of endotoxemia in awake sheep. Am Rev Respir Dis 1990; 142:775–781.

38. Bone RC, et al. A second large controlled clinical study of E5, a monoclonal antibody to endotoxin: result of a prospective, multicenter, randomized, controlled trial. Crit Care Med 1995; 23(6):99–1005.

39. Brigham KL, Meyrick B. Endotoxin and lung injury. Am Rev Respir Dis 1986; 133:913–927.

40. Gnidec AG, Sibbald WJ, Cheung H, Metz CA. Ibuprofen reduces the progression of permeability edema in an animal model of hyperdynamic sepsis. J Appl Physiol 1988; 65:1024–1032.

41. Wheeler AP, Hardie WD, Bernard GR. The role of cyclooxygenase products in lung injury induced by tumor necrosis factor in sheep. Am Rev Respir Dis 1992; 145:632–639.

42. Bernard GR, Reines HD, Halushka PV, et al. Prostacyclin and thromboxane A2 formation is increased in human sepsis syndrome. Effects of cyclooxygenase inhibition. Am Rev Respir Dis 1991; 144:1095–1101.

43. Bernard GR, Wheeler AP, Russell JA, Schein R, Summer WR, Steinberg KP, Fulkerson WJ, Wright PE, Christman BW, Dupont WD, Higgins SB, Swindell BB. The effects of ibuprofen on the physiology and survival of patients with sepsis. The Ibuprofen in Sepsis Study Group. N Engl J Med 1997; 336:912–918.

44. Debets JMH, Kampmeijer R, van der Linden MPMH, Buurman WA, van der Linden CJ. Plasma tumor necrosis factor and mortality in critically ill septic patients. Crit Care Med 1989; 17:489–494.

45. Casey LC, Balk RA, Bone RC. Plasma cytokine and endotoxin levels correlate with survival in patients with the sepsis syndrome. Ann Intern Med 1993; 119:771–778.

46. Pinsky MR, Vincent JL, Deviere J, Alegre M, Kahn RJ, Dupont E. Serum cytokine levels in human septic shock. Relation to multiple-system organ failure and mortality. Chest 1993; 103:565–575.

47. Zeni F, Freeman B, Natanson C. Anti-inflammatory therapies to treat sepsis and septic shock: a reassessment. Crit Care Med 1997; 25:1095–1100.

48. Fisher CJ Jr, Slotman GJ, Opal SM, et al. Initial evaluation of human recombinant inter-leukin-1 receptor antagonist in the treatment of sepsis syndrome: a randomized, open-label, placebo-controlled multicenter trial. The IL-1RA Sepsis Syndrome Study Group. Crit Care Med 1994; 22:12–21.

49. Fisher CJJ, Dhainaut JFA, Opal SM, et al. Recombinant human interleukin-1 receptor antagonist in the treatment of patients with sepsis syndrome: results from a randomized, double-blind, placebo-controlled trial. JAMA 1994; 271:1836–1843.

50. Kietzmann D, Kahl R, Muller M, Buchardi H, Kettler D. Hydrogen peroxide in expired breath condensate of patients with acute respiratory failure and with ARDS. Intensive Care Med 1993; 19:78–81.

51. Morris PE, Bernard GR. Significance of glutathione in lung disease and implications for therapy. Am J Med Sci 1994; 307:119–127.

52. Bernard GR, Wheeler AP, Arons MM, Morris PE, Paz HL, Russell JA, Wright PE. A trial of antioxidants N-acetylcysteine and procysteine in ARDS. The Antioxidant in ARDS Study Group. Chest 1997; 112:164–172.

53. Christman BW, Lefferts PL, King GA, Snapper JR. Role of circulating platelets and granu-locytes in PAF-induced pulmonary dysfunction in awake sheep. J Appl Physiol 1988; 64:2033–2041.

54. Christman BW, Lefferts PL, Blair IA, Snapper JR. Effect of platelet-activating factor receptor antagonism on endotoxin-induced lung dysfunction in awake sheep. Am Rev Respir Dis 1990; 142:1272–1278.

55. Olson NC, Joyce PB, Fleisher LN. Role of platelet-activating factor and eicosanoids dur-ing endotoxin-induced lung injury in pigs. Am J Physiol 1990; 258:H1674–1686.

56. Dhainaut JF, Tenaillon A, Letulzo Y, et al. Platelet activating factor receptor antagonist BN 52021 in the treatment of severe sepsis: a randomized, double-blind, placebo-con-trolled, multi-center, clinical trial. Crit Care Med 1994; 22:1720–1728.

57. Radermacher P, Santak B, Becker H, Falke KJ. Prostaglandin E1 and nitroglycerin reduce pulmonary capillary pressure but worsen ventilation-perfusion distributions in patients with adult respiratory distress syndrome. Anesthesiology 1989; 70:601–606.

58. Melot C, Lejeune P, Leeman M, Moraine JJ, Naeije R. Prostaglandin E1 in the adult respi-ratory distress syndrome. Benefit for pulmonary hypertension and cost for pulmonary gas exchange. Am Rev Respir Dis 1989; 139:106–110.

59. Holcroft JW, Vassar MJ, Weber CJ. Prostaglandin E1 and survival in patients with the adult respiratory distress syndrome. A prospective trial. Ann Surg 1986; 203:371–378.

60. Bone RC, Slotman G, Maunder R, et al. Randomized double-blind, multicenter study of prostaglandin E1 in patients with the adult respiratory distress syndrome. Prostaglandin E1 Study Group. Chest 1989; 96:114–119.

61. Slotman GJ, Kerstein MD, Bone RC, et al. The effects of prostaglandin E1 on non-pul-monary organ function during clinical acute respiratory failure. The Prostaglandin E1 Study Group. J Trauma 1992; 32:480–488; discussion 488–489.

62. Abraham E, Park YC, Covington P, Conrad SA, Schwartz M. Liposomal prostaglandin E1

in acute respiratory distress syndrome: a placebo-controlled, randomized, double-blind, multicenter clinical trial. Crit Care Med 1996; 24:10–15.

63. Van Heerden PV, Blythe D, Webb SA. Inhaled aerosolized prostacyclin and nitric oxide as selective pulmonary vasodilators in ARDS – a pilot study. Anaesth Intensive Care 1996; 24:564–568.

64. Zwissler B, Kemming G, Habler O, Kleen M, Merkel M, Haller M, Briegel J, Welte M, Peter K. Inhaled prostacyclin (PGI2) versus inhaled nitric oxide in adult respiratory distress syndrome. Am J Respir Crit Care Med 1996; 154:1671–1677.

65. Walmrath D, Schneider T, Schermuly R, Olschewski H, Grimminger F, Seeger W. Direct comparison of inhaled nitric oxide and aerosolized prostacyclin in acute respiratory distress syndrome. Am J Respir Crit Care Med 1996; 153:991–996.

66. Frazee LA, Neidig JA. Ketoconazole to prevent acute respiratory distress syndrome in critically ill patients. Ann Pharmacotherapy 1995; 29:784–786.

67. Williams JG, Maier RV. Ketoconazole inhibits alveolar macrophage production of inflammatory mediators involved in acute lung injury (adult respiratory distress syndrome). Surgery 1992; 112: 270–277.

68. Slotman GJ, Burchard KW, D'Arezzo A, Gann DS. Ketoconazole prevents acute respiratory failure in critically ill surgical patients. J Trauma 1988; 28:648–654.

69. Yu M, Tomasa G. A double-blind, prospective, randomized trial of ketoconazole, a thromboxane synthetase inhibitor, in the prophylaxis of the adult respiratory distress syndrome. Crit Care Med 1993; 21:1635–1642.

70. Schade UF. Pentoxifylline increases survival in murine endotoxin shock and decreases formation of tumor necrosis factor. Circ Shock 1990; 31:171–181.

71. Sigurdsson GH, Youssef H. Effects of pentoxifylline on hemodynamics, gas exchange and multiple organ platelet sequestration in experimental endotoxic shock. Acta Anaesthesiol Scand 1993; 37:396–403.

72. Zabel P, Wolter DT, Schonharting MM, Schade UF. Oxpentifylline in endotoxaemia. Lancet 1989; 2:1474–1477.

73. Martich GD, Parker MM, Cunnion RE, Suffredini AF. Effects of ibuprofen and pentoxifylline on the cardiovascular response of normal humans to endotoxin. J Appl Physiol 1992; 73:925–931.

74. Montravers P, Fagon JY, Gilbert C, Blanchet F, Novara A, Chastre J. Pilot study of cardiopulmonary risk from pentoxifylline in adult respiratory distress syndrome. Chest 1993; 103:1017–1022.

75. Lee CT, Fein AM, Lippmann M, Holtzman H, Kimbel P, Weinbaum G. Elastolytic activity in pulmonary lavage fluid from patients with adult respiratory-distress syndrome. N Engl J Med 1981; 304:192–196.

76. McGuire WW, Spragg RG, Cohen AB, Cochrane CG. Studies on the pathogenesis of the adult respiratory distress syndrome. J Clin Invest 1982; 69:543–553.

77. Suter PM, Suter S, Girardin E, Roux-Lombard P, Grau GE, Dayer JM. High bronchoalveolar levels of tumor necrosis factor and its inhibitors, interleukin-1, interferon, and elastase, in patients with adult respiratory distress syndrome after trauma, shock, or sepsis. Am Rev Respir Dis 1992; 145:1016–1022.

78. Idell S, Kucich U, Fein A, et al. Neutrophil elastase-releasing factors in bronchoalveolar lavage from patients with adult respiratory distress syndrome. Am Rev Respir Dis 1985; 132:1098–1105.

79. Weiland JE, Davis WB, Holter JF, Mohammed JR, Dorinsky PM, Gadek JE. Lung neutrophils in the adult respiratory distress syndrome. Clinical and pathophysiologic significance. Am Rev Respir Dis 1986; 133:218–225.

80. Wewers MD, Herzyk DJ, Gadek JE. Alveolar fluid neutrophil elastase activity in the adult respiratory distress syndrome is complexed to alpha-2-macroglobulin. J Clin Invest 1988; 82:1260–1267.

81. Tenholder MF, Rajagopal KR, Phillips YY, et al. Urinary desmosine excretion as a marker of lung injury in the adult respiratory distress syndrome. Chest 1991; 100:1385–1390.

82. Gossage JR, Kuratomi Y, Davidson JM, Lefferts PL, Snapper JR. Neutrophil elastase inhibitors, SC-37698 and SC-39026, reduce endotoxin-induced lung dysfunction in awake sheep. Am Rev Respir Dis 1993; 147:1371–1379.

83. Rinaldo JE. The adult respiratory distress syndrome. In Current pulmonology (Vol. 15), ed DF Tierney, Mosby-Year Book, St. Louis, 1994, pp. 137–156.

84. Anonymous. American College of Chest Physicians/Society of Critical Care Medicine Consensus Conference: definitions for sepsis and organ failure and guidelines for the use of innovative therapies in sepsis. Crit Care Med 1992; 20:864–874.

85. Pepe PE, Potkin RT, Reus DH, Hudson LD, Carrico CJ. Clinical predictors of the adult respiratory distress syndrome. Am J Surg 1982; 144:124–130.

86. Fowler AA, Hamman RF, Good JT, et al. Adult respiratory distress syndrome: risk with common predispositions. Ann Intern Med 1983; 98:593–597.

87. Wheeler AP, Swindell B, Carroll F, et al. The lung in sepsis: data from the ibuprofen human sepsis multicenter trial. Chest 1993; 104:56S [Abstract].

88. Fein AM, Lippmann M, Holtzman H, Eliraz A, Goldberg SK. The risk factors, incidence, and prognosis of ARDS following septicemia. Chest 1983; 83:40–42.

89. Bernard GR, Artigas A, Brigham KL, et al. The American-European Consensus Conference on ARDS. Definitions, mechanisms, relevant outcomes, and clinical trial coordination. Am J Respir Crit Care Med 1994; 149:818–824.

90. Weiss SM, Hudson LD. Outcome from respiratory failure. Crit Care Clin 1994; 10:197–215.

91. Bartlett RH, Hirschl RB. Liquid ventilation in ARDS. Acta Anaesthesiologica Scandinavica. Suppl 1997; 111: 68–69.

11

Nosocomial Pneumonia in ARDS

Ahmed Bahammam and R. Bruce Light

Introduction

Pneumonia is the most common infectious complication of ARDS, with published occurrence rates ranging from 15% to 70% during the period of endotracheal intubation for respiratory support.[1-3] This highly variable incidence of nosocomial pneumonia in ARDS likely relates to variability in the physician's awareness of the problem, diagnostic criteria and use of antibiotics, as well as to differences in patient population and nursing and infection control standards. An important cause of intensive care morbidity, it has also become increasingly clear that pneumonia in ARDS is strongly associated with mortality.[4] Of nosocomial infections, it has long been established that pneumonia is the leading cause of excess mortality, and in ARDS patients in particular it has been reported that patients developing pneumonia have mortality rates nearly triple that of those who do not. Although it may be that this association of nosocomial pneumonia with poor prognosis is not causal in nature, it nevertheless has led to speculation that nosocomial pneumonia is a major cause of sepsis, multiple organ system failure, and death in patients surviving acute illness precipitating ARDS. Limiting the effect of nosocomial pneumonia on outcome in ARDS requires careful attention to the principles of infection control for prevention, vigilance in diagnosis of the infection when it occurs, and appropriate antimicrobial therapy. All three of these aspects of management of pneumonia in ARDS patients involve elements of controversy. We point these out in this chapter even as we outline suggested approaches that we believe are practical without being simplistic.

Microbiology

In mechanically ventilated patients with and without ARDS, the most frequently isolated pathogens causing nosocomial pneumonia are the aerobic and facultatively anaerobic gram-negative bacilli. Although comprising 40% to 60% of all pneumonias in ventilated patients, the distribution of gram-negative species in different units is highly variable. *Staphylococcus aureus,* although seen less often now than in the past, is still a common cause of nosocomial pneumonia, together with other gram-positive bacteria accounting for about 30% of recovered isolates. Anaerobic bacteria do not appear to play a very significant role in ventilator-associated pneumonia in ARDS patients.

In recent years many ICUs have witnessed the emergence of nosocomially transmitted strains of more antimicrobial resistant gram-negative organisms as important causes of pneumonia. In many ICUs *Pseudomonas aeroginosa* is the most common pathogen. This hardy organism is a strictly aerobic, nonfermentative gram-negative bacillus, which requires minimal growth factors and is able to survive in both distilled water and in many antiseptic solutions. In the hospital environment, it has been identified in respiratory therapy equipment, disinfectants, sinks, mops, and flowers. Acinetobacter spp., nonfermenting gram-negative bacilli commonly found in soil and water, on latex gloves, and on human skin, have also become significant pathogens in some centers. Important sources of this bacterium include respiratory equipment, room air humidifiers, and intravenous catheters. Another organism seen with increasing frequency in ICU practice is *Stenotrophomonas maltophilia.* Few data are available describing the risk factors for acquisition and infection with this organism, but it seems that respiratory equipment and hands of the intensive care personnel, as with other resistant gram negatives, are the most important routes of transmission.

Some evidence suggests that infections which are polymicrobial and those which involve organisms such as Pseudomonas spp. and Acinetobacter spp., which are likely to be both hospital acquired and relatively resistant to antimicrobials, are associated with higher mortality rates than infections due to endogenous microflora such as *Staphylococcus aureus* and Enterobacteriaceae.[5] Although it seems likely that this is related at least in part to greater intrinsic pathogenicity and antimicrobial resistance of these organisms, it is also true that there is a greater probability of their occurrence in more severe and protracted illness.

Pathogenesis

Patients with ARDS are at increased risk for developing pneumonia for four general reasons: increased access of potentially pathogenic organisms to the lower respiratory tract; impairment of normal respiratory host defenses; associated medical conditions; and the presence of invasive devices needed for intensive respiratory support. The routes by which organisms can gain access to the lower respiratory tract are hematogenous spread, inhalation from ambient air, exogenous penetration, and aspi-

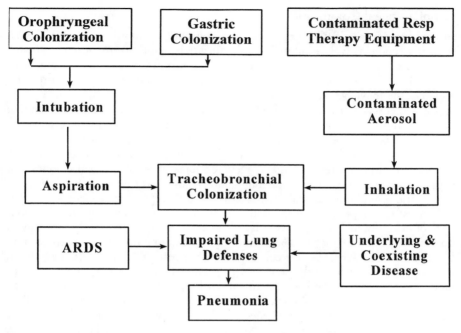

Figure 11.1. Pathogenesis of nosocomial pneumonia in ARDS.

ration. Of these, aspiration is by far the most important in the genesis of nosocomial pneumonia (Figure 11.1). Substantially less frequently, organisms reach the lung as aerosols generated by contaminated respiratory therapy equipment; hematogenous spread of organisms to the lung is probably uncommon in this setting. However, even after potentially virulent organisms are present in the lower respiratory tract, the development of clinical pneumonia generally implies abnormality of respiratory host defenses. It is known that a majority of healthy adults aspirate to some degree during sleep, but because of the efficiency of an array of host defenses, pneumonia occurs only infrequently. As we shall see, some or all of these protective mechanisms are impaired to some extent in patients with ARDS.

Microbial Colonization

Although in some cases of acute nosocomial pneumonia colonization of the tracheo-bronchial tree prior to the onset of apparent active infection cannot be demonstrated, more often colonization precedes infection.[3] Potential sources of lower respiratory tract colonizers include oropharyngeal and upper gastrointestinal tract colonization and direct contamination of the endotracheal tube itself from caregivers or respiratory therapy equipment.

Oropharyngeal Colonization

In healthy individuals, the oropharynx is colonized by a mostly anaerobic normal flora that competitively inhibits local colonization by other organisms of greater pathogenic potential. In addition, the nose, pharynx, and larynx subserve a mechanical barrier function and provide mucociliary clearance of particulate matter and microbes that have been deposited within the upper respiratory tract, aided by upper airway secretions which contain bactericidal enzymes, IgA, and lactoferrin limiting bacterial replication. Enteric gram-negative bacilli are normally absent in the oropharynx because of the efficacy of these mechanisms, and *Staphyococcus aureus* colonization is limited to the anterior nares. Hospitalized patients in general and ICU patients in particular have markedly elevated rates of oropharyngeal colonization with enteric gram negatives, a phenomenon strongly associated with presence of nasogastric or endotracheal tubes, increasing severity of the illness, longer duration of hospitalization, prior or concomitant use of antibiotics, and advanced age. About 25% of critically mechanically ventilated patients are colonized by the first day of hospitalization, and 40% to 60% become colonized during the first week thereafter.[6] In most cases the source of this colonization is the patient's own enteric microflora; however, in 15% or more the source is exogenous, from respiratory therapy equipment or the hands of personnel.[7] In establishing colonization, bacteria bind to mucosal epithelial cells, adhering to cell receptors via surface appendages called adhesins. This process has been likened to a lock-in-key interaction and is relatively irreversible and organism specific.[8] One factor that may play an important role in protecting the airway from adherence by gram negatives is the glycoprotein fibronectin. Although this glycoprotein is a receptor for gram-positive bacteria binding, it appears to cover airway receptors for gram-negative bacteria and its removal unmasks these receptors. Some organisms have the capacity to degrade fibronectin, which could expose potential bacterial binding sites.

Gastric Colonization

The role of the upper gastrointestinal tract as a source of oropharyngeal and tracheal colonization with enteric gram negatives is controversial. That colonization of the stomach with potential pathogens can and does occur in ventilated patients is not disputed. Multiple factors are known to predispose to gastric colonization including increased age, malnutrition, antibiotic use, intrinsic gastrointestinal disease, and increased gastric pH. The stomach is normally sterile when its pH is very low (< 2) and as gastric pH increases, colonization increases.[9] Critically ill patients in intensive care units are prone to have higher gastric pH because they are often receiving prophylaxis for upper gastrointestinal bleeding with agents that reduce gastric acidity, or continuous tube feeding which increases gastric pH and supports bacterial growth.[10] Several centers have reported an association between oropharyngeal colonization and lung infection with a particular organism and gastric colonization with the same organism, but others have been unable to replicate this finding. The suggestion of those finding such an association has been that the stomach can act as a reservoir for colonization of the oropharynx and trachea and aspiration into the lungs, and that prevention of such colonization reduces the risk of nosocomial pneumonia; this contention has also been supported by the results of some controlled clinical trials but refuted by others. More and larger trials are ongoing to try to resolve this issue; however, in our opinion, the differences in study findings likely relate to intercenter differences in practice and patient population resulting in different levels of importance being ascribed to particular routes of infection and colonization.

Contamination of Respiratory Therapy Equipment

All patients with ARDS require respiratory therapy devices which have their own role in the pathogenesis of respiratory tract infections in that they provide a direct route by which exogenous pathogens can reach the tracheobronchial tree of the ventilated patient. Direct contamination of the endotracheal tube can occur from suction equipment or the hands of caregivers if good aseptic technique is not maintained. Medication nebulizers can also be contaminated by the hands of caregivers, oxygen sources or entrained room air, use of contaminated water to fill the reservoir, or inadequate sterilization of equipment and can produce bacterial aerosols leading to environmental contamination or cross contamination between patients. Similar routes of exogenous contamination can occur with ventilator tubing, humidification cascades in the ventilator, and resuscitation bags kept at the bedside. Reports of outbreaks of pneumonia attributable to preventable exogenous contamination from such sources continue to appear regularly, and most active intensive care units experience groupings of such infections requiring an infection control investigation from time to time.

Ventilator humidification systems and tubing also often develop significant microbial colonization with organisms that originate from the patients' oropharynx or from prior tracheobronchial colonization. This has led to a long-running debate about the relationship between nosocomial pneumonia and the frequency with which ventilator circuit changes are performed. Recently available data indicate that tubing colonization does not increase the risk of pneumonia in ventilated patients and that frequent circuit changes do not reduce infection rates.[11] Presumably, this is because in most cases the source of circuit contamination is the patient's own respiratory tract colonization, which already places the patient at a risk of developing pneumonia that would not be affected by circuit changes.

Host Factors Predisposing to Infection

Endotracheal Intubation and Aspiration

Endotracheal intubation not only bypasses the mechanical and chemical barriers between the oropharynx and the trachea, but also permits continual leakage of small amounts of contaminated upper airway secretions around the cuff of the endotracheal tube into the trachea.[12] Irritation produced by the tube itself provokes mucus secretion that leads to the pooling of secretions both above the cuff and in the trachea below. Intubated patients may also have direct mechanical injury to the airway epithelium that reduces the efficiency of the mucocilliary mechanism, and the endotracheal tube cuff also mechanically blocks mucociliary clearance. Thus, even with regular endotracheal suctioning, some accumulation of contaminated airway secretions cannot be completely eliminated, and this likely helps to promote airway colonization. Finally, some nosocomial pathogens colonizing the airway produce glycocalyx, a molecular cement used by bacteria to attach to each other and to the polyvinyl chloride surface of the endotracheal tube, forming a biofilm in which organisms are sequestered from both antibiotics and immunologic defenses.[13]

Pulmonary and Systemic Changes in ARDS Predisposing to Infection

The higher incidence of nosocomial pneumonia in ARDS patients compared to other mechanically ventilated patients is probably primarily related to impairment of host defenses in the ARDS lung (Table 11.1). Several intrinsic changes occur in the lung in ARDS patients that result in impairment of phagocytic function, reduction in mucociliary clearance, increase in mucosal colonization, and enhancement of bacterial growth. The insult that produced the lung injury leading to ARDS, in addition to damaging the pulmonary endothelial and epithelial barriers, also damages alveolar type II cells, reducing surfactant production and reducing its contribution to antibacterial defense. Pulmonary edema fluid also interferes with the antibacterial function of surfactant by dilution and by changing its functional characteristics, as well as interfering with alveolar macrophage function. Elastase, the predominant protease in the airway of patients with ARDS, can proteolytically cleave protective antibodies, reduce the beat frequency of human cilia, and remove fibronectin from epithelial cell surfaces, thereby exposing more receptors for bacterial adherence.[14] In addition, the underlying acute illness and any coexisting illnesses may themselves be risk factors for both colonization and pneumonia. In particular, acidosis, malnutrition, and shock all negatively affect host immune function. Extrapulmonary infections also affect the lung's ability to clear a bacterial challenge by depressing pulmonary polymorphonuclear cell recruitment. Therapeutic interventions used in ARDS patients also may have unwanted effects promoting infection: corticosteroids producing relative immunosuppression; high concentrations of oxygen causing damage to airway epithelium and reducing mucociliary clearance; and sedatives and muscle relaxants reducing upper airway defenses against aspiration and reducing the patient's ability to contribute to secretion clearance by deep breathing, coughing, and turning.

Diagnosis

The diagnosis of nosocomial pneumonia in patients with ARDS can be problematic. Commonly used diagnostic criteria for nosocomial pneumonia, such as those of the Centers for Disease Control (CDC), involve various combinations of clinical, laboratory, and radiographic evidence of infection such as (1) radiographic appearance of a new or progressive pulmonary infiltrate, (2) fever, (3) leukocytosis, (4) purulent tra-

Table 11.1 Systemic and pulmonary changes
associated with ARDS that favor infection

Impairment of phagocytic cell function

Edema
Local hypoxia
Loss of surfactant
Acidosis
Malnutrition
Oxygen therapy
Shock
Inflammatory mediators
Corticosteroids
Extrapulmonary infection

Reduced mucociliary clearance effectiveness

Endotracheal intubation
Increased elastase
Oxygen therapy
Drugs: sedatives, muscle relaxants, anticholinergics

Reduced mucosal defenses against colonization

Endotracheal intubation
Damage to bronchial mucosa from suctioning
Increased elastase
Malnutrition

Enhanced bacterial growth

Alveolar hemorrhage
Increased intra-alveolar protein concentration

cheobronchial secretions, and (5) tracheal aspirate gram stain showing more than 25 leukocytes and less than 10 squamous epithelial cells per low power field with recovery of a potential pathogen.[15] Although these clinical criteria are virtually diagnostic of the presence of pneumonia in the absence of underlying lung disease, acute lung injury itself can cause a radiographic infiltrate, fever, leukocytosis, or purulent sputum, and prolonged intubation or chemical tracheobronchitis can increase the leukocyte count in the tracheal aspirate. With coincident airway colonization, it can be difficult to differentiate infection from colonization. In ventilated patients with acute respiratory failure it has been suggested that use of these clinical criteria leads to substantial overdiagnosis of pneumonia and hence unnecessary treatment. In patients dying with ARDS, however, postmortem studies have shown that pneumonia is a frequent histologic finding (69%) which was often not recognized antemortem (43%).[4]

Thus, in ARDS the diagnosis of pneumonia using this aggregate of clinical criteria at a single point in time may be neither sensitive nor specific.

Because of these difficulties with the clinical definition of nosocomial pneumonia in ARDS and other mechanically ventilated patients, in recent years considerable effort has been expended in seeking more accurate diagnostic methods. The definitive diagnostic test, tissue diagnosis in the form of an open lung biopsy, has a very limited role in this setting. Although clearly useful in the diagnosis of the underlying cause of ARDS-like lung disease when this is in doubt, particularly in the immunocompromised host, for the diagnosis of pneumonia in established ARDS the morbidity associated with lung biopsy and the availability of other diagnostic techniques make it a method of last resort. Attempts to make this diagnosis with greater accuracy and to overcome the problem of upper airway colonization have therefore focused mainly on the collection of samples from the tracheobronchial tree, either through a bronchoscope or by blindly using an endotracheal catheter, using quantitative culture methods to establish a quantitative "diagnostic threshold" for the presence of pneumonia.

Nonbronchoscopic Techniques

The advantage of these methods over bronchoscopic ones are that they are less invasive, less costly, less likely to compromise gas exchange during the procedure, and are readily available both to the nonbronchoscopist clinician and to patients with small endotracheal tubes. The disadvantage is that there is no opportunity for airway visualization, leading to an inherent potential for sampling error.

Endotracheal Aspiration (EA)

Aspiration through the endotracheal tube is the easiest, cheapest, and most readily available technique in most intensive care units for obtaining respiratory secretions for microbiologic analysis. When used qualitatively (that is, an organism is either present or absent) to try to establish an etiologic diagnosis in patients in whom a diagnosis of pneumonia has been made on clinical grounds, this technique is very sensitive, but it is notoriously nonspecific when compared to quantitative techniques using samples collected directly from the lower airways. However, recent work using quantitative culture of endotracheal aspiration specimens, using a diagnostic threshold for pneumonia of 100,000 colony-forming units(cfu)/mL for a particular pathogen instead of simple qualitative culture, showed that its specificity can be improved to a level comparable to quantitative bronchoscopic techniques without compromising its sensitivity.[16–18] To a considerable extent, this work validates the current practice of most clinical microbiology laboratories that report endotracheal aspirate culture results as heavy, moderate, or light growth; > 10^5 cfu/mL corresponds roughly to moderate to heavy growth, which are the levels usually considered potentially clinically significant in patients not already being treated with antibiotics, and numbers of bacteria at this order of magnitude are also the minimal requirement to yield a gram stain showing moderate to heavy numbers of bacteria (or > 2+ on a

0–3+ scale). There is also evidence that larger numbers of PMNs and evident intra-cellular organisms in PMNs are strongly associated with the presence of parenchymal lung infection.[19] If future work confirms these findings, the EA technique with quantitative or possibly semiquantitative culture together with careful assessment of the gram stain may continue to hold its current place as the initial bacteriologic diagnostic tool for suspected pneumonia in ventilated patients.

Other Techniques

Three other "blind " sampling techniques for quantitative bacteriology have been described: (1) protected specimen brushing, (2) nonprotected bronchoalveolar lavage, and (3) protected bronchoalveolar lavage. Several studies have shown that blind sampling is statistically comparable to some bronchoscopic methods; however, none of these methods has been tested against quantitative EA sampling. Although none have yet become widely used, further investigation is clearly warranted.

Nonculture methods that have been used to try to increase the specificity of the diagnosis of pneumonia have included looking for antibody-coated bacteria or elastin fibers in EA or bronchoscopic samples. The antibody-coated bacteria test depends on the assumption that bacteria involved in active infection will be coated with host antibodies and colonizing bacteria will not. Tracheal aspirates or bronchoalveolar lavage (BAL) effluent are stained with fluorescein-labeled antibody against human gamma globulin, and the number of bacteria present taking up the label are estimated. Although initial results are encouraging, this test is not widely available and remains a research tool. Similarly, microscopic examination of respiratory secretions for elastin fibers in respiratory secretions has been reported to be of use in the diagnosis of necrotizing pneumonia but has yet to be widely adopted.[19] Although presence of these fibers is likely specific for lung necrosis, its specificity for pneumonia in the setting of ARDS, in which necrotic lung is commonly found, is likely inadequate.

Bronchoscopic Techniques

Over the last decade fiber-optic bronchoscopy, combined with protected specimen brushing (PSB) or BAL for sampling distal airway secretions, has seen increasing use in the diagnosis of the ventilator-associated pneumonia, in an attempt to overcome the problem of confusing tracheobronchial colonization for infection. Although the procedure can be performed safely in all but the most severely ill intubated patients, ARDS patients are often in this latter category. It should not, therefore, be undertaken without careful consideration of possible alternative diagnostic approaches and risk versus benefit. In ARDS the main risk is worsening hypoxemia; however, pneumothorax due to barotrauma or from sampling catheter injury can occur, and significant bleeding is occasionally seen. Risk of encountering one of these complications of bronchoscopy is significantly increased in patients requiring high levels of PEEP (> 10 cm H_2O) and/or high FiO_2 ($> 70\%$) to maintain arterial oxygenation and in those with a bleeding diathesis. Reasonable precautions to ensure safety, in addition to careful case selection, include (1) performance by an experienced operator to minimize duration of procedure, (2) assistant familiar with the procedure to continuously watch all patient monitors, (3) adequate sedation of the patient and paralysis if needed, (4) FiO_2 of 1.0 during procedure, (5) oxygen saturation monitored continuously with pulse oximetry, (6) exhaled tidal volume monitored during procedure; inspiratory volume increased, if necessary, to compensate for leaks, and (7) PEEP reduced as much as oxygen saturation permits during procedure. In addition to these precautions, physicians doing bronchoscopy in ICU settings should ensure that adequate disinfection procedures are in place for their equipment. Problems with inadequate cleaning of scopes, both mechanical manual cleaning and subsequent disinfection in automated cleaning machines, have been widely reported and have led to both patient-to-patient transmission of pathogens and to outbreaks of pseudoinfection.

Protected Specimen Brush (PSB)

The PSB consists of a telescoping double catheter that houses a sterile brush which can be extended beyond the distal end of the telescoped catheter. The outer cannula is occluded distally by a gelatin or wax plug that is expelled as the brush is extended, thus minimizing contamination of the brush in the upper airway. The specimen obtained is small (0.01–0.001 mL), but usually free of upper airway contamination. The brush is cut off and placed into 1 mL of sterile physiologic solution and sent for quantitative culture. The most widely accepted diagnostic threshold for pneumonia for PSB is 1,000 colony-forming units (cfu) per 1 mL.[20] In the absence of prior antimicrobial therapy, PSB has been shown to have excellent diagnostic specificity (> 90%), with somewhat lower sensitivity (70% to 80%) likely attributable to the small sample size and sampling region of the lung. Unfortunately, prior use of antibiotics significantly reduces both the sensitivity and specificity of PSB cultures. False positives may be due to airway colonization with antimicrobial resistant organisms, and false negatives result from partial treatment of infection and antibiotic effect in the small specimen. One additional disadvantage of PSB is the time it takes to obtain quantitative culture results (around 48 hours).

Bronchoalveolar Lavage (BAL)

BAL is a well-established bronchoscopic technique with proven efficacy in the diagnosis of pulmonary infiltrates in immunocompromised patients that has only more recently been applied to the diagnosis of pneumonia in ventilated patients. The procedure is performed by wedging the tip of the bronchoscope into a segmental bronchus, then flooding that segment with aliqouts (100–200 mL) of sterile physiologic solution; the effluent is then aspirated and analyzed. Although providing a broader reflection of the lung bacterial content than PSB, BAL is subject to a greater risk of contamination from the upper airway, which may occur in up to a third of specimens. In an attempt to minimize this problem, the initial effluent return is normally discarded. Quantitative culture thresholds for BAL diagnosis of pneumonia are less well defined than for PSB, with reported values ranging from 1000 cfu/mL to 100,000 cfu/mL or greater;[20] this problem appears to be compounded by relatively poor quantitative reproducibility of positive cultures.[21] Microscopy of the BAL effluent may provide rapid identification of some patients with pneumonia and allow early institution of specific antimicrobial therapy.

On gram stain, both presence of high semiquantitative grading of a predominant bacterial morphotype and presence of organisms within macrophages or PMNs are associated with parenchymal lung infection. BAL is probably more sensitive than PSB for the diagnosis of pneumonia, but somewhat less specific, although this depends somewhat on the diagnostic threshold selected. Although prior or current antimicrobial therapy reduces diagnostic accuracy of BAL, sensitivity is less reduced than with PSB.

Protected BAL (PBAL) is a refinement of BAL designed to reduce the likelihood of upper airway bacterial contamination while maintaining the superior diagnostic sensitivity of BAL. This technique is performed using a balloon-tipped catheter inserted through the suction channel of the bronchoscope and wedged in the orifice of a subsegmental bronchus by inflating the balloon positioned at the distal end. BAL is performed through the uncontaminated irrigation lumen of the catheter. Although experience is limited, it appears that PBAL does yield a less contaminated specimen than BAL, with diagnostic sensitivity similar to PSB using a quantitative diagnostic threshold of 10,000 cfu/mL. As with BAL the specimen obtained is large enough to permit rapid diagnosis by microscopic examination.

An Approach to the Diagnosis of Pneumonia in ARDS

Due to the high incidence and difficulty in the diagnosis of pneumonia in ARDS patients, considering the possibility that this complication has occurred should be on the ICU team's agenda at least daily. The following parameters should be monitored closely: gas exchange, volume and nature of pulmonary secretions, temperature, and WBC count. Because of the high incidence of both pneumonia and other pulmonary complications in ARDS, daily chest radiographs are probably justified until the patient is clearly past the phase of critical illness. However, radiographic diagnosis of pneumonia in the first week is exceedingly difficult because pneumonia and other processes such as atelectasis, alveolar hemorrhage, as well as low-pressure edema itself all produce airspace consolidation that may be patchy or asymmetric. Later in the course of ARDS, when the radiographic appearance becomes more interstitial, new or evolving areas of consolidation due to pneumonia may be more easily seen. With any deterioration in gas exchange or the chest radiograph, increase in the volume or purulence of respiratory secretions, or increase in temperature or WBC, pneumonia should be considered and a differential diagnosis constructed. In Figure 11.2 an algorithmic approach to this problem is shown, in which detection of one of these markers for possible pulmonary or systemic infection is designated step 1.

Step 2 is the initial collection and consideration of information to support the construction of a differential diagnosis. This initial evaluation should include a detailed clinical examination, chest x-ray, blood culture, endotracheal aspirate for gram stain and quantitative or semiquantitative culture, and specimens for whatever alternative sepsis sites can be identified. When the presentation is one of systemic signs of inflammation together with evidence that the lung may be its source, the leading considerations are pneumonia versus other pulmonary processes like atelectasis, congestive heart failure, and the fibroproliferative phase of ARDS. Alterna-

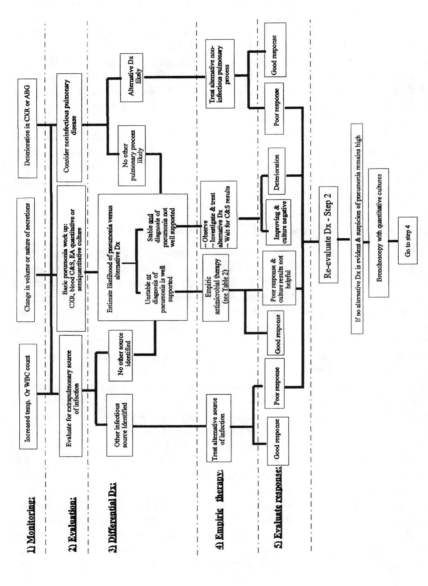

Figure 11.2. A stepwise approach to the diagnosis and management of suspected nosocomial pneumonia in ARDS.

tively, if the presentation is predominantly one of systemic signs of infection without supporting evidence for a pulmonary source, infections at other sites are the leading considerations along with noninfectious causes of fever.

Step 3 is considering the differential diagnosis and estimating the relative probability of each possibility identified. Careful application of this step is crucial to avoiding unnecessary empiric antimicrobial therapy, and also to avoid expensive and unnecessary invasive investigations and radiographic studies. Although diagnostic uncertainty is the main thing that is certain at this point in this exercise, a thorough and thoughtful approach to listing potential sources of the problem and estimating their relative probabilities, followed by selective stepwise investigation, is preferable to pursuit of certainty using a nonselective investigative strategy or shotgun empiric therapy.

Step 4 is selection and application of an empiric treatment approach based on the differential diagnosis. Often, this does not imply antimicrobial therapy. If the patient's condition is relatively stable with respect to cardiovascular and respiratory status, and if a reasonably high probability noninfectious diagnosis can be made, therapy aimed at that diagnosis can be prescribed and empiric antibiotics withheld. For example, if chest radiography findings together with absence of purulent secretions containing large numbers of bacteria suggest that CHF or atelectasis are likelier than pneumonia as an explanation for infiltrates and gas exchange deterioration and low-grade fever, therapy directed at these entities can be given and antibiotic withheld. The presumptive diagnosis is then reevaluated over the next 24 to 48 hours, with the added information of how the patient has fared during that time, along with the results of cultures, sent initially. Similarly, if the initial evaluation does not point to the lung as an explanation for elevated temperature and WBC, but other likely sources of sepsis are identified, such as central lines or possible abscess at a surgical site, in stable patients antimicrobials can be withheld while lines are changed and cultured or imaging performed to look for the abscess. If the clinical probability of pneumonia seems high *or* if the patient is unstable, empiric therapy appropriate for both pneumonia and any other identified potential source of sepsis should be started.

In the 24 to 48 hours following a decision regarding the empiric therapeutic plan, the response of the patient is carefully evaluated (step 5), and if the response is less than adequate, step 2 is revisited to determine whether with time and with more available laboratory information a diagnostic possibility has emerged that was not previously evident. If nosocomial pneumonia remains a leading diagnostic candidate but without definite support from endotracheal aspirate microscopy and bacteriology, bronchoscopy with quantitative bacteriology is a reasonable next step.

Antimicrobial Therapy

Although it is important to recognize that the diagnosis of nosocomial pneumonia in ARDS patients is imprecise and overuse of empiric antimicrobial therapy can lead to unnecessary complications and cost, it is also true that this group of patients has a high incidence of pneumonia caused by virulent organisms associated with a rapidly progressive course and high mortality rate. Prompt and appropriate antimicrobial therapy for these infections can significantly improve survival.[22,23] The key steps in ensuring that the negative impact of infectious complications are minimized are first, deciding when to employ empiric antimicrobial therapy; second, selecting antimicrobials that are appropriate for the patient and for the situation; and third, tailoring subsequent therapy in accordance with culture results and the clinical course.

Pharmacologic Considerations

An ideal antimicrobial regimen for nosocomial pneumonia would be a regimen without important toxicities which is rapidly bactericidal for the common nosocomial pathogens, with little propensity for inducing antimicrobial resistance, and which attains high and sustained antimicrobial activity in respiratory secretions. Although all of the agents currently available have significant limitations in one or more of these areas, the mainstay of therapy for nearly all nosocomial pneumonias are beta-lactam antibiotics, which are relatively safe, with a good therapeutic index. They are bactericidal and kill organisms in a time-dependent fashion, which means they require frequent dosing and make it particularly important not to miss a dose of therapy. Their concentration in the respiratory secretions is less than 50% of their serum level, but this is nevertheless usually sufficient for bactericidal activity against most pathogens.

Aminoglycosides, in contrast, are bactericidal, but have a killing effect that is concentration dependent with a significant postantibiotic effect, which means they can be given less frequently, possibly even as a single daily dose. Aminoglycoside levels in pulmonary secretions are generally only 10% to 15% of simultaneously measured serum levels. As their ratio of therapeutic to toxic level is relatively small, it is difficult using conventional dosing regimens to safely reach serum levels that will achieve good therapeutic concentrations in the lung. In addition, the acidic pH of the pneumonic lung reduces the efficacy of aminoglycosides. These pharmacologic considerations have two main implications for the use of these drugs in treating pneumonia. First, when the aminoglycoside is considered to be a key part of the selected regimen, as is usually the case in treating *Pseudomonas aeruginosa* or other resistant gram-negative infection, the aminoglycoside should be dosed to achieve the highest peak serum levels consistent with safety. One way to do this is to prolong the dosing interval while increasing the dose;[24] it is our practice to dose aminoglycosides once daily in this setting in most patients. Second, aminoglycosides should never be used as the sole agent for the treatment of pneumonia. This affects the selection of concomitant agents in choosing empiric therapy, because a second agent likely to be effective against gram negatives must be included, which is not the case with infections at most other sites.

The third group of antimicrobials used frequently in the treatment of nosocomial pneumonia in the ICU is the fluoroquinolones. They are bactericidal and possess a pronounced postantibiotic effect. Their penetration into the lung is excellent with concentrations that equal or exceed serum concentrations. One of the big advantages of quinolones is the availability of oral formulations of these drugs, which make them very valuable in the convalescence stage. The disadvantage of quinolones is the propensity for the development of microbial resistance, especially if they are used as monotherapy. For this reason, we believe these agents should be used as presumptive or empiric therapy only under exceptional conditions (e.g., multiple drug allergies, patient known to be colonized with resistant pathogen), and even when a diagnosis has been established their use should be limited to cases where no other good therapeutic option exists.

Empiric Therapy

Empiric antimicrobial therapy is warranted for suspected nosocomial pneumonia when the patient's cardiovascular or respiratory status is unstable or threatens survival in the short term, or when the diagnosis of pneumonia is not substantially in doubt. The initial choice of antimicrobial regimen should take into account the presence and degree of immunosuppression, prior use of antibiotics (as this will increase the risk of infection with relatively resistant pathogens), gram stain and previous culture results, the length of stay in the intensive care unit before the development of pneumonia, and knowledge of locally endemic organisms and their resistance patterns. In general, in a patient sick enough to warrant immediate empiric therapy the initial regimen should always include agents active against enteric gram-negative bacilli and *Staphylococcus aureus*, and also against relatively resistant gram negatives such as Pseudomonas spp. in patients at risk because of a long ICU stay, prior antibiotic therapy, immunosuppression, or high local incidence of such infection. A beta-lactam alone is likely sufficient in stable patients with less severe pneumonia; in more severely ill patients, including most patients with ARDS, a beta-lactam combined with an aminoglycoside is the usual first choice. For patients at lower risk of resistant gram negatives, second- or third-generation cephalosporins such as cefuroxime, cefotaxime, or ceftriaxone are useful choices, combining coverage for most Enterobacteriacae with adequate gram-positive coverage. For suspected Pseudomonas or other resistant gram negatives, active antipseudomonal beta-lactams include the third-generation cephalosporins ceftazidime and cefoperazone; the antipseudomonal penicillin piperacillin; the carbapenems imipenem with cilastatin or meropenem; and the monobactam aztreonam. If specific contraindications to aminoglycoside use exist, another approach is to combine a beta-lactam with a fluoroquinolone (e.g., ciprofloxacin). The need for the aminoglycoside should be reassessed at 48 to 72 hours, once cultural results are available. As most of these beta-lactams and quinolones have reasonable activity against *Staphylococcus aureus*, an additional agent to cover this important pathogen is usually not necessary except in patients in whom methicillin-resistant *Staphylococcus aureus* (MRSA) is suspected, in which case addition of vancomycin should be considered. Some suggested empiric antimicrobial regimens are shown in Table 11.2.

Specific Antimicrobial Therapy

When culture results are available, therapy should be tailored to the organism isolated and its sensitivity pattern. Some suggested regimens are shown in Table 11.3. All antibiotics should be administered intravenously initially. Patients with ARDS are often seriously ill for such a lengthy period that a full antimicrobial treatment course for pneumonia is completed by the parenteral route. However, if the patient improves and is stable enough to leave the unit before completing the antibiotic course, a shift to oral therapy may be possible. The chosen oral antibiotic need not be from the same class as the preceding parenteral agent as long as it has been shown to be active against the isolated organism. Little good quality information on the necessary duration of therapy exists; however, we generally suggest a 2-week total treatment course for infections due to susceptible community-acquired organisms (Streptococcal spp., *Moraxella catarrhalis,* or *Hemophilus influenzae*), and 3 weeks for infections due to susceptible Enterobacteriacae or *Staphylococcus aureus* without overt complications such as abscess or empyema. A minimum of 3 weeks up to 4 to 6 weeks is suggested for resistant infections such as *Pseudomonas aeruginosa* or more susceptible infections associated with suppurative complications, depending on the clinical course.

Assessing the Response to Therapy

Radiographic changes may persist for a long time in ARDS patients, so repeated chest radiographs are useful only in demonstrating whether or not infiltrates are worsening on therapy. Response to therapy must therefore be judged using a constellation of clinical features including clinical and laboratory signs of active infection (temperature, mental alertness, hemodynamic stability, white blood cell and platelet count) and findings specific to the lung (quality and quantity of endotracheal secretions and trend in gas exchange). Frequent changes in therapy based only on absence of prompt and dramatic improvement are generally not useful. A change in therapy should be based on both failure to improve clinically and isolation of an organism for which the selected antibiotic is ineffective. Use of follow-up quantitative cultures of respiratory secretion to assess response has been suggested;[25] however, there is not yet sufficient supportive evidence, particularly in ARDS patients, to warrant a recommendation for this.

Prevention

Considering the serious effect of nosocomial pneumonia on the prognosis of ARDS patients, the difficulty in diagnosing it, and the limited success of treatment, preven-

Table 11.2. Empiric therapy for nosocomial pneumonia[a]

Patient group	Recommended regimen	Alternative
Low risk of resistant gram negative	Cefotaxime: 2g Q8h or ceftriaxone: 2g Q24h AND Gentamicin 1.5 mg/kg Q8h or 4–5 mg/kg Q24h[b] or aztreonam 1–2 g Q8h	Ciprofloxacin 400 mg Q12h AND Gentamicin or aztreonam
High risk of resistant gram negative (e.g., Pseudomonas and Acinetobacter)	Ceftazidime: 1–2 g Q8h or piperacillin/tazobactam 3.375 g Q6h AND Gentamicin or aztreonam	Ciprofloxacin AND Gentamicin or antipseudo-monal beta-lactam
Legionella spp. infection suspected	Add erythromycin 1 g Q6h	Ciprofloxacin 400 mg Q8h

[a]Doses shown are for patients with normal renal function and may require adjustment in presence of renal insufficiency.
[b]The aminoglycoside selected for adjunctive therapy may vary depending on local gram-negative susceptibility patterns. Monitoring of aminoglycoside levels for dose adjustment is strongly advised.

tion is clearly crucial. Reason to believe that this infection can be prevented can be found in numerous studies of specific interventional strategies and in the observation that reported rates of nosocomial pneumonia in mechanically ventilated patients range from 5% to 6% to as high as 70% to 80%. Although some of these differences may relate to differing patient populations or diagnostic criteria, we believe that much is attributable to real differences in standards of care. Pneumonia rates are generally lower in units with well-trained, full-time medical staff and nursing staff specifically trained for ICU work, working with an adequate nurse-to-patient ratio (preferably 1:1 for ARDS patients), and an active and aggressive infection control program. In addition to these general measures for overall standard of care, a number of specific measures to reduce pneumonia risk in ventilated patients are available.

General Patient Care

Body Position

Placing mechanically ventilated patients in the semirecumbent position (30–45 degree) or upright position is an effective prophylactic measure in those who can tolerate it because it minimizes the aspiration of gastric contents to lower airways,[26] especially during enteral feeding using gastric tubes.

Although difficult to document, it seems reasonable to expect prolonged immobility to cause dependent accumulation of edema fluid and respiratory secretions and impairment of normal mucociliary function, increasing the risk of atelectasis and

Table 11.3. Specific therapy[a]

Organism	Recommended regimen	Comments
Gram-positive organisms		
Streptococcus pneumoniae and other non-enterococcal streptococci	Penicillin G 2 million units IV Q4h	If allergic to penicillins, alternative agents for gram-positives include clindamycin or vancomycin.
Staphylococcus aureus	Nafcillin or cloxacillin 1–2 g IV Q4h	
Methicillin-resistant *Staphylococcus aureus*	Vancomycin 1 g IV Q12h	
Gram-negative organisms		
Enterobacteriaceae (e.g., *E. coli*, Klebsiella spp.)	Cefotaxime or ceftriaxone AND Gentamicin	Gentamicin may be stopped after a few days as the patient improves, or omitted if the infection is not severe.
Pseudomonas and Acinetobacter spp.	Ceftazidime or imipenem or piperacillin/tazobactam AND Gentamicin	Patients doing well after the first week of IV therapy may be switched to oral ciprofloxacin 750 mg Q12h to complete a 3-week course.
Legionella spp.	Erythromycin 1 g Q6h ± rifampin 600 mg po Q24h OR Ciprofloxacin 400 mg IV Q8h	When stable, erythromycin 500 mg po Q6h

[a]Where not shown, doses are those shown in Table 11.2. Doses given here are for patients with normal renal function and may require adjustment in the presence of renal insufficiency. The aminoglycoside selected for adjunctive therapy may vary depending on local gram-negative susceptibility patterns. Monitoring of aminoglycoside levels for dose adjustment is strongly advised.

pneumonia. Continuous lateral rotational therapy, in which patients are placed on beds that turn on their longitudinal axes intermittently or continuously, has recently been reported to be potentially useful in avoiding these problems,[27] although it remains to be seen if this approach will be practical in ARDS patients. Nevertheless, it seems advisable to minimize the tendency for dependent secretion accumulation as much as possible using the methods immediately at hand. In most units this means frequent side-to-side turning of patients in bed, even intermittent turning to the prone position, as well as minimizing the use of deep sedation or muscle relaxants, unless absolutely required for effective ventilation and oxygenation.

Airway Care

Mechanically ventilated patients lose their ability to clear respiratory secretions, a problem made worse by sedation and muscle relaxants. For that reason frequent gentle suctioning is recommended for all intubated patients. There are two types of suctioning catheters: the standard single catheter and the closed multiuse catheter. There is no known significant difference in the incidence of pneumonia between the two systems; however, the closed multiuse system may be more convenient.[28]

To reduce the risk of aspiration, good mouth care should be part of daily nursing routine, the oropharynx should be suctioned prior to deflation of cuffs on endotracheal tubes, and the endotracheal tube cuff should be checked frequently for cuff pressure and adequacy of seal. A new technique using an endotracheal tube fitted with a separate dorsal lumen that allows continuous suctioning of subglottic secretions has recently been reported to decrease the incidence of pneumonia in mechanically ventilated patients.[29] If these results can be replicated, this may come into wider use; meanwhile, it serves to remind us of the need for provision of adequate and frequent suctioning and secretion mobilization.

The relationship between nosocomial pneumonia and frequency of ventilatory circuit changes has been debated for many years; however, based on the currently available data, it would appear that the only time ventilator circuits need to be changed is if they leak or if they are visibly soiled, provided all other appropriate infection control procedures are maintained.[11]

Nutrition

Although specific data on ARDS patients are lacking, ample evidence suggests an adverse effect of malnutrition on respiratory tract host defenses, the corollary being that nutritional intervention might reduce the risk of pneumonia. Enteral feeding is superior to total parenteral nutrition if it can be given effectively because stimulation of the intestinal mucosa by feeding may enhance the immune system. However, when tube feeding is used, it is important to minimize the risk of aspiration by proper positioning of the patient, verifying appropriate placement of the feeding tube, assessing the patient's intestinal motility, and adjusting the rate and volume of infusion to avoid regurgitation. In patients being ventilated using an orotracheal tube and fed by the gastric route, we recommend use of an orogastric rather than a nasogastric tube to reduce the likelihood of sinusitis, which in some series has been associated with pneumonia. In patients who do not tolerate feeding via an intragastric tube, placement of a tube in the jejunum is generally effective and has been reported to reduce the risk of aspiration and pneumonia.[30]

Infection Control and Surveillance

By carefully following infection rates and the frequency of occurrence of particular pathogens in an ICU, the infection control team may be alerted to problems such as the occurrence of new reservoirs or increased incidence of cross infection. Continuous surveillance for nosocomial pneumonia is of fundamental importance in ICU practice, permitting the calculation of an ICU-specific pneumonia rate and identification of changes in that rate which might require further epidemiologic investigation.[31] Any increase in the incidence of a particular organism over the baseline rate, or a predominance of antimicrobial resistant water-borne gram negatives such as *Pseudomonas aeruginosa*, *Pseudomonas cepacia*, or Acinetobacter spp. signals an infection control problem that is potentially correctable. Application of such surveillance and infection control programs has been shown to reduce nosocomial pneumonia rates.[32]

Conventional infection control measures have relied primarily on decreasing person-to-person spread of pathogens (exogenous infection) and also aim in a simple way to halt progression from colonization to infection by attention to aseptic techniques and early removal of invasive devices (Table 11.4). These important measures may virtually eliminate acquisition of exogenous pathogens if followed strictly. However, because virtually all patients are colonized with potentially pathogenic microorganisms on admission to the ICU, these measures cannot be expected to eliminate all infections.

The value of performing routine surveillance cultures of airway secretions in ventilated patients is controversial because of their low predictive value as a result of airway colonization. But these cultures may help in the detection of colonization by potentially pathogenic organisms, which may prompt the initiation of infection control measures and help in the selection of appropriate antimicrobial therapy if an infection occurs. Our practice is to order respiratory secretion cultures in the general ICU population only when there is clinical suspicion of pneumonia, performing surveillance cultures about twice weekly only in patients at particularly high risk of pneumonia, a category that includes most ARDS patients.

Experimental Control Measures

Role of Gastric pH

Critically ill patients in the ICU are frequently given agents for prophylaxis against gastrointestinal bleeding that may increase gastric pH. Considerable attention has been paid to the association between gastric alkalinization and pneumonia in critically ill patients in the past few years. Several studies have documented that the administration of antacids and H_2 receptor blockers for prevention of stress bleeding in critically ill patients is associated with gastric bacterial overgrowth.[9,33] Sucralfate, a cytoprotective agent that has little effect on gastric pH and may have its own bactericidal properties, has been suggested as a substitute for antacids and H_2 receptor blockers.[34,35] Clinical trials comparing the risk of pneumonia in patients receiving sucralfate to that in patients receiving antacids and H_2 receptor blockers have yielded highly variable results which are not easily explained. Some studies show marked reduction in pneumonia rates with sucralfate and others show no differences.[36] Further studies to clarify this issue are in progress, however. In the interim we would point out that sucralfate is nontoxic, cheap, and as effective for prophylaxis as the other agents, and on that basis can be recommended even if its effects on bacterial colonization are illusory. Other suggested approaches to minimizing bacterial colonization in the stomach include acidification of tube feedings and intermittent rather than continuous feedings, but neither of these measures has yet

Table 11.4. Conventional infection control measures in the ICU

Surveillance

Identify reservoirs (colonized and infected patients and environmental contamination).

Education and awareness programs

Reducing cross contamination among patients

Hand washing before and after patient contact
Aseptic technique
Barrier precautions (gloves and gowns) for patients colonized with highly resistant pathogens
No transfer of equipment between patients
Proper disinfection between patients

Reducing progression from colonization to infection

Extubation and removal of nasogastric tube as clinically indicated
Proper removal of ventilator tubing condensate
Frequent endotracheal suctioning as required using aseptic technique and sterile solutions
to rinse the catheter

Modify host risk

Treat underlying disease.
Minimize unnecessary antibiotic use.

been shown to influence the incidence of nosocomial pneumonia and cannot, therefore, be recommended.[37–39]

Prophylactic Antimicrobials

In the 1970s attempts to use polymyxin B topically to suppress colonization of the oropharynx and gastrointestinal tract were initially successful in reducing nosocomial pneumonia rates, but with prolonged use led to the emergence of antimicrobial-resistant strains that were associated with increased mortality when pneumonia supervened.[40] More recently a strategy termed selective decontamination of digestive tract (SDD) has received much investigative attention. Based on the hypothesis that antimicrobial prophylaxis using oral and parenteral antimicrobials that eliminate or reduce potentially pathogenic organisms, without altering the anaerobic flora of the digestive tract, would result in fewer infections, different forms of SDD were initially used in the early 1980s with substantial success to prevent bacterial infection in patients with granulocytopenia. A modified regimen for use in mechanically ventilated patients consists of a combination of topical nonabsorbable antibiotics (polymyxin B, tobramycin, and amphotericin B or nystatin) in both paste and liquid form, achieving concentrations in saliva and feces high enough to abolish the carriage of potentially pathogenic organisms, with the addition of an injectable antibiotic (cefotaxime) given in the first 4 days after admission to control primary endogenous infection. Most clinical trials of SDD have demonstrated a decrease in the rates of nosocomial respiratory tract infection; however, none has yet demonstrated a reduction in length of hospital stay, major morbidity, or mortality.[41] Cost/benefit is also a significant issue because these regimens are extremely expensive. Few of these studies have systematically addressed the potential of this regimen to promote antimicrobial resistance, which proved to be a major problem in the earlier studies of polymyxin B prophylaxis. For all of these reasons, we do not recommend routine use of any prophylactic antimicrobial regimen, including SDD, in the ICU in general or in ARDS patients in particular for the purpose of preventing nosocomial pneumonia.

Summary

Nosocomial pneumonia is a common occurrence in mechanically ventilated ARDS patients and is associated with surprisingly high morbidity and mortality rates. The fundamentals of managing nosocomial pneumonia in ARDS patients are attention to the principles of infection control for prevention, vigilance in diagnosis of pneumonia, and appropriate antimicrobial therapy.

References

1. Niederman MS, Fein AM. Sepsis syndrome, the adult respiratory distress syndrome and nosocomial pneumonia. Clin Ches Med 1990; 11:633–656.
2. Sutherland KR, Steinberg KP, Maunder RJ, et al. Pulmonary infection during the acute respiratory distress syndrome. Am J Respir Crit Care Med 1995; 152:550–556.
3. Delclaux C, Roupie E, Blot F, et al. Lower respiratory tract colonization and infection during severe acute respiratory distress syndrome. Am J Respir Crit Care Med 1997; 156:1092–1098.
4. Bell RC, Coalson JJ, Smith JD, et al. Multiple organ system failure and infection in ARDS. Ann Intern Med 1983; 99:293–298.
5. Fagon JY, Chastre J, Hanse AJ, et al. Nosocomial pneumonia in ventilated patients: a cohort study evaluating attributable mortality and hospital stay. Am J Med 1993; 94:281–288.
6. Johanson WG, Pierce AK, Sanford JP, et al. Nosocomial respiratory infections with gram-negative bacilli. The significance of colonization of the respiratory tract. Ann Int Med 1972; 77:701–706.
7. Rogers CJ, Van Saene HK, Suter PM, et al. Infection control in critically ill patients: effect of selective decontamination of the digestive tract. Am J Hosp Pharm 1994; 51:631–648.

8. Niederman MS. Bacterial adherence as a mechanism of airway colonization. Eur J Microbiol Infec Dis 1989; 8:15–20.
9. Atherton ST, White DJ. Stomach as a source of bacteria colonising the respiratory tract during artificial ventilation. Lancet 1978; 2(8097):968–969.
10. Pingleton SK, Hinthorn DR, Liu C. Enteral nutrition in patients receiving mechanical ventilation. Multiple sources of tracheal colonization include the stomach. Am J Med 1986; 80:827–832.
11. Kollef MH, Shapiro SD, Fraser VJ, et al. Mechanical ventilation with or without 7-day circuit changes. Ann Int Med 1995; 123:168–174.
12. Seegobin RD, Hasselt GL. Aspiration beyond endotracheal cuffs. Can Anaes Soc J 1986; 33:273–279.
13. Sottile RD, Marrie TJ, Prough DS, et al. Nosocomial pulmonary infection: possible etiologic significance of bacterial adhesion to endotracheal tubes. Crit Care Med 1986; 14:265–270.
14. Sibille Y, Reynolds HY. Macrophages and polymorphonuclear neutrophils in lung defense and injury. Am Rev Respir Dis 1990; 141:471–501.
15. Garner J, Jarvis W, Emori TG, et al. CDC definitions for nosocomial infections. J Infect Control 1988; 16:128–140.
16. Torres A, Martos A, Bellasca J, et al. Specificity of endotracheal aspiration, protected specimen brush, and bronchoalveolar lavage in mechanically ventilated patients. Am Rev Respir Dis 1993; 147:952–957.
17. Marquette CH, Georges H, Wallet F, et al. Diagnostic efficacy of endotracheal aspirates with quantitative bacterial cultures in intubated patients with suspected pneumonia. Comparison with protected specimen brush. Am Rev Respir Dis 1993; 148:138–144.
18. Papazian L, Thomas P, Garbe L, et al. Bronchoscopic or blind sampling techniques for the diagnosis of ventilator-associated pneumonia. Am J Respir Crit Care Med 1995; 152:1982–1991.
19. Salata RA, Lederman MM, Shlaes DM, et al. Diagnosis of nosocomial pneumonia in intubated, intensive care unit patients. Am Rev Respir Dis 1987; 135:426–432.
20. Baselski V, El-Torky M, Coalson JJ, et al. The standardization of criteria for processing and interpreting laboratory specimens in patients with suspected ventilator-associated pneumonia. Chest 1992; 102:571S–579S.
21. Gerbeaux P, Ledory V, Boussuges A, et al. Diagnosis of nosocomial pneumonia in mechanically ventilated patients. Repeatability of the bronchoalveolar lavage. Am J Respir Crit Care Med 1998; 157:76–80.
22. Torres A, Anzar R, Gatell JM, et al. Incidence, risk and prognosis factors of nosocomial pneumonia in mechanically ventilated patients. Am Rev Respir Dis 1990; 142:523–528.
23. Celis R, Torres A, Gatell JM. Nosocomial pneumonia: a multivariate analysis of risk and prognosis. Chest 1988; 93:318–324.
24. Prins JM, Buller HR, Kuijper EJ, et al. Once versus thrice daily gentamicin in patients with serious infections. Lancet 1993; 341:38–44.
25. Montraves P, Fagon JY, Chastre J, et al. Follow-up protected specimen brushes to assess treatment in nosocomial pneumonia. Am Rev Respir Dis 1993; 147:38–44.
26. Torres A, Serra-Batlles J, Rose E, et al. Pulmonary aspiration of gastric contents in patients receiving mechanical ventilation: the effect of body position. Ann Int Med 1992; 116:540–543.

27. Sahn SA. Continuous lateral rotational therapy and nosocomial pneumonia. Chest 1991; 99:1263–1267.
28. Deppe SA, Kelly JW, Thoi LL, et al. Incidence of colonization, nosocomial pneumonia and mortality in critically ill patients using Trach Care closed system: prospective randomized study. Crit Care Med 1990; 18:1389–1393.
29. Rello J, Sonora R, Jubert P, et al. Pneumonia in intubated patients: role of respiratory airway care. Am J Respir Crit Care Med 1996; 154:111–115.
30. Montecalvo MA, Steger KA, Farber HW, et al. Nutritional outcome and pneumonia in critical care patients randomized to gastric versus jejunal tube feedings. Crit Care Med 1992; 20:1377–1387.
31. Maloney SA, Jarvis WR. Epidemic nosocomial pneumonia in the intensive care unit. Clin Chest Med 1995; 16:209–223.
32. Haley RW, Culver DH, White JW, et al. The efficacy of infection surveillance and control programs in preventing nosocomial infections in US hospitals. Am J Epidemiol 1985; 121:182–205.
33. Craven DE, Dascher FD. Nosocomial pneumonia in intubated patients: role of gastric colonization. Eur J Microbiol Infect Dis 1989; 8:40–50.
34. Driks MR, Craven DE, Celi R, et al. Nosocomial pneumonia in intubated patients given sucralfate as compared with antacids or H_2 blockers. N Engl J Med 1987; 317:1376–1382.
35. Prod'hom G, Leuenberger PH, Koerfer J, et al. Nosocomial pneumonia in mechanically ventilated patients receiving antacids, ranitidine or sucralfate as prophylaxis for stress ulcer. Ann Intern Med 1994; 120:653–662.
36. Cook DJ, Reeve BK, Guyatt GH, et al. Stress ulcer prophylaxis in critically ill patients. Resolving discordant meta-analyses. JAMA 1996; 275:308–314.
37. Bonten MJM, Gaillard CA, van der Hulst R, et al. Intermittent enteral feeding: the influence on respiratory and digestive tract colonization in mechanically ventilated intensive care unit patients. Am J Respir Crit Care Med 1996; 154:394–399.
38. Spilker CA, Hinthorn DR, Pingleton SK. Intermittent enteral feeding in mechanically ventilated patients. The effect on gastric pH and gastric cultures. Chest 1996; 110:243–248.
39. Heyland D, Bradley C, Mandell LA. Effect of acidified enteral feedings on gastric colonization in the critically ill patient. Crit Care Med 1992; 20:1388–1394.
40. Feeley TW, Du Moulin GC, Hedley-Whyte J, et al. Aerosol polymyxin and pneumonia in seriously ill patients. N Engl J Med 1975; 293:471–475.
41. Duncan RA, Steger KA, Craven DE. Selective decontamination of the digestive tract: risks outweigh benefits for intensive care unit patients. Sem Respir Infect 1993; 8:308–324.

12

Resolution and Repair of Acute Lung Injury

Russell Bowler, Chrystelle Garat, and Michael A. Matthay

Introduction

Successful recovery of lung function after acute lung injury requires that the repair process occur in an orderly and controlled sequence similar to that of other injured tissues.[1] First, the excess alveolar fluid and soluble proteins must be removed from the airspaces. Second, the excess soluble and insoluble proteins must be cleared from the alveoli. Third, alveolar epithelial type II cells must repopulate the denuded epithelial barrier. Fourth, the edematous and fibrotic interstitium must shrink and reconstitute its normal matrix. Fifth, the injured and obstructed endothelium must be recanalized to restore normal blood flow to the lung. Sixth, all of the nonessential cells that participated in the repair process must die and their cellular debris must be cleared. Failure of any one of these processes will result in persistent lung injury with fibrosing alveolitis and nonresolving respiratory failure.

This chapter reviews what is known about the recovery of normal lung function after acute lung injury. The first section reviews the mechanisms responsible for removal of alveolar edema fluid. The second section discusses the fibrosing alveolitis that develops as a response to acute lung injury with an emphasis on the role of extracellular matrix proteins in this process. The third section describes the potential contribution of growth factors in remodeling of the vascular endothelium, the interstitium, and the alveolar epithelial barrier. The clinical manifestations and significance of these recovery phases is considered as well.

Removal of Excess Alveolar Fluid and Protein

The alveolar epithelium serves as a functional barrier between the air-filled alveolus and the lung interstitium and pulmonary capillaries. Normally, there are tight intercellular junctions between the type I alveolar cells; these junctions are relatively impermeable to macromolecules and electrolytes.[2] Gas exchange depends on maintaining a dry alveolus that is in communication with the conducting airways. By instilling isosmolar physiologic solutions directly into the distal airspaces of small and large animals, it has been possible to measure water, solute, and protein transport from the alveoli in both normal and pathologic conditions.

If the alveolar barrier were only a passive barrier, then transport of fluid across the alveolar epithelial barrier would depend on hydrostatic and osmotic pressure gradients. Transport across the alveolar epithelium could then be modeled with the following equation: $Q_{(A)} = K_{(A)}[(P_{(if)} - P_{(alv)} - \mu_{(As)}(\pi_{(ifs)} - \pi_{(alvs)})]$ where $K_{(A)}$ is the hydraulic conductance across the alveolar epithelium, $P_{(if)}$ and $P_{(alv)}$ are the hydrostatic pressures in the interstitial space and alveolar space, respectively, $\mu_{(As)}$ is a permeability constant for the alveolar epithelium, and $_{(ifs)}$ and $_{(alv)}$ are the osmotic concentrations in the interstitial and alveolar spaces.[3] However, recent evidence indicates that active ion transport is critical for regulating fluid balance across the alveolar epithelium.

The primary force driving alveolar fluid clearance is active sodium transport by alveolar type II cells. Sodium is absorbed by apical channels in alveolar type II cells. Recent evidence indicates that sodium uptake in alveolar epithelial type II cells occurs, at least in part, through ENaC, an amiloride-sensitive sodium channel.[4] Next Na-K-ATPase pumps sodium into the interstitial space across the basolateral membrane of type II cells[4-7] (Figure 12.1). Water clearance follows the osmotic gradient created by the sodium transport. New evidence suggests that much of the water may move through transmembrane water channels.[4,8-10] Based on recent data, it appears that much of the water transport may occur across alveolar epithelial type I cells,[11] whereas the sodium transport may occur primarily across alveolar epithelial type II cells.

The clearance of edema fluid from the distal airspaces to the interstitium is largely independent of the protein gradient between the airspace and vascular compartment.[12,13] In fact, alveolar fluid clearance occurs against a rising alveolar protein concentration experimentally (Table 12.1) and clinically (Table 12.2). In addition, clearance occurs in the absence of ventilation[14,15] and blood flow.[15-17]

In dogs,[18] rats,[19,20] sheep,[17] and human lungs[15,21] beta-adrenergic agents have been shown to double the rate of alveolar fluid clearance, although this does not occur in all species.[22] The beta-agonist effect is mediated by cAMP and results from increased uptake of sodium across the apical epithelial membrane.[7] These results correlate well with experimental studies in normal lungs that show enhanced alveolar liquid clearance associated with an increase in endogenous catecholamines.[20]

In acute lung injury, the endothelial barrier must be injured for the edema fluid to enter the interstitium. Once edema fluid accumulates in the interstitium, the edema fluid may enter the airspaces simply because interstitial pressure rises sufficiently to

ALVEOLAR LIQUID REABSORPTION
DEPENDS ON ACTIVE NA⁺TRANSPORT

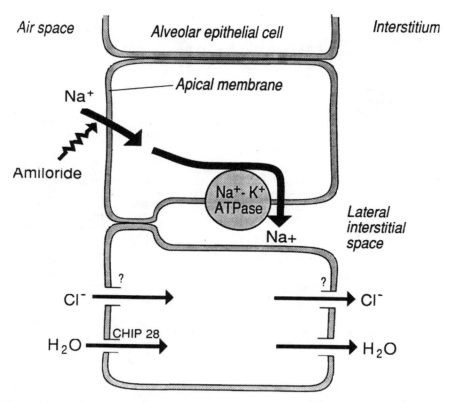

Figure 12.1. Schematic diagram that provides a model of net alveolar liquid reabsorption based on sodium (Na^+) uptake across the apical membrane of alveolar type II cells followed by extension into the interstitium by Na-K-ATPase. Chloride and water follow the osmotic gradient created by vectorial sodium transport to maintain electrical and osmotic neutrality. CHIP 28 refers to the first water channel that was discovered (aquaporin 1). Recent evidence suggests a considerable fraction of transcellular water transport across alveolar epithelial type I cells (see text and Dobbs et al.[11]). These cells have abundant quantities of aquaporin 5 on the apical membrane.

cause focal breaks in the distal airway or alveoli epithelial junctions.[3,23] This usually occurs when interstitial lung water has increased by 20% to 30%. The ability of the lung to hold interstitial edema fluid appears to increase with lung distension. Alternatively, there may be direct injury to the alveolar epithelial cells resulting in transla-

Table 12.1 Alveolar liquid clearance in sheep as reflected by progressive concentrations of protein in the air spaces of the lung

| Time (h) | ALVEOLAR PROTEIN CONCENTRATION (g/100 mL) | | Lung liquid clearance (% of instilled) |
	Initial[a]	Final[a]	
4	6.3 ± 0.6	8.4 ± 0.6	33
12	5.9 ± 0.4	10.2 ± 1.2	59
24	6.4 ± 0.6	12.9 ± 1.9	76

Data as mean ± S.D.
[a]$P < 0.05$ compared to other groups.
Source: Matthay MA, Berthiaume Y, Staub NC. Long-term clearance of liquid and protein from the lungs of unanesthetized sheep. Appl Physiol 1985; 59(3):928–934. Reprinted with permission.

Table 12.2 Resolution of alveolar edema in patients with acute pulmonary edema

| Classification of edema | No. | ALVEOLAR PROTEIN CONCENTRATION (g/100 mL) | |
		Initial	Final
Hydrostatic	15	3.3 ± 1.0	4.8 ± 2.3[a]
Increased permeability	9	4.7 ± 0.9	6.8 ± 1.6[a]

Data as mean ± S.D.
[a]$P < 0.05$.
Source: Matthay MA, Wiener-Kronish JP. Intact epithelial barrier function is critical for the resolution of alveolar edema in humans. Am Rev Resp Dis 1990; 142(6 Pt 1):1250–1257.

tion of interstitial edema into the airspaces, as occurs in acid aspiration[24] or in gram-negative pneumonia[25] (Figure 12.2).

Other mechanisms may be important in regulating fluid clearance in acute lung injury. Transforming growth factor-alpha (TGF-alpha) is present in human edema fluid from patients with acute lung injury[26] and accelerates fluid clearance by increasing sodium uptake by alveolar epithelial cells.[27] Interestingly, new evidence indicates that several other noncatecholamine dependent factors can increase alveolar fluid clearance including epidermal growth factor,[28] endotoxin and exotoxin,[20,29] and tumor necrosis factor.[30] Increased alveolar fluid clearance may be associated with alveolar type II cell hyperplasia.[31] In the severely injured alveolar epithelium, these mediators may be unable to stimulate adequate fluid clearance if injury to the epithelial tight junctions is extensive.

The capacity to remove alveolar fluid may have prognostic implications. In one study, patients who demonstrated the ability to remove alveolar fluid had significantly decreased mortality[32] (Figure 12.3). Alveolar fluid clearance was calculated

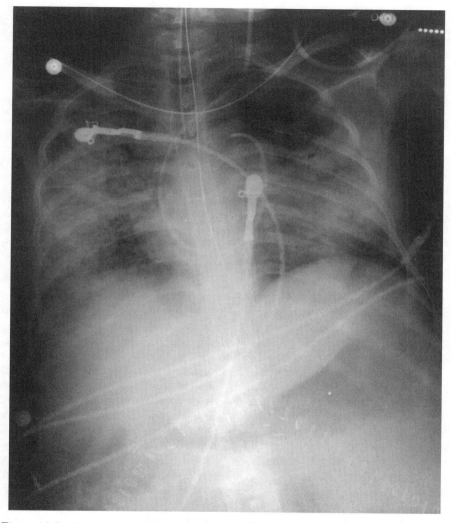

Figure 12.2. Anterior-posterior chest radiograph illustrating early pulmonary radiographic changes of acute lung injury in a 55-year-old man with gram-negative sepsis following abdominal surgery. The patient had severe hypoxemia ($PaO_2 = 59$ mmHg on an $FiO_2 = 0.9$ with positive end-expiratory pressure of 12 cm H_2O). The pulmonary arterial wedge pressure was normal.

from the progressive concentration of alveolar protein in the edema fluid in the first 12 hours after intubation. The ability to remove fluid was also associated with clinical improvement as measured by reduction in the alveolar-arterial oxygen difference, the extent of pulmonary edema on chest radiograph, and a decreased mortality. Fur-

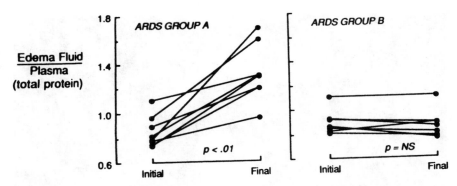

Figure 12.3. Individual data points are shown for the initial and final pulmonary edema fluid-to-plasma total protein concentration in 9 ARDS patients who clinically improved (group A) compared to 7 ARDS patients who did not clinically improve (group B). The mean time interval between the initial and final sample was similar between group A (6.8 ± 5.1 hours) and group B (5.4 ± 4.1 hours) patients. (Adapted with permission from the American Thoracic Society; see Matthay and Wiener-Kronish.[32])

ther studies are under way in larger numbers of patients with active lung injury to test the prognostic value of this index of alveolar fluid clearance.

Until recently, the mechanisms of alveolar protein clearance were poorly understood. In sheep, dogs, rabbits, as well as humans, protein is cleared at 1% to 2% per hour. The half-time of albumin clearance from the alveolar space to plasma is approximately 48 hours.[33,34] The majority of albumin instilled in distal airspaces is cleared as an intact molecule.[34] In a study of protein clearance in rabbits and humans, smaller proteins such as cyanocobalamin and insulin were cleared at a faster rate than larger proteins such as albumin and immunoglobulin.[35] Additional studies with nocodazole, which inhibits microtubules and therefore transcytosis, and monensin, which inhibits acidification of intracellular organelles and therefore endocytosis, have demonstrated that these two pathways do not account for the majority of albumin and immunoglobulin clearance from the airspace.[36] In the normal lung, macrophages also appear to play a minor role in protein clearance because < 1% of instilled albumin is found within airspace in phagocytic cells.[34] Thus most alveolar protein is removed from the uninjured lungs as an intact molecule by a paracellular route. These data might best apply to the resolution of hydrostatic or cardiogenic pulmonary edema. However, in patients with acute lung injury, protein may precipitate out of solution and then require engulfment and degradation by alveolar macrophages, a process that would be slow and might in fact be one of the reasons recovery from severe acute lung injury occurs slowly in many patients.

Unlike the lung endothelial barrier, the alveolar epithelial barrier can continue to function reasonably well under a variety of pathologic conditions. For example, when

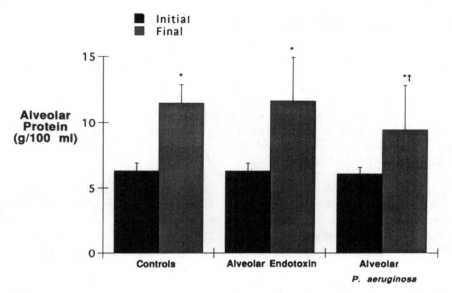

Figure 12.4. Alveolar protein concentration ratio increases as an index of alveolar fluid clearance. The presence of alveolar endotoxin does not significantly impair the alveolar clearance of fluid, but there was a mild decrease with live *Pseudomonas aeruginosa*.
*p < 0.05 for initial concentration compared to final concentration.
†p < 0.05 for the final concentration of live *Pseudomonas aeruginosa* compared to final concentration of control and endotoxin.

endotoxin is given intravenously or within the distal airspaces, there is little epithelial barrier injury and protein transport and alveolar liquid clearance remain near normal, even though there is a marked increase in lung vascular permeability.[37] Even when live *Pseudomonas aeruginosa* is instilled into the airspaces[25] or intravenously,[38] there is evidence of preserved alveolar epithelium function, except in severe epithelial injury (Figure 12.4). The alveolar epithelium may remain intact despite extensive chemoattraction of neutrophils into the airspaces. In normal humans, instillation of leukotriene B4 into the airspaces produces neutrophil chemotaxis into the airspace, but does not change protein permeability.[39] Various other experimental models of acute lung injury that produce moderately severe epithelial and endothelial damage, including oleic acid[40] and hyperoxia,[41] have shown persistent alveolar fluid removal. Because clinical acute lung injury always involves alveolar flooding with protein-rich edema fluid,[32,42] it is clear that a breakdown in the alveolar barrier with subsequent alveolar flooding is a major pathogenic step in the development of clinical and experimental acute lung injury.

Fibrosing Alveolitis in Acute Lung Injury

Pulmonary fibrosis is characterized by alterations in the quantity and organization of the extracellular matrix of the lung. The increase in matrix results from a proliferation and "activation" of fibroblasts with increased production and deposition of a variety of extracellular matrix molecules including fibronectin, collagen, laminin, and elastin.[43] Detailed biochemical, histologic (Figure 12.5), and electron micrograph studies of humans dying of ARDS have shown that alveolar fibrosis develops early, even before interstitial fibrosis.[44] Although the characteristic matrix accumulation in pulmonary fibrosis has been well described, the underlying pathogenic mechanisms driving this dysregulated process are not well understood.[45–47]

In this section, we describe the proteins that have been identified in the alveolar space during acute lung injury and their possible role in the fibrosing alveolitis which develops in many patients (Figure 12.6). Interestingly, in a recent clinical study at our institution, markedly elevated levels of procollagen peptide III, a biochemical marker of collagen synthesis, are present in high levels in the pulmonary edema fluid on day 1 after the onset of clinical acute lung injury, in contrast to control patients with hydrostatic pulmonary edema.[48] These results indicate that the process of fibrosing alveolitis following acute lung injury begins very early in the course of clinical acute lung injury. In addition, in two studies, patients with higher levels of procollagen peptide III were associated with a higher risk of nonsurvival, suggesting that release of this molecule may be an early biologic marker of the severity of acute lung injury.[42,48]

Fibrin and Fibrinogen

Fibrinogen is secreted by mesenchymal cells and is the precursor of fibrin. Fibrin has been detected within hyaline membranes in patients dying with the adult respiratory distress syndrome (ARDS)[49] and within the interstitium and alveolar spaces in fibrosing alveolitis.[44,50] Persistent fibrin deposition in alveoli during acute injury is a pathologic hallmark of ARDS. The removal of fibrin is probably required for full restoration of normal tissue architecture.[51,52]

Previous studies have suggested that alveolar epithelial cells may actively participate in controlling fibrin clearance from the alveolar spaces. Purified alveolar epithelial cells were found to secrete substantial quantities of urokinase-type plasminogen activator (uPA) and plasminogen activator inhibitor-1 (PAI-1), and alveolar epithelial cells express cell surface receptors for uPA.[53,54] The ability of alveolar epithelium to promote local fibrinolysis has several important implications for the pathogenesis of inflammatory tissue injury and subsequent fibrosis. When attached to damaged alveolar walls, fibrin can prevent normal reepithelialization of denuded basement membranes. In an effort to provide a new epithelial barrier to the damaged alveolar walls, the alveolar epithelial cells may migrate over the fibrin mass, thereby incorporating this inflammatory matrix into the alveolar interstitium (Figure 12.7). Also, the

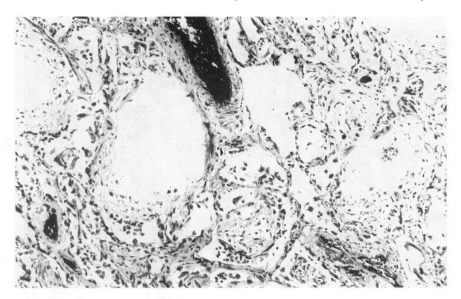

Figure 12.5. Light microscopy of a lung sample from a 45-year-old patient with acute lung injury from primary pneumonia 2 weeks after the onset of clinical lung injury. There is marked loss of normal alveolar histology, which is replaced with intra-alveolar fibrosis. There is minimal interalveolar fibrosis. (Courtesy of Martha Warnock, M.D., Department of Pathology, University of California at San Francisco.)

fibrin network provides an adhesive surface, promoting alveolar collapse and stacking up of adjacent alveolar walls that often leads to a thick, fibrotic scar.[52]

Clinical studies of patients with acute lung injury demonstrate important alterations in fibrin metabolism. Both urokinase and small amounts of tissue plasminogen activator are detectable in the lavage of patients with acute lung injury; however, functional fibrinolytic activity remains significantly depressed from days 3 to 14 after the initial injury.[55] Surprisingly, immunochemical assays reveal normal levels of urokinase and tissue plasminogen activator despite low fibrinolytic activity.[56] The diminished fibrinolytic activity in lavage fluid is most likely secondary to enhanced expression of plasminogen-activator inhibitor type 1 (PAI-1).[55,56]

Fibronectin

Fibronectin represents the earliest known and by far the best studied adhesive protein component of extracellular matrix involved in cell attachment and chemotaxis.[57,58] This 540-kD glycoprotein is a dimer of two similar polypeptide chains. Each polypeptide subunit is made up of repeating modular domains; these include two cell-binding domains (Arg-Gly-Asp; RGD tripeptide) in addition to the unique mod-

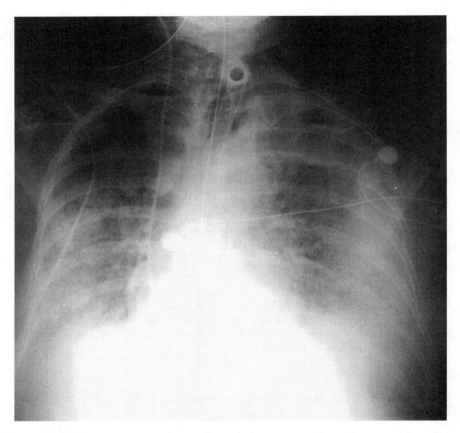

Figure 12.6. Anterior-posterior chest radiograph demonstrating late pulmonary radiographic changes in acute lung injury. A 50-year-old woman developed severe acute lung injury following acute pancreatitis and aspiration of gastric contents. There was a marked decrease in lung compliance. The chest radiograph taken 4 weeks after the onset of acute lung injury demonstrates diffuse ground glass bilateral infiltrates compatible with fibrosing alveolitis. A pulmonary arterial catheter was inserted to manage right ventricular failure secondary to pulmonary hypertension. A tracheostomy was placed because of the patient's prolonged ventilatory failure.

ules interacting with collagen, heparin, and fibrin.[59] Also, fibronectin exists as a soluble dimer in the blood plasma, as well as a component of the fibrous extracellular matrix, and in the basement membrane. Plasma fibronectin accumulates in the lung during the early phase of lung injury[44,60] and could play an important role in connective tissue cell proliferation, fibroblast and epithelial migration, and provisional matrix formation.[61]

We reported that fibronectin (soluble and insoluble) was the most potent stimulus for the early phase of alveolar epithelial cell motility and wound repair using a novel in vitro alveolar epithelial wound model.[62] Also, local production of cellular fibronectin by fibroblasts, alveolar macrophages, and alveolar type II cells could also contribute to the proliferative process.[63] It was also reported that lung steady-state fibronectin mRNA level is increased from hamsters with bleomycin-induced fibrosis.[64] Furthermore, in situ hybridization studies indicated that fibronectin gene expression is increased in alveolar macrophages, as well as in fibroblasts in areas of airspace fibrosis.[65]

The mechanism of increased fibronectin production is incompletely understood. However, some connections between extracellular matrix biology and cytokine/growth factor–mediated cellular responses have been reported in recent years.[66,67] Most extracellular matrix molecules are made up of multiple molecules and contain variable numbers of epidermal growth factor–like domains that are potentially capable of regulating cell proliferation. It is well established that activation of the epidermal growth factor receptor stimulates collagen and glycosaminoglycan synthesis by mesenchymal cells.[68,69]

Fibronectin may act synergistically with other growth factors. Fibronectin-mediated cell adhesion substantially synergizes the action of platelet-derived growth factor to trigger cytoplasmic alkalization, via the platelet-growth factor receptor. This apparent synergism between fibronectin (and its receptor) and platelet-derived growth factor (and its receptor) has functional consequences associated with altered cellular phenotype.[70]

Collagens

The backbone of extracellular matrix is normally composed predominantly of collagens.[71,72] Depending on the source of extracellular matrix, the collagens may be represented by fibrillar (type I, II, III), nonfibrillar (e.g., type IV), or the so-called FACIT collagens (Fibril-Associated Collagens with Interrupted Triple helices) in various combinations thereof.[73] Type I collagen forms a relatively rigid, linear fibrillar network, whereas type IV collagen is assembled into a complex network, found mainly in basement membranes.

Pulmonary fibrosis is associated with an increase in peripheral lung collagen, abnormalities in the ultrastructural appearance and spatial distribution of collagen fibers, and alterations in proportions of collagen types.[74] An increased ratio of type I to type III collagen mRNA in a 3–4 to 1 ratio was observed within 1 to 3 days after bleomycin instillation in bleomycin-sensitive mice.[75] Also, clinical studies have shown increased lung collagen content in patients who died with ARDS.[76] As early as 3 days after the onset of acute lung injury, high levels of collagen precursors (procollagen III) in bronchoalveolar lavage fluid correlate with an increased risk of death,[42] presumably related to increased alveolar fibrosis. Interestingly, lungs from patients dying with idiopathic pulmonary fibrosis (IPF) showed similar biochemical alterations.[77]

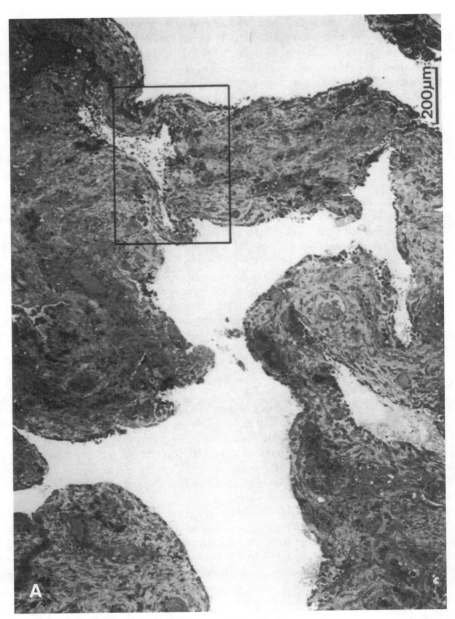

Figure 12.7. The lung at necropsy of a 32-year-old man who died 18 days after drug-induced acute lung injury. Massive tissue plates replace the delicate septal structure. (A) Light microscopy of the lung. (B) Four times magnification of previous framed area. Note

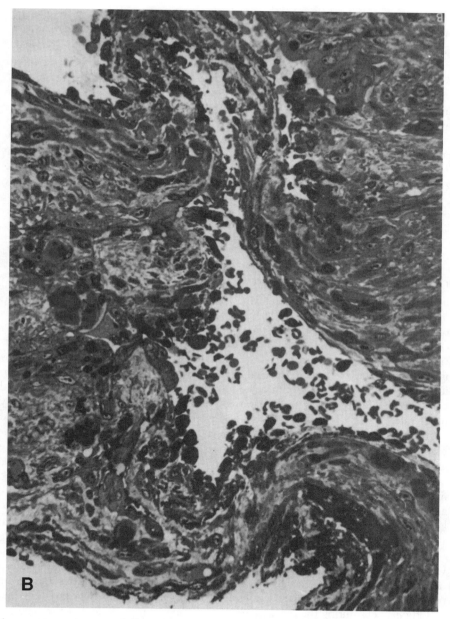

the prominent interstitial fibrosis in contrast to the intra-alveolar fibrosis in Figure 12.5. (Reproduced with permission from W.B. Saunders Company; see Bachofen and Weibel.[49])

Relatively little is known about the contribution of altered matrix degradation to the pathogenesis of pulmonary fibrosis. Alterations in level of collagenase and collagenase inhibitors have been described in patients with ARDS and IPF. Gadek et al.[78] have reported an increase in levels of interstitial collagenase in lavage of patients with IPF. Also, an increase in type I and type III collagenolytic activity has been found in lavage from patients with ARDS.[79] Matrix degradation at sites of alveolar inflammation could contribute in more subtle ways to matrix reorganization. For example, protease and oxidants released in excess of local inhibitors and antioxidants could degrade protein involved in the regulation of fiber assembly, disrupt type IV collagen aggregates important for basal membrane integrity, or degrade surfactant apoproteins, thereby contributing to alveolar collapse. New work indicates that metalloproteinases are present in the inflammatory edema fluid of patients with acute lung injury, suggesting the hypothesis that the release of gelatinase B and other matrix-degrading molecules may contribute to the breakdown of the alveolar epithelial barrier.[80,81]

Mesenchymal Cellular Changes

In addition to exudation of fluid and protein, acute lung injury results in substantial increases in inflammatory, mesenchymal, endothelial, and epithelial cells, as shown in detailed morphologic studies.[44] Often there is also extensive necrosis or apoptosis of type I alveolar cells. The regenerating epithelial cells are type II alveolar epithelial cells, as well as a single layer of (metaplastic) stratified squamous epithelial cells, particularly in areas of severe fibrosis (Figure 12.8). Several molecules secreted by macrophages may play a role in regulating alveolar type II cell proliferation in vivo including hepatocyte and keratinocyte growth factor.[82] Mesothelial and subpleural cells also proliferate during the reparative phase of acute lung injury.[83] In the early proliferative stage (3–14 days), activated myofibroblasts double in number[60,84] and migrate through intra-alveolar spaces through gaps in the epithelial basement membrane. Next, they attach to the luminal side of the epithelial basement membrane and begin to produce extracellular elements. The process of intra-alveolar fibrosis was observed in three different patterns: budding connecting alveolar walls, diffuse fibrosis that obliterated the alveolar space, and broad-based areas attached to the alveolar wall underneath the hyaline membrane. The tissue area ratio of intra-alveolar to interstitial fibrosis peaked at 3 to 1 at 15 days and then gradually decreased to 1 to 1.

A major mystery in the resolution of acute lung injury has been how these activated, recruited cells are cleared from the lung. One possible explanation is controlled cellular death, or apoptosis. One study has shown that lavage fluid from patients with acute lung injury causes increased cell death of lung fibroblasts and endothelial cells during the repair stage.[46] There appear to be at least several mediators; one is heat stable, and the other is heat labile. Cell death appeared to be independent of TNF-alpha. Although the morphologic changes during endothelial cell death were similar to the pattern characteristic of apoptosis, the mediators remain

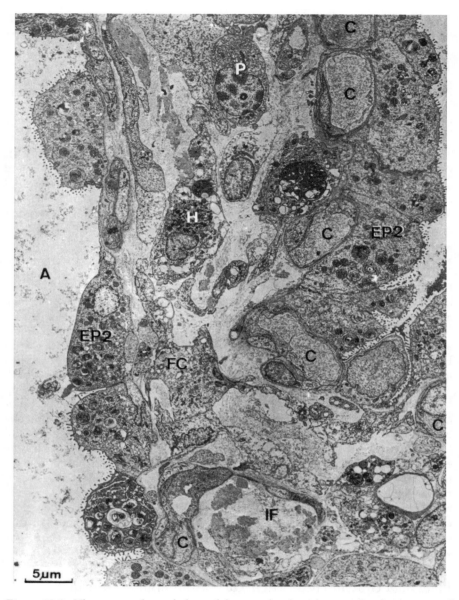

Figure 12.8. Ultrastructural morphology of the interalveolar septum in the chronic stage of acute lung injury. Note the alveolar epithelial transformation (EP2) on both sides of the septum, the abundance of interstitial cells and fibers (IF), and the low capillary density (C); (A), alveolar space; (FC), fibrocyte; (H), histiocyte; (P), plasmacyte. (Reproduced with permission from W.B. Saunders Company; see Bachofen and Weibel.[49])

unknown. These findings should be regarded with caution because there was significantly more DNA synthesis during the repair stage, and the morphologic changes during fibroblast cell death were not typical. Further work needs to be done to elucidate the mechanisms of cell death during recovery from acute lung injury.

Growth Factors

This final section considers growth factors relevant to acute lung injury (Table 12.3). Although much has been learned about the possible role of growth factors in injury and repair of acute lung injury, most of the data are circumstantial. Nevertheless, the availability of newer experimental models including transgenic knockout mice will make it possible to test the role of specific growth factors in the pathogenesis and recovery from acute lung injury.

Platelet Derived Growth Factor (PDGF)

Investigators have found that the bronchoalveolar lavage of patients with ARDS contained both growth-promoting activity in lung fibroblasts and migration-promoting activity in human foreskin fibroblasts compared with patients being ventilated for other reasons.[85] The lavage fluid possessed bioactivity similar to known growth factors and was shown to replace the activity of epidermal-derived growth factor (EGF), PDGF, and insulinlike growth factor (IGF). Several authors have immunopurified lavage fluid and found significant bioactivity for PDGF.[45,47,85] The target cells of PDGF are cells that have PDGF receptors such as fibroblasts, vascular smooth muscle cells, as well as mesenchymal, epithelial, and endothelial cells. PDGF also stimulates extracellular matrix deposition.[86] Some controversy exists about the size of the bioactive protein. Certain authors have identified PDGF at 14 kD;[45,85] yet other authors have found the majority of immunoreactive PDGF at 38–40 kD.[47] This discrepancy may be explained because PDGF is composed of two peptide chains (A&B) linked by disulfide bonds. The 14 kD peptide may actually be a single peptide strand secreted constitutively by lung fibroblasts that have migrated into the alveolar space.[87] The additional observation that the 38–40 kD size PDGF-BB peaks at 3 to 6 days after injury, corresponding to the highest biologic activity of the BAL,[47] suggests that significant modification of the protein occurs at different stages of acute lung injury. The factors which influence the type of PDGF that are secreted remain unknown.

Epidermal Growth Factor (EGF) and Transforming Growth Factor-Alpha (TGF-Alpha)

EGF is a small polypeptide of 6 kD and a mitogen for both mesenchymal and epithelial cells.[88–91] It acts synergistically with both insulin and PDGF to promote mitosis.[92] Also, we recently reported that EGF simulates an increase in mammary epithelial

Table 12.3 Growth factors in repair and resolution of acute lung injury[a]

Growth factor	Origin	Activity
Platelet derived growth factor	Platelet	Fibroblast proliferation and migration; matrix deposition
Epidermal growth factor	Fibroblast Macrophage	Increased alveolar fluid removal; type II cell proliferation
Transforming growth factor-α	Macrophage	Increased alveolar fluid removal; promotes growth of type II pneumocytes and other lung cells
α-thrombin	BAL	Fibroblast growth
Insulin-like growth factor	Macrophage	Fibroblast proliferation and migration
Basic fibroblast growth factor	Macrophage, epithelial type II cell	Fibroblast and endothelial cell proliferation and migration
Vascular endothelial growth factor	Alveolar type II cell	Endothelial cell proliferation and migration
Hepatocyte growth factor	Fibroblast	Proliferation and migration of type II cells
Keratinocyte growth factor	Fibroblast	Proliferation of alveolar type II cells
Interleukin-1	Fibroblast	Proliferation and migration of mesenchymal cells
Tumor necrosis factor	Macrophage	Neutrophil migration
Transforming growth factor-β	Macrophage, fibroblast	Proliferation of fibroblasts, smooth muscle cells, epithelial cells, fibroblasts

[a]See text for references.

cell motility and wound closure with a morphologic transformation of the cells and modifications in cell-cell and cell-substrate adhesion systems.[93]

Control of cellular proliferation after lung injury is thought to involve complex autocrine/paracrine interactions between epithelial and interstitial cells in pulmonary tissues. There is increasing evidence that epidermal factor family members, including EGF and TGF-alpha, are mediators of lung repair. EGF and TGF-alpha have pleiotropic effects on cell proliferation and gene expression, and bind to the EGF receptor, which transmits intracellular signals in cells.[94] In addition, activation of the EGF receptor stimulates collagen and glycosaminoglycan synthesis by mesenchymal cells.[68,69] TGF-alpha is synthesized and released by alveolar macrophages and platelets within the lung after stimulation by lipopolysaccharides, supporting a potential role of TGF-alpha in response to infection.[95] Also, TGF-alpha mRNA synthesis has been shown to increase in epithelial cells in rats after bleomycin-induced pulmonary fibrosis.[96] Korfhagen et al.[97] generated transgenic mice in which human TGF-alpha was expressed in the lung in an epithelial cell-specific manner. These mice developed pulmonary fibrosis, demonstrating that TGF-alpha produced by the lung epithelium can cause a fibroproliferative response in the interstitium and pleural surface.

Transforming Growth Factor-Beta (TGF-Beta)

A central event in tissue repair is the release of cytokines in response to injury. Several lines of evidence point to transforming growth factor-beta (TGF-beta) as a critical cytokine that initiates and terminates tissue repair and whose sustained production underlies the development of tissue fibrosis.[98] TGF-beta is a multifunctional cytokine that was isolated from platelets and characterized just over 10 years ago. In mammals, the cytokine has three isoforms: TGF-beta-1, -2, and -3. These three TGF-beta isoforms are present in the normal lung. During the "inflammatory" phase (days 1 and 3) of bleomycin-induced injury, there was an increase in the mRNA and protein expression of all three TGF-beta isoforms in the injured areas, most prominently in parenchymal cells and alveolar macrophages.[99] In contrast, Khalil et al.[100] found an increase of active TGF-beta-1 secreted by macrophages, whereas quantities of TGF-beta-2 and TGF-beta-3 were unchanged. Based on in vitro studies, TGF-beta has been shown to induce the synthesis of many extracellular matrix molecules including fibronectin, type I collagen, and tenascin.[101,102] The principal cellular source of TGF-beta includes alveolar macrophages,[103] bronchial epithelial cells,[104] fibroblasts,[105] endothelial cells,[106] and type II alveolar epithelial cells.[100] Recent work has demonstrated that TFG-beta-1 can be regulated by the pulmonary epithelial integrin alpha-v beta-6 through latency-associated peptide (LAP). This provides a new mechanism for the development of pulmonary fibrosis in experimental lung injury in mice from bleomycin because this method of lung injury upregulates alpha-v beta-6, an effect that in turn leads to upregulation of TGF-beta-1 through LAP. Mice that do not express alpha-v beta-6 do not develop pulmonary fibrosis following intratracheal instillation of bleomycin.[107]

Hepatocyte Growth Factor (HGF)

HGF is a heterodimeric heparin-binding growth factor that has been shown to be an important growth factor in the liver and kidney after injury and compensatory growth.[107] By immunocytochemistry, HGF was found in rat and human pulmonary airway epithelium and macrophages, but not in alveolar epithelial cells.[108] However, HGF has recently been reported to stimulate rat alveolar type II cell DNA synthesis in primary culture, suggesting its role as a potential paracrine growth factor.[109,110] Also, Yanagita et al.[111] demonstrated increased HGF gene expression after acid instillation into adult rat lung. Interestingly, hepatocyte growth factor/scatter factor (HGF/SF) has been shown to enhance wound closure by influencing migration and spreading using an in vitro T84 intestinal epithelial cell model.[112]

Interestingly, recent work from clinical studies at our institution indicate that HGF levels are significantly higher in the pulmonary edema fluid from patients with acute lung injury than control patients with hydrostatic pulmonary edema.[82,113] In addition, HGF levels were significantly higher in the edema fluid of patients with acute lung injury who did not survive compared to those patients who survived. One explanation for this finding may be that HGF is released in greater levels from patients with more severe injury, or alternatively, that somehow HGF itself compounds the systemic and pulmonary injury associated with acute lung injury. The former explanation seems more likely given the apparent predominant reparative effects of HGF.

Keratinocyte Growth Factor (KGF)

KGF is 28 kD heparin-binding growth factor secreted by lung fibroblasts with properties similar to HGF.[114] KGF, like HGF, stimulates alveolar type II cell DNA synthesis and proliferation. Because antibodies blocking KGF diminish this effect, KGF is a component of alveolar epithelial repair. From in vitro studies it appears that the majority of stimulating activity to type II cells is KGF and HGF, but this activity requires a serum cofactor which is unidentified.

Interestingly, pretreatment of rats with KGF can markedly attenuate experimental acute lung injury from hyperoxia, acid aspiration, and bleomycin.[115] The mechanism(s) by which KGF prevents acute lung injury is incompletely understood at present, but there are several interesting possibilities. First, in vitro data indicate that KGF can increase surfactant production. Second, KGF can decrease epithelial injury by inducing antioxidant mechanisms. Third, recent in vitro data from our laboratory indicate that KGF can enhance alveolar epithelial cell wound healing by up-regulating type II cell motility. Finally, additional recent in vivo data from our laboratory indicate that KGF can induce a sustained up regulation of alveolar epithelial fluid clearance in rats, at least in part by increasing the total number of alveolar epithelial type II cells.[116]

Tumor Necrosis Factor-Alpha (TNF-Alpha)

It is generally assumed that the infiltration of inflammatory cells and the proliferation of interstitial cells associated with fibrosis are related to an overproduction of cytokines. Tumor necrosis factor-alpha is a cytokine with both inflammatory and fibrogenic activities.[117] TNF-alpha mRNA and protein have been detected in lungs from patients with idiopathic pulmonary fibrosis[118] and in lungs from mice with pulmonary fibrosis elicited by exposure to bleomycin.[119] However, the pathogenic mechanisms responsible for TNF-alpha overexpression by alveolar epithelial cells in human pulmonary fibrosis are not clearly understood. Recently, Miyazaki et al.[120] produced transgenic mice in which TNF-alpha was expressed in the lungs for a prolonged period. These mice had hyperplasia of type II alveolar epithelial cells. The progressive accumulation of fibroblasts in the alveolar wall was associated with the deposition of collagen and progressive destruction of alveolar structures. More importantly, TNF-alpha induces monocytes[121] and endothelial cells[122] to release interleukin-1, a mitogenic factor for fibroblasts.[123] Interestingly, clinical studies indicate that biologically active interleukin-1 (IL-1) is present in high quantities in bronchoalveolar lavage fluid[80] or in pulmonary edema fluid[81] from patients with clinical lung injury.

Many investigators have identified additional factors within the acutely injured alveolus that induce mitogenesis, migration, and secretion of extracellular matrix, including insulinlike growth factor,[45] basic fibroblast growth factor (bFGF),[124] alpha-thrombin,[125] angiogenesis growth factor,[91] as well as IL-1. Activated alveolar macrophages may be a major source of these peptides and have been shown to secrete TGF-alpha,[95] IL-6,[126] insulinlike growth factor I,[127] and bFGF.[124] Alveolar epithelial cells also appear to be important in controlling fibroblast growth and may lose the ability to inhibit fibroblast-blast proliferation late in the course of ARDS.[128] Some growth factors such as bFGF can also be found in alveolar basement membrane[129] and may be released during acute injury, thereby stimulating additional growth. Once activated, mesenchymal interstitial cells may even be able to proliferate with no exogenous growth factors.[45]

As is the case with most growth systems, there also appear to be factors in lavage fluid that inhibit mesenchymal cell replication and migration.[85] Candidates include prostaglandins from alveolar macrophages[130] and interleukins (e.g., IL-6) from mesenchymal cells.[131]

In addition to controlled mesenchymal cell growth, reestablishing patency of the microcirulation by neoangiogenesis is essential to recovery of the alveolus.[132] Similar to the epithelial and mesenchymal cells, neoangiogenesis bioactivity requires both proliferation and migration of endothelial cells. There are at least two humoral factors present in bronchoalveolar lavage fluid from patients with ALI that have this bioactivity. One appears identical to the well-characterized endothelial cell growth factor bFGF; the other is a 150-kD nonheparin-binding protein that mediates endothelial cell migration and attachment in vitro and growth of new vessels in vivo.[91] Recently, Maniscalco et al.[133] discovered a vascular endothelial growth factor (VEGF) that promotes endothelial cell repair. VEGF is a 42-kD heparin-binding peptide secreted by alveolar type II cells recovering from acute lung injury. Other factors that might be related to neoangiogenesis include lung ornithine decarboxylase activity and polyamine (putrescine, spermidine, and spermine) content which correlate with the number and surface area of capillary endothelial cells.[134]

Summary

In the past 15 years, much has been learned about the repair and resolution of clinical acute lung injury. The response to acute lung injury is a complex pathophysiologic process that often results in impaired lung function. Alveolar edema fluid clearance is driven by active sodium transport across the alveolar epithelium, a process that can be up-regulated by catecholamine-dependent and -independent mechanisms. Water is probably primarily transported through transcellular water channels, perhaps primarily in alveolar epithelial type I cells, following the osmotic gradient created by vectorial transport of sodium from the apical to the basolateral surface of alveolar epithelial type II cells. Soluble protein is probably removed by restricted diffusion, whereas insoluble proteins probably require alveolar macrophage engulfment and clearance. Large macromolecules such as fibrin, collagen, and immunoglobulins are cleared by undetermined mechanisms. Recruitment, activation, and disappearance of inflammatory and mesenchymal cells are orchestrated by a host of growth factors that are just beginning to be identified. Considerable progress has been made in understanding some of the signals that regulate programmed cell death (apoptosis) as well as the regeneration of normal alveolar epithelial cells and capillary endothelial cells.

Understanding the basic mechanisms of alveolar fluid transport and alveolar epithelial repair may aid in developing more effective treatment strategies in the future. For example, the capacity of beta-adrenergic stimulation to increase net sodium and fluid transport has raised the possibility that beta-agonist therapy might be used to hasten the resolution of clinical alveolar edema. Also, the use of alveolar epithelial mitogens, such as keratinocyte growth factor, might be used clinically to enhance alveolar epithelial repair in patients with clinical acute lung injury.

References

1. Marinelli WA, Henke CA, Harmon KR, Hertz MI, Bitterman PB. Mechanisms of alveolar fibrosis after acute lung injury. Clin Chest Med 1990; 11(4):657–672.
2. Schneeberger E, Lynch R. Structure, function, and regulation of cellular tight junctions. Am J Physiol 1992; 262:L647–L661.
3. Staub NC. Alveolar flooding and clearance. Am Rev Respir Dis Crit Care 1983; 127 (5 Pt 2):S44–S51.
4. Matthay MA, Folkesson HG, Verkman AS. Salt and water transport across alveolar and distal airway epithelia in the adult lung. Am J Physiol (Lung Cell & Mol) 1996; 270: L487–L503.
5. Nici L, Dowin R, Jamieson JD, Ingbar DH. Upregulation of rat type II pneumocyte nakatase during hyperoxic lung injury. Am J Physiol (Lung) 1991; 261:L307–L314.
6. Saumon G, Basset G. Electrolyte and fluid transport across the mature alveolar epithelium. J Appl Physiol 1993; 74:1–15.
7. Matalon S, Benos D, Jackson RM. Biophysical and molecular properties of amiloride-inhibitable sodium channel in alveolar epithelial cells. Am J Physiol 1996; 271:L1–L22.
8. Folkesson HG, Matthay MA, Hasegawa H, Kheradmand F, Verkman AS. Transcellular water transport in lung alveolar epithelium through mercury-sensitive water channels. Proc Natl Acad Sci 1994; 91(11):4970–4974.
9. Carter EP, Matthay MA, Farinas J, Verkman AS. Transalveolar osmotic and diffusional water permeability in intact mouse lung measured by a novel surface fluorescence method. J Gen Physiol 1996; 108:133–142.
10. Carter EP, Umenishi F, Matthay MA, Verkman AS. Developmental changes in water permeability across the alveolar barrier in perinatal rabbit lung. J Clin Invest 1997; 100:1071–1078.

11. Dobbs LD, Gonzales R, Matthay MA, Carter EP, Allen C, Verkman AS. Highly water-permeable type I alveolar epithelial cells confer high water permeability between the air-space and vasculature in rat lung. Proc Natl Acad Sci USA 1998; 95:2991–2996.

12. Matthay MA, Berthiaume Y, Staub NC. Long-term clearance of liquid and protein from the lungs of unanesthetized sheep. J Appl Physiol 1985; 59(3):928–934.

13. Effros RM, Hacker A, Silverman P, Hukkanen J. Protein concentrations have little effect on reabsorption of fluid from isolated rat lungs. J Appl Physiol 1991; 70(1):416–422.

14. Sakuma T, Pittet JF, Jayr C, Matthay MA. Alveolar liquid and protein clearance in the absence of blood flow or ventilation in sheep. J Appl Physiol 1993; 74(1):176–185.

15. Sakuma T, Okaniwa G, Nakada T, Nishimura T, Fujimura S, Matthay MA. Alveolar fluid clearance in the resected human lung. Am J Respir Crit Care Med 1994; 150(2):305–310.

16. Matthay MA, Landolt CC, Staub NC. Differential liquid and protein clearance from the alveoli of anesthetized sheep. J Appl Physiol 1982; 53(1):96–104.

17. Berthiaume Y, Staub NC, Matthay MA. Beta-adrenergic agonists increase lung liquid clearance in anesthetized sheep. J Clin Invest 1987; 79(2):335–343.

18. Berthiaume Y, Broaddus VC, Gropper MA, Tanita T, Matthay MA. Alveolar liquid and protein clearance from normal dog lungs. J Appl Physiol 1988; 65(2):585–593.

19. Jayr C, Garat C, Meignan M, Pittet JF, Zelter M, Matthay MA. Alveolar liquid and protein clearance in anesthetized ventilated rats. J Appl Physiol 1994; 76(6):2636–2642.

20. Pittet JF, Wiener-Kronish JP, McElroy MC, Folkesson HG, Matthay MA. Stimulation of lung epithelial liquid clearance by endogenous release of catecholamines in septic shock in anesthetized rats. J Clin Invest 1994; 94(2):663–671.

21. Sakuma T, Folkesson HG, Suzuki S, Okaniwa G, Fujimura S, Matthay MA. Beta-adrenergic agonist stimulated alveolar fluid clearance in ex vivo human and rat lungs. Am J Resp Crit Care Med 1997; 155:506–512.

22. Smedira N, Gates L, Hastings R, Jayr C, Sakuma T, Pittet JF, Matthay MA. Alveolar and lung liquid clearance in anesthetized rabbits. J Appl Physiol 1991; 70(4):1827–1835.

23. Cottrell TS, Levine OR, Senior RM, Wiener J, Spiro D, Fishman AP. Electron microscopic alterations at the alveolar level in pulmonary edema. Circ Res 1967; 21(6):783–797.

24. Folkesson HG, Matthay MA, Hebert CA, Broaddus VC. Acid aspiration-induced lung injury in rabbits is mediated by interleukin-alpha-8–dependent mechanisms. J Clin Invest 1995; 96:107–116.

25. Wiener-Kronish JP, Sakuma T, Kudoh I, Pittet JF, Frank D, Dobbs L, Vasil ML, Matthay MA. Alveolar epithelial injury and pleural empyema in acute P. aeruginosa pneumonia in anesthetized rabbits. J Appl Physiol 1993; 75(4):1661–1669.

26. Chesnutt A, Kheradmand F, Folkesson HG, Alberts M, Matthay MD. Soluble transforming growth factor-α is present in pulmonary edema fluid of patients with acute lung injury. Chest 1997; 111:652–656.

27. Folkesson HG, Pittet JF, Nitenberg G, Matthay MA. Transforming growth factor-α increases alveolar liquid clearance in anesthetized ventilated rats. Am J Physiol (Lung Cell Mol Physiol) 1996; 271:L236–L244.

28. Borok Z, Hami A, Danto SI, Lubman RL, Kim K-J, Chandall ED. Effects of epidermal growth on alveolar epithelial junctional permeability and active sodium transport. Am J Physiol 1996; 270:L599–L565.

29. Garat C, Rezaigmia S, Meignan M, D'Ortho M, Harp A, Matthay MA, Jayr C. Alveolar endotoxin increases alveolar liquid clearance in rats. J Appl Physiol 1995; 79:2021–2028.
30. Rezaiguia S, Garat C, Meignan M, Matthay MA, Jayr C. Acute bacterial pneumonia in rats increases alveolar epithelial fluid clearance by a tumor necrosis-alpha-dependent mechanism. J Clin Invest 1997; 99:325–335.
31. Nitenberg F, Folkesson H, Osorio O, Cohen-Gold J, Matthay M. Alveolar epithelial ligand clearance is markedly increased 10 days following acute lung injury from bleomycin. Am J Respir Crit Care Med 1995; 151:A620.
32. Matthay MA, Wiener-Kronish JP. Intact epithelial barrier function is critical for the resolution of alveolar edema in humans. Am Rev Respir Dis 1990; 142(6 Pt 1):1250–1257.
33. Gorin AB, Stewart PA. Differential permeability of endothelial and epithelial barriers to albumin flux. J Appl Physiol 1979; 47(6):1315–1324.
34. Berthiaume Y, Albertine KH, Grady M, Fick G, Matthay MA. Protein clearance from the air spaces and lungs of unanesthetized sheep over 144 h. J Appl Physiol 1989; 67(5):1887–1897.
35. Hastings RH, Grady M, Sakuma T, Matthay MA. Clearance of different-sized proteins from the alveolar space in humans and rabbits. J Appl Physiol 1992; 73(4):1310–1316.
36. Hastings RH, Wright JR, Albertine KH, Ciriales R, Matthay MA. Effect of endocytosis inhibitors on alveolar clearance of albumin, immunoglobulin G, and SP-A in rabbits. Am J Physiol 1994; 266(5 Pt 1):L544–L552.
37. Wiener-Kronish JP, Albertine KH, Matthay MA. Differential responses of the endothelial and epithelial barriers of the lung in sheep to *Escherichia coli* endotoxin. J Clin Invest 1991; 88(3):864–875.
38. Pittet JF, Wiener-Kronish JP, Serikov V, Matthay MA. Resistance of the alveolar epithelium to injury from septic shock in sheep. Am J Respir Crit Care Med 1995; 151(4):1093–1100.
39. Martin TR, Pistorese BP, Chi EY, Goodman RB, Matthay MA. Effects of leukotriene B4 in the human lung. Recruitment of neutrophils into the alveolar spaces without a change in protein permeability. J Clin Invest 1989; 84(5):1609–1619.
40. Wiener-Kronish JP, Broaddus VC, Albertine KH, Gropper MA, Matthay MA, Staub NC. Relationship of pleural effusions to increased permeability pulmonary edema in anesthetized sheep. J Clin Invest 1988; 82(4):1422–1429.
41. Garat C, Meignan M, Matthay MA, Luo DF, Jayr C. Alveolar epithelial fluid clearance mechanisms are intact after moderate hyperoxic lung injury in rats. Chest 1997; 111:1381–1388.
42. Clark JG, Milberg, JA, Steinberg KP, Hudson LD. Type III procollagen peptide in the adult respiratory distress syndrome: association of increased peptide levels in bronchoalveolar lavage fluid with increased risk for death. Ann Intern Med 1995; 122(1):17–23.
43. Crouch E. Pathobiology of pulmonary fibrosis. Am J Physiol 1990; 259(4 Pt 1):L159–L184.
44. Fukuda Y, Ishizaki M, Masuda Y, Kimura G, Kawanami O, Masugi Y. The role of intraalveolar fibrosis in the process of pulmonary structural remodeling in patients with diffuse alveolar damage. Am J Pathol 1987; 126(1):171–182.
45. Bitterman PB. Pathogenesis of fibrosis in acute lung injury. Am J Med 1992; 92(6A): 39S–43S.
46. Polunovsky VA, Chen B, Henke C, Snover D, Wendt C, Ingbar DH, Bitterman PB. Role of mesenchymal cell death in lung remodeling after injury. J Clin Invest 1993; 92(1):388–397.

47. Walsh J, Absher M, Kelley J. Variable expression of platelet-derived growth factor family proteins in acute lung injury. Am J Respir Cell Mole Biol 1993; 9(6):637–644.

48. Chesnutt A, Matthay MA, Tibayan F, Clark J. Early detection of type III procollagen peptide in acute lung injury: pathogenetic and prognostic significance. Am J Resp Crit Care Med 1997; 156:840–845.

49. Bachofen A, Weibel ER. Alterations of the gas exchange apparatus in adult respiratory insufficiency associated with septicemia. Am Rev Respir Dis Crit Care 1977; 116(4):589–615.

50. Kuhn CD, Boldt J, King TE Jr, Crouch E, Vartio T, McDonald JA. An immunohistochemical study of architectural remodeling and connective tissue synthesis in pulmonary fibrosis. Am Rev Respir Dis Crit Care 1989; 140(6):1693–1703.

51. Senior RM, Skogen WF, Griffin GL, Wilner GD. Effects of fibrinogen derivatives upon the inflammatory response. Studies with human fibrinopeptide B. J Clin Invest 1986; 77(3):1014–1019.

52. Burkhardt A. Alveolitis and collapse in the pathogenesis of pulmonary fibrosis. Am Rev Respir Dis Crit Care 1989; 140(2):513–524.

53. Gross TJ, Simon RH, Sitrin RG. Expression of urokinase-type plasminogen activator by rat pulmonary alveolar epithelial cells. Am J Respir Cell Mol Biol 1990; 3(5):449–456.

54. Simon RH, Gross TJ, Edwards JA, Sitrin RG. Fibrin degradation by rat pulmonary alveolar epithelial cells. Am J Physiol 1992; 262(4 Pt 1):L482–L488.

55. Idell S, Koenig KB, Fair DS, Martin TR, McLarty J, Maunder RJ. Serial abnormalities of fibrin turnover in evolving adult respiratory distress syndrome. Am J Physiol 1991; 261 (4 Pt 1):L240–L248.

56. Bertozzi P, Astedt B, Zenzius L, Lynch K, LeMaire F, Zapol W, Chapman H Jr. Depressed bronchoalveolar urokinase activity in patients with adult respiratory distress syndrome. N Engl J Med 1990; 322(13):890–897.

57. Limper AH, Roman J. Fibronectin. A versatile matrix protein with roles in thoracic development, repair and infection. Chest 1992; 101(6):1663–1673.

58. Mosher DJ, Sottile J, Wu C, McDonald JA. Assembly of extracellular matrix. Curr Opin Cell Biol 1992; 4(5):810–818.

59. Damsky CH, Werb Z. Signal transduction by integrin receptors for extracellular matrix: cooperative processing of extracellular information. Curr Opin Cell Biol 1992; 4(5):772–781.

60. Durr RA, Dubaybo BA, Thet LA. Repair of chronic hyperoxic lung injury: changes in lung ultrastructure and matrix. Exp Mol Pathol 1987; 47(2):219–240.

61. McDonald JA. Receptors for extracellular matrix components. Am J Physiol 1989; 257(6 Pt 1):L331–L337.

62. Garat C, Kheradmand F, Albertine K, Agnost V, Folkesson H, Meignan M, Matthay M. Soluble and insoluble fibronectin increases alveolar epithelial wound healing in vitro. Am J Physiol (Lung Cell and Mol) 1996; 271:L844–L853.

63. Sage H, Farin FM, Striker GE, Fisher AB. Granular pneumocytes in primary culture secrete several major components of the extracellular matrix. Biochem 1983; 22(9):2148–2155.

64. Raghow R, Lurie S, Seyer JM, Kang AH. Profiles of steady state levels of messenger RNAs coding for type I procollagen, elastin, and fibronectin in hamster lungs undergoing bleomycin-induced interstitial pulmonary fibrosis. J Clin Invest 1985; 76(5):1733–1739.

65. Adachi K, Yamauchi K, Bernaudin JF, Fouret P, Verrans VJ, Crystal RG. Evaluation of

fibronectin gene expression by in situ hybridization. Differential expression of the fibronectin gene among populations of human alveolar macrophages. Am J Pathol 1988; 133(2):193–203.

66. Ruoslahti E, Yamaguchi Y. Proteoglycans as modulators of growth factor activities. Cell 1991; 64(5):867–869.

67. Thiery JP, Boyer B. The junction between cytokines and cell adhesion. Curr Opin Cell Biol 1992; 4(5):782–792.

68. Silver MH, Murray JC, Pratt RM. Epidermal growth factor stimulates type-V collagen synthesis in cultured murine palatal shelves. Differentiation 1984; 27(3):205–208.

69. Pisano MM, Greene RM. Epidermal growth factor potentiates the induction of ornithine decarboxylase activity by prostaglandins in embryonic palate mesenchymal cells: effects on cell proliferation and glycosaminoglycan synthesis. Dev Biol 1987; 122(2):419–431.

70. Schwartz MA, Lechene C. Adhesion is required for protein kinase C–dependent activation of the Na+/H+ antiporter by platelet-derived growth factor. Proc Natl Acad Sci 1992; 89(13):6138–6141.

71. Davidson JM. Biochemistry and turnover of lung interstitium. Eur Respir J 1990; 3(9): 1048–1063.

72. Vuorio E, de Crombrugghe B. The family of collagen genes. Ann Rev Biochem 1990; 59:837–872.

73. Shaw LM, Olsen BR. FACIT collagens: diverse molecular bridges in extracellular matrices. Trends Biochem Sci 1991; 16(5):191–194.

74. Clark JG, Kuhn CD, McDonald JA, Mecham RP. Lung connective tissue. Int Rev Connective Tissue Res 1983; 10:249–331.

75. Harrison JH Jr, Hoyt DG, Lazo JS. Acute pulmonary toxicity of bleomycin: DNA scission and matrix protein mRNA levels in bleomycin-sensitive and -resistant strains of mice. Mole Pharmacol 1989; 36(2):231–238.

76. Zapol WM, Trelstad RL, Coffey JW, Tsai I, Salvador RA. Pulmonary fibrosis in severe acute respiratory failure. Am Rev Respir Dis Crit Care 1979; 119(4):547–554.

77. Kirk JM, Heard BE, Kerr I, Turner-Warwick M, Laurent GJ. Quantitation of types I and III collagen in biopsy lung samples from patients with cryptogenic fibrosing alveolitis. Collaborative Relative Res 1984; 4(3):169–182.

78. Gadek JE, Kelman JA, Fells G, Weinberger SE, Horwitz AL, Reynolds HY, Fulmer JD, Crystal RG. Collagenase in the lower respiratory tract of patients with idiopathic pulmonary fibrosis. N Engl J Med 1979; 301(14):737–742.

79. Christner P, Fein A, Goldberg S, Lippmann M, Abrams W, Weinbaum G. Collagenase in the lower respiratory tract of patients with adult respiratory distress syndrome. Am Rev Respir Dis Crit Care 1985; 131(5):690–695.

80. Pugin J, Ricou K, Steinberg K, Suter P, Martin TR. Proinflammatory activity in bronchoalveolar lavage fluids from patients with ARDS, a prominent role for interleukin-1. Am J Resp Crit Care Med 1996; 153:1850–1856.

81. Pugin J, Verghese G, Widmer MC, Matthay MA. The alveolar space is the site of intense inflammatory and profibrobrotic reactions in the early phase of ARDS. Crit Care Med 1999; in press.

82. Verghese GM, McKormick-Shannon K, Mason RJ, Matthay MA. Hepatocyte growth factor and keratinocyte growth factor in the pulmonary edema fluid of patients with acute lung injury. Am J Resp Crit Care Med 1998; 158:386–394.

83. Adamson IY, Bakowska J, Bowden DH. Mesothelial cell proliferation: a nonspecific response to lung injury associated with fibrosis. Am J Respir Cell Mole Biol 1994; 10(3):253–258.

84. Thet LA, Parra SC, Shelburne JD. Sequential changes in lung morphology during the repair of acute oxygen-induced lung injury in adult rats. Exper Lung Res 1986; 11(3):209–228.

85. Snyder LS, Hertz MI, Peterson MS, Harmon KR, Marinelli WA, Henke CA, Greenheck JR, Chen B, Bitterman PB. Acute lung injury. Pathogenesis of intraalveolar fibrosis. J Clin Invest 1991; 88(2):663–673.

86. Lynch SE, Nixon JC, Colvin RB, Antoniades HN. Role of platelet-derived growth factor in wound healing: synergistic effects with other growth factors. Proc Natl Acad Sci 1987; 84(21):7696–7700.

87. Fabisiak JP, Absher M, Evans JN, Kelley J. Spontaneous production of PDGF A-chain homodimer by rat lung fibroblasts in vitro. Am J Physiol 1992; 263(2 Pt 1):L185–L193.

88. Carpenter G, Cohen S. Epidermal growth factor. Ann Rev Biochem 1979; 48:193–216.

89. Leslie CC, McCormick-Shannon K, Cook JL, Mason RJ. Macrophages stimulate DNA synthesis in rat alveolar type II cells. Am Rev Respir Dis Crit Care 1985; 132(6):1246–1252.

90. Chiang CP, Nilsen-Hamilton M. Opposite and selective effects of epidermal growth factor and human platelet transforming growth factor-beta on the production of secreted proteins by murine 3T3 cells and human fibroblasts. J Biol Chem 1986; 261(23):10478–10481.

91. Henke C, Fiegel V, Peterson M, Wick M, Knighton D, McCarthy J, Bitterman P. Identification and partial characterization of angiogenesis bioactivity in the lower respiratory tract after acute lung injury. J Clin Invest 1991; 88(4):1386–1395.

92. Shipley GD, Childs CB, Volkenant ME, Moses HL. Differential effects of epidermal growth factor, transforming growth factor, and insulin on DNA and protein synthesis and morphology in serum-free cultures of AKR-2B cells. Cancer Res 1984; 44(2):710–716.

93. Matthay MA, Thiery JP, Lafont F, Stampfer F, Boyer B. Transient effect of epidermal growth factor on the motility of an immortalized mammary epithelial cell line. J Cell Sci 1993; 106(3):869–878.

94. Reynolds FH Jr, Todaro GJ, Fryling C, Stephenson JR. Human transforming growth factors induce tyrosine phosphorylation of EGF receptors. Nature 1981; 292(5820):259–262.

95. Madtes DK, Raines EW, Sakariassen KS, Assoian RK, Sporn MB, Bell GI, Ross P. Induction of transforming growth factor-alpha in activated human alveolar macrophages. Cell 1988; 53(2):285–293.

96. Madtes DK, Busby HK, Strandjord TP, Clark JG. Expression of transforming growth factor-alpha and epidermal growth factor receptor is increased following bleomycin-induced lung injury in rats. Am J Respir Cell Mole Biol 1994; 11(5):540–551.

97. Korfhagen TR, Swantz RJ, Wert SE, McCarty JM, Kerlakian CB, Glasser SW, Whitsett JA. Respiratory epithelial cell expression of human transforming growth factor-alpha induces lung fibrosis in transgenic mice. J Clin Invest 1994; 93(4):1691–1699.

98. Border WA, Ruoslahti E. Transforming growth factor-beta in disease: the ark side of tissue repair. J Clin Invest 1992; 90(1):1–7.

99. Santana A, Saxena B, Noble NA, Gold LI, Marshall BC. Increased expression of transforming growth factor beta isoforms (β1, β2, β3) in bleomycin-induced pulmonary fibrosis. Am J Respir Cell Mole Biol 1995; 13(1):34–44.

100. Khalil N, O'Connor RN, Flanders KC, Shing W, Whitman CI. Regulation of type II alve-

olar epithelial cell proliferation by TGF-beta during bleomycin-induced lung injury in rats. Am J Physiol 1994; 267(5 Pt 1):L498–L507.

101. Ignotz RA, Massague J. Transforming growth factor-beta stimulates the expression of fibronectin and collagen and their incorporation into the extracellular matrix. J Biol Chem 1986; 261(9):4337–4345.

102. Hoyt DG, Lazo JS. Alterations in pulmonary mRNA encoding procollagens, fibronectin and transforming growth factor-beta precede bleomycin-induced pulmonary fibrosis in mice. J Pharmacol Exp Ther 1988; 246(2):765–771.

103. Denholm EM, Rollins SM. Expression and secretion of transforming growth factor-beta by bleomycin-stimulated rat alveolar macrophages. Am J Physiol 1993; 264(1 Pt 1):L36–L42.

104. Sacco O, Romberger D, Rizzino A, Beckmann JD, Rennard SI, Spurzem JR. Spontaneous production of transforming growth factor-beta 2 by primary cultures of bronchial epithelial cells. Effects on cell behavior in vitro. J Clin Invest 1992; 90(4):1379–1385.

105. Kelley J, Fabisiak JP, Hawes K, Absher M. Cytokine signaling in lung: transforming growth factor-beta secretion by lung fibroblasts. Am J Physiol 1991; 260(2 Pt 1):L123–L128.

106. Phan SH, Gharaee-Kermani M, Wolber F, Ryan US. Stimulation of rat endothelial cell transforming growth factor-beta production by bleomycin. J Clin Invest 1991; 87(1):148–154.

107. Munger JS, Huang X, Kawakatsu H, Griffiths M, Dalton S, Wu J, Pittet JF, Kaminski N, Garat C, Matthay MA, Rifkin DB, Sheppard D. The integrin αVB6 binds and activates latent TGB1: a mechanism for regulating pulmonary inflammation and fibrosis. Cell 1999; in press.

108. Matsumoto K, Nakamura T. Hepatocyte growth factor: molecular structure, roles in liver regeneration, and other biological functions. Crit Rev Oncogenesis 1989; 3:27–54.

109. Panos RJ, Bak PM, Simone WS, Rubin JS, Smith LJ. Intratracheal instillation of kerotinocyte growth factor decreases hyperoxia-induced mortality in rats. J Clin Invest 1995; 96:2026–2033.

110. Shiratori M, Michalopoulos G, Shinozuka H, Singh G, Ogasawara H, Katyal SL. Hepatocyte growth factor stimulates DNA synthesis in alveolar epithelial type II cells in vitro. Am J Respir Cell Mole Biol 1995; 12(2):171–180.

111. Yanagita K, Matsumoto K, Sekiguchi K, Ishibashi H, Niho Y, Nakamura T. Hepatocyte growth factor may act as a pulmotrophic factor on lung regeneration after acute lung injury. J Biol Chem 1993; 268(28):21212–21217.

112. Nusrat A, Parkos CA, Bacarra AE, Godowski PJ, Delp-Archer C, Rosen EM, Madara JL. Hepatocyte growth factor/scatter factor effects on epithelia. Regulation of intercellular junctions in transformed and nontransformed cell lines, basolateral polarization of c-met receptor in transformed and natural intestinal epithelia, and induction of rapid wound repair in a transformed model epithelium. J Clin Invest 1994; 93(5):2056–2065.

113. Matthay MA, Conner EJ, Ware L, Verghese G. β-adrenergic markers of acute lung injury. In The Adult Respiratory Disease Syndrome. S. Matalon, JI Sznajder (eds). New York, Plenum Publishers, 1998, pp. 207–214.

114. Panos RJ, Rubin JS, Csaky KG, Aaronson SA, Mason RJ. Keratinocyte growth factor and hepatocyte growth factor/scatter factor are heparin-binding growth factors for alveolar type II cells in fibroblast-conditioned medium. J Clin Invest 1993; 92(2):969–977.

115. Matushak GM, Lechner AJ. Targeting the alveolar epithelium in acute lung injury: Ker-

atinocyte growth factor and regulation of the alveolar epithelial barrier. Crit Care Med 1995; 24:905–907.

116. Wang Y, Folkesson HG, Jayr C, Ware LB, Matthay MA. Keratinocyte growth factor induces a sustained upregulation of alveolar liquid clearance over 5 days in rats. FASEB J 1998; 12:40A.

117. Piguet PF, Grau GE, Vassalli P. Subcutaneous perfusion of tumor necrosis factor induces local proliferation of fibroblasts, capillaries, and epidermal cells, or massive tissue necrosis. Am J Pathol 1990; 136(1):103–110.

118. Piguet PF, Ribaux C, Karpuz V, Grau GE, Kapanci Y. Expression and localization of tumor necrosis factor-alpha and its mRNA in idiopathic pulmonary fibrosis. Am J Pathol 1993; 143(3):651–655.

119. Piguet PF, Collart MA, Grau GE, Kapanci Y, Vassalli P. Tumor necrosis factor/cachectin plays a key role in bleomycin-induced pneumopathy and fibrosis. J Exper Med 1989; 170(3):655–663.

120. Miyazaki Y, Araki K, Vesin C, Garcia C, Kapanci Y, Whitsett JA, Piguet PF, Vassalli P. Expression of a tumor necrosis factor-alpha transgene in murine lung causes lymphocytic and fibrosing alveolitis. A mouse model of progressive pulmonary fibrosis. J Clin Invest 1995; 96(1):250–259.

121. Bachwich PR, Chensue SW, Larrick JW, Kunkel SL. Tumor necrosis factor stimulates interleukin-1 and prostaglandin E2 production in resting macrophages. Biochem Biophys Res Commun 1986; 136(1):94–101.

122. Nawroth PP, Bank I, Handley D, Cassimeris J, Chess L, Stern D. Tumor necrosis factor/cachectin interacts with endothelial cell receptors to induce release of interleukin-1. J Exper Med 1986; 163(6):1363–1375.

123. Palombella VJ, Yamashiro DJ, Maxfield FR, Decker SJ, Vilcek J. Tumor necrosis factor increases the number of epidermal growth factor receptors on human fibroblasts. J Biol Chem 1987; 262(5):1950–1954.

124. Henke C, Marinelli W, Jessurun J, Fox J, Harms D, Peterson M, Chiang L, Doran P. Macrophage production of basic fibroblast growth factor in the fibroproliferative disorder of alveolar fibrosis after lung injury. Am J Pathol 1993; 143(4):1189–1199.

125. Tani K, Yasuoka S, Ogushi F, Asada K, Fujisawa K, Ozaki T, Sano N, Ogura T. Thrombin enhances lung fibroblast proliferation in bleomycin-induced pulmonary fibrosis. Am J Respir Cell Mole Biol 1991; 5(1):34–40.

126. Jordana M, Richards C, Irving LB, Gauldie J. Spontaneous in vitro release of alveolar-macrophage cytokines after the intratracheal instillation of bleomycin in rats. Characterization and kinetic studies. Am Rev Respir Dis Crit Care 1988; 137(5):1135–1140.

127. Rom WN, Basset P, Fells GA, Nukiwa T, Trapnell BC, Crysal RG. Alveolar macrophages release an insulin-like growth factor I–type molecule. J Clin Invest 1988; 82(5):1685–1693.

128. Young L, Adamson IY. Epithelial-fibroblast interactions in bleomycin-induced lung injury and repair. Environ Health Perspect 1993; 101(1):56–61.

129. Folkman J, Klagsburn M. Angiogenic factors. Science 1987; 235(4787):442–447.

130. Bitterman PB, Wewers MD, Rennard SI, Adelberg S, Crystal RG. Modulation of alveolar macrophage-driven fibroblast proliferation by alternative macrophage mediators. J Clin Invest 1986; 77(3):700–708.

131. Kohase M, Henriksen-DeStefano D, May LT, Vilcek J, Sehgal PB. Induction of beta 2-

interferon by tumor necrosis factor: a homeostatic mechanism in the control of cell proliferation. Cell 1986; 45(5):659–666.

132. Jones R, Langleben D, Reid L. Patterns of remodeling of the pulmonary circulation in acute and subacute lung injury. In The pulmonary circulation and acute lung injury, ed S Said, Futura, Mount Kisco, NY, 1985, pp. 137–188.

133. Maniscalco WM, Watkins RH, Finkelstein J, Campbell, N, Campbell MH. Vascular endothelial growth factor mRNA increases in alveolar epithelial cells during recovery from oxygen injury. Am J Respir Cell Mole Biol 1995;13:377–386.

134. Thet LA, Parra SC, Shelburne JD. Repair of oxygen-induced lung injury in adult rats. The role of ornithine decarboxylase and polyamines. Am Rev Respir Dis Crit Care 1984; 129(1):174–181.

13

Multiple System Organ Failure

Ari Uusaro and James A. Russell

Introduction

Multiple system organ failure (MSOF) is important in management of patients who have ARDS for several reasons. First, MSOF is the most common *cause* of death of patients who have ARDS.[1] Furthermore, development of multiple system organ dysfunction is a *predictor* of death of patients who have ARDS.[2] Second, ARDS is basically the expression of lung failure in critically ill patients who have multiple system organ failure. That is, ARDS and MSOF are inextricably linked and are not really separate issues. Third, MSOF is extremely costly. Indeed, a significant portion of any ICU budget is spent on patients who have MSOF because of the intensity and duration of support.

This chapter reviews what MSOF is, why it is important, how it occurs, and how it can be predicted. The clinical management of organ failure is presented in Chapter 9 on total patient care. Here we first review several definitions of MSOF. We then describe the epidemiology of MSOF in ARDS. Then, the pathophysiology of MSOF is presented, especially the role(s) of tissue hypoxia as a cause of MSOF. Finally, we evaluate several methods to predict MSOF.

Definitions of Multiple System Organ Failure

The definitions of organ failure versus organ dysfunction require clarification. Organ failure is organ dysfunction of such severity that life support is required. Organ failure is associated with significant morbidity and mortality. Organ dysfunction defines the dynamic process of organ dysfunction, which ranges from mild to extreme.[3] Mild

Table 13.1. Multiple system organ failure/dysfunction scoring systems

Organ system	Fry (ref. 4)	Knaus (ref. 5)	Marshall (ref. 6)	Hebert (ref. 7)	Le Gall (ref. 8)	Vincent (ref. 9)
Respiratory	X	X	X	X	X	X
Cardiovascular		X	X	X	X	X
Renal	X	X	X	X	X	X
Hepatic	X		X	X	X	X
Neurologic		X	X	X	X	X
Coagulation		X	X	X	X	X
Gastrointestinal	X					

Note: Most organ system dysfunction scoring systems use similar variables to assess respiratory (PaO_2/FiO_2), renal (creatinine), hepatic (bilirubin), coagulation (platelets), and neurologic (Glasgow Coma score) dysfunction. Cardiovascular dysfunction is assessed by different methods in different scoring systems. Gastrointestinal dysfunction is not assessed in recently described scoring systems.

to moderate organ dysfunction may not result in clinical findings (e.g., mildly to moderately elevated serum creatinine).

Several scoring systems for multiple organ dysfunction syndrome are shown in Table 13.1.[4–9] An example of dichotomous (organ failure present/absent) classification of organ failures is shown in Table 13.2. An example of a classification of the severity of organ failures that uses 5 grades of severity is shown in Table 13.3.

There are many initiating events of MSOF such as shock, sepsis, trauma, aspiration, and pancreatitis. Sepsis is the most frequent initiator of MSOF.[10] Indeed, in patients who have ARDS, it has been found that abdominal sepsis is the most common source of sepsis that precedes ARDS. Nosocomial pneumonia is the most common cause of sepsis after development of ARDS. Nosocomial pneumonia often progresses to MSOF.[11]

Epidemiology of Multiple System Organ Failure in ARDS

High morbidity, high mortality, and high costs emphasize the importance of MSOF. The mortality of MSOF ranges from 20% to 100% depending on the number of organ failures. In general, there is a direct association between the number of organ failures and mortality (Figure 13.1). Regarding costs of MSOF, it is estimated that up to half of ICU costs are spent on care of patients who have MSOF.[12–17]

ARDS can occur as single organ failure without multiple system organ failure. Usually, direct injury to the lung, such as by viral pneumonia, near-drowning, and aspiration of gastric contents, leads to ARDS without other organ dysfunction, at least at the onset. Thus ARDS is the primary injury and MSOF occurs as a complication of ARDS.[18] Suchyta and colleagues[19] found that aspiration pneumonia-induced ARDS had a significantly lower mortality than did other causes of ARDS.

Table 13.2. A dichotomous organ system failure scoring system (OSF)

I. **Respiratory failure** (presence of one or more of the following):
   A. Respiratory rate $\leq$ 5/min or $\geq$ 49/min
   B. $PaCO_2 \geq$ 50 mmHg
   C. $AaDO_2 \geq$ 350 mmHg ($AaDO_2 = 713 \times FiO_2 - PaCO_2 - PaO_2$)
   D. Dependent on ventilator on the fourth day of OSF; not applicable for the initial 72 hours of OSF
II. **Cardiovascular failure** (presence of one or more of the following):
   A. Heart rate $\leq$ 54/min
   B. Mean arterial blood pressure $\leq$ 49 mmHg
   C. Ventricular tachycardia and/or ventricular fibrillation
   D. Serum pH $\leq$ 7.24 with $PaCO_2$ of $\leq$ 49 mmHg
III. **Renal failure** (presence of one or more of the following)[a]:
   A. Urine output $\leq$ 479 mL/24 h or $\leq$ 159 mL/8 h
   B. Serum BUN $\geq$ 100 mg/100 mL
   C. Serum creatinine $\geq$ 3.5 mg/100 mL
IV. **Neurologic failure:**
   Glasgow Coma score $\leq$ 6 (in the absence of sedation at any point in day)
V. **Hematologic failure** (presence of one or more of the following):
   A. WBC $\leq$ 1,000/mm^3
   B. Platelets $\leq$ 20,000/mm^3
   C. Hematocrit $\leq$ 20%

Note: $AaDO_2$ = alveolar–arterial oxygen difference.
[a]Excluding patients on chronic dialysis before hospital admission.
Source: Knaus WA, Draper EA, Wagner DP, Simmerman JE. Prognosis in acute organ-system failure. Ann Surg 1985; 202:685–693.

Alternatively, ARDS can occur as a component of multiple system organ failure.[18] Most often, ARDS as a component of MSOF occurs when ARDS is caused by a systemic insult such as severe sepsis, multiple trauma, severe shock, and severe pancreatitis. Several studies showed that sepsis was significantly more common in patients who had ARDS who died of nonrespiratory causes compared with patients who died of respiratory failure who had ARDS.[1,11,19,20]

The incidence of MSOF during the course of ARDS varies from 25% to almost 100%.[1,11,19–29] The incidence of MSOF in patients who have ARDS appears to be related to the underlying cause of ARDS. MSOF is the most common cause of death if ARDS is caused by nonpulmonary sepsis. Ferring and Vincent[1] found that MSOF was the cause of death in 33 of 67 nonsurvivors who had ARDS. Varying incidence of MSOF is also due in part to different definitions of ARDS and different definitions of organ failure. The case mix of ARDS (e.g., mainly medical vs. mainly surgical), the timing of study of ARDS (e.g., early vs. late ARDS), and the year of the study (e.g., 1980–1995) also influence the findings in these studies.

Table 13.3. A scoring system using multiple severity grades

Organ system	SCORE			
	1	2	3	4
Respiratory PaO₂/FiO₂, mmHg	< 400	< 300	< 200 (Respiratory support)	< 100 (Respiratory support)
Cardiovascular Hypotension	MAP < 70 mmHg	Dopamine < 5 or dobutamine (any dose)	Dopamine > 5 or epinephrine ≤ 0.1 or norepinephrine ≤ 0.1	Dopamine > 15 or epinephrine > 0.1 or norepinephrine > 0.1
Renal Creatinine, mg/dL (μmol/L) or urine output	1.2–1.9 (110–170)	2.0–3.4 (171–299)	3.5–4.9 (300–440) or < 500 mL/day	> 5.9 (> 440) or < 200 mL/day
Neurologic Glasgow Coma score	13–14	10–12	6–9	< 6
Hepatic Bilirubin, mg/dL (μmol/L)	1.2–1.9 (20–32)	2.0–5.9 (33–101)	6.0–11.9 (102–204)	> 12.0 (> 204)
Coagulation Platelets × 10³/mm³	< 150	< 100	< 50	< 20

Note: Adrenergic drugs infused for at least 1 hour (doses are in μg/kg/min). A score of 1 indicates mild organ dysfunction and a score of 4 indicates the most severe organ failure. Normal organ function gives a score of 0. The worst value for each organ system is recorded on each day.
Source: Vincent J-L, Moreno R, Takala J, Willatts S, De Mendonca A, Bruining H, Reinhart CK, Suter PM, Thijs LG. The SOFA (Sepsis-related Organ Failure Assessment) score to describe organ dysfunction/failure. Intensive Care Med 1996; 22:707–710.

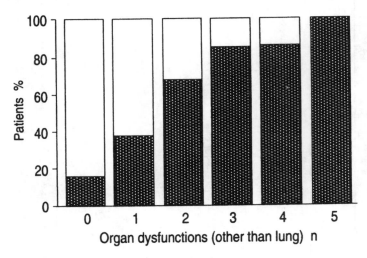

Figure 13.1. Percentage of survivors (open column) and nonsurvivors (gray column) for each number of organ dysfunctions in patients with ARDS.[1]

Clinicians recognize that multiple system organ failure generally follows a common course: cardiovascular and lung dysfunction usually occur early, and hepatic, intestinal, neurologic, coagulation, and renal dysfunction usually occur later.[12] This pattern of organ dysfunction was found in a prospective study of patients who had ARDS.[22]

The contribution of different individual organ dysfunctions (e.g., hepatic vs. renal vs. coagulation) in patients with ARDS to morbidity and mortality is unclear. Table 13.4 shows ranges of the incidence of nonpulmonary organ failure in patients with ARDS. In general, renal and cardiovascular failure are the most common organ dysfunction associated with ARDS.

Refractory respiratory failure is not the most common cause of death of patients who have ARDS (Table 13.5).[18–29] Some studies suggest that refractory hypoxemia is more commonly the cause of death if ARDS is caused by pneumonia. Six representative studies from the 1980s and 1990s found that respiratory failure was the cause of 16% to 57% of deaths. Some studies[1,11] found that about 1 out of 6 patients who have ARDS die of refractory hypoxemia. Suchyta and colleagues[19] found that refractory hypoxemia causes 40% of deaths, and they had a large proportion of patients whose ARDS was caused by pneumonia. Similarly, Ferring and Vincent[1] found that refractory hypoxemia was the leading cause of death if ARDS was caused by pneumonia.

Organ failure scoring is widely used in randomized controlled trials (RCT) of new therapy in ARDS. It is used to assess baseline comparability of treatment and placebo groups.[25,28,30] Organ scoring has also been used to exclude patients from study who have severe MSOF and are unlikely to benefit from intervention.[31] With one exception,[28] to date, randomized controlled trials designed to improve lung function and oxygenation have failed to find improved survival with new therapy for patients who

Table 13.4. Incidence of organ failure in patients who had ARDS

Organ failure	Incidence (%)
Renal	13–55
Hepatic	12–95
Central nervous system	0–30
Cardiovascular	6–54
Gastrointestinal	7–30
Hematologic	0–5

Sources: Compiled from Dorinsky PM, Gadek JE. Mechanisms of multiple nonpulmonary organ failure in ARDS. Chest 1989; 96:885–892. Gattinoni L, Bombino M, Pelosi P, Lissoni A, Pesenti A, Fumagalli R, Tagliabue M. Lung structure and function in different stages of severe adult respiratory distress syndrome. JAMA 1994; 271:1772–1779. Gregory TJ, Steinberg KP, Spragg R, Gadek JE, Hyers TM, Longmore WL, Moxley MA, Cai G-Z, Hite RD, Smith RM, Hudson LD, Crim C, Newton PP, Mitchell BR, Gold AL. Bovine surfactant therapy for patients with acute respiratory distress syndrome. AM J Respir Crit Care Med 1997; 155:1309–1315. Knaus WA, Sun X, Hakim RB, Wagner DP. Evaluation of definitions for adult respiratory distress syndrome. Am J Respir Crit Care Med 1994; 150:311–317.

have ARDS.[21,25,30,31] Perhaps this is because patients with ARDS often die from causes other than lung failure. Hence new therapies may not improve survival if they only improve lung function and oxygenation. Recently, organ failure scoring has also been used to assess outcome of treatment in RCTs. For example, Bernard and colleagues[32] found that antioxidants decreased the development of MSOF compared to placebo in patients who had ARDS.

Table 13.5. Causes of death of patients who had ARDS

Study	No. of deaths (mortality %)	CAUSE OF DEATH (%)						
		Respiratory	MSOF	Sepsis	Cardiac	CNS	Hem	Other
Montgomery[11]	32 (68)	16	NA	34	19	22	3	6
Suchyta[19]	113 (53)[a]	40	NA	28	19	7		6
Amato[28]	30 (57)	23	NA	43				33
Anzueto[21]	288 (40)	31	26	23	10			10
Ferring[1]	67 (52)	16	49		15	10	4	4
Suchyta[29]	28 (55)	57	NA	29	7	3		4

[a]Of nonsurvivors, 33% had MSOF.

Pathophysiology of MSOF

The pathophysiology of multiple organ dysfunction is multifactorial. Because shock and arterial hypoxemia are common in ARDS, because tissues require oxygen for maintenance of function, and because prolonged cell hypoxia leads to cell death, it has been hypothesized that tissue hypoxia is an important cause of multiple system organ failure in ARDS. However, it is now clear that a systemic inflammatory response triggered by an initiating event is fundamentally important to the genesis of MSOF. As discussed in Chapter 4, several cascades of inflammatory mediators are triggered by such initiating events as sepsis, shock, and multiple trauma. Mediators of inflammation cause multiple system organ injury, which becomes expressed initially as organ dysfunction, which if progressive develops into organ failure. The evidence to support inflammation as the fundamental pathophysiology of multiple system organ failure includes molecular, cellular, whole animal, and clinical studies. Because inflammation was covered in detail in Chapter 4, we cover only tissue hypoxia as a potential cause of MSOF now.

Tissue Hypoxia and Multiple System Organ Failure

Cells require a continuous supply of oxygen to synthesize adenosine triphosphate (ATP). If cellular oxygen supply is limited, oxidative ATP synthesis decreases and ATP is then synthesized by anaerobic glycolysis[33] associated with acid production and detrimental change in the redox state of the cell. Aerobic metabolism is crucial to cell survival and organ function. Hence adequate delivery of oxygen to cells is fundamentally important.

Oxygen delivery (DO_2) is the product of cardiac output and arterial oxygen content as shown here:

$$DO_2 = CO \times CaO_2 \times 10$$

where CO = cardiac output (L/minute), CaO_2 = arterial oxygen content (mL/100 mL).
Arterial oxygen content is calculated as:

$$CaO_2 = (Hb \times 1.34 \times SaO_2) + (PaO_2 \times 0.0031)$$

where Hb = hemoglobin concentration, SaO_2 = arterial oxygen saturation, and PaO_2 = partial pressure of oxygen. Dissolved oxygen ($PaO_2 \times 0.0031$) is approximately 1% of total of oxygen content and can usually be ignored in the clinical setting. Examination of these equations demonstrates that DO_2 can become inadequate due to decreased hemoglobin (anemia), inadequate blood flow (perfusion), or extreme arterial desaturation (hypoxemia).

Anemia lowers oxygen-carrying capacity of the blood. In chronic anemia, increased cardiac output and decreased blood viscosity prevent tissue hypoxia at rest.[34] Acute relatively severe anemia did not induce tissue hypoxia in patients undergoing minor surgery or in healthy volunteers.[35] Acute anemia was compensated for by increased cardiac output and by increased utilization of oxygen.[35] In critically ill patients the optimum hemoglobin or hematocrit is not known.[36] If tissue perfusion is adequate, experimental studies indicate that very low hematocrit levels are well tolerated.[37] However, the effects of anemia on tissue oxygenation in critically ill patients are not simple because several factors change affinity of hemoglobin for oxygen and consequently change unloading capacity of oxygen from hemoglobin at the tissue level. Hydrogen ion (acidosis), carbon dioxide, fever, and increased 2,3-diphosphoglycerate (2,3 DPG) decrease affinity of hemoglobin for oxygen and shift the oxyhemoglobin dissociation curve to the right.[38] The rightward shift increases oxygen availability to tissues at a given oxygen tension. Although some evidence indicates that critically ill patients tolerate moderate anemia without increased mortality or morbidity, outcome may be worse for anemic critically ill patients who have impaired cardiovascular reserve.[39]

Recent clinical trial evidence suggests a more conservative transfusion strategy decreases transfusion requirements and may improve outcome.[39] Transfusion of packed erythrocytes increases oxygen delivery but does not increase oxygen consumption,[40,41] possibly because oxygen demand is already met by DO_2 and possibly because erythrocytes are rigid, occlude the microcirculation, and may even cause tissue hypoxia.

Inadequate perfusion may be due to decreased total cardiac output, inappropriate distribution of flow between organs, and mismatching of oxygen supply to demand within organs. Inadequate cardiac output is due to hypovolemic, cardiogenic, or obstructive shock. Maldistribution of flow between or within organs is frequently seen in ARDS and sepsis.

Perfusion Distribution between Organs

ARDS and its therapy, such as mechanical ventilation, alter perfusion distribution between organs. Mechanical ventilation and therapy such as sedation and paralysis change blood flow, oxygen delivery, and oxygen consumption to respiratory muscles. In ARDS, increased respiratory muscle work increases oxygen demand and oxygen consumption of respiratory muscles. Increased oxygen demand must be met by increased respiratory muscle blood flow to avoid anaerobic metabolism.[42,43] Cardiogenic shock increases respiratory muscle oxygen demand, and as a result the respiratory muscles receive about 21% of cardiac output during spontaneous breathing.[44] Following institution of paralysis and mechanical ventilation, respiratory muscle blood flow falls to the normal 3% of cardiac output.[44] Indirect evidence from human studies suggests this redistribution of blood flow to respiratory muscles arises in part from splanchnic circulation. More specifically, Mohsenifar and colleagues found that gastric mucosal perfusion as measured by gastric mucosal pH_i predicted success of weaning.[45] Patients who had gastric mucosal pH_i decrease during weaning had increased risk of failure to wean. This suggests that blood flow was diverted from gut to respiratory muscles causing gastric mucosal acidosis in patients who failed to wean.

Respiratory support (i.e., PEEP) of patients who have ARDS may change global blood flow and also blood flow distribution between organs. Although PEEP increases arterial oxygen tension, PEEP may decrease oxygen delivery because PEEP may decrease cardiac output.[46] PEEP also changes distribution of blood flow between organs in animal models of critical illness.[47–51] Positive pressure ventilation reduces gut and hepatic blood flow.[48,50] High levels of PEEP (> 20 cm H_2O) decrease hepatic, renal, pancreatic, and colonic blood flow while brain and cardiac perfusion are maintained.[49] Sepsis modifies the PEEP-induced changes in organ perfusion such that PEEP only decreases hepatic, pancreatic, and splenic blood flow in septic sheep. Volume resuscitation does not restore normal blood flow distribution.[49] Hypocapnia decreases hepatic arterial blood flow without affecting hepatic function, and mild hypercapnia increases hepatic blood supply.[52] It is not clear how PEEP changes blood flow distribution between organs in human ARDS.

The splanchnic circulation is important in the regulation of circulating blood volume and systemic blood pressure.[53] In acute hypovolemia, splanchnic blood volume and blood flow are markedly reduced to maintain perfusion of heart and brain.[54–56] However, splanchnic circulation appears to be hyperdynamic in normovolemic stable patients who have ARDS.[57] In general, hypovolemic models of endotoxic shock find decreased splanchnic blood flow, and hyperdynamic models of endotoxic shock find increased splanchnic blood flow.[58,59] In healthy humans, a bolus of endotoxin roughly doubles splanchnic blood flow without changing heart rate or blood pressure.[60] Similarly, septic patients have nearly double normal splanchnic blood flow.[61,62]

Perfusion Distribution within Organs

ARDS and sepsis impair the normal distribution of perfusion *within organs* such as heart, kidneys, and gut and also alter the normal redistribution of blood flow that occurs in hemorrhagic shock. Abnormal distribution of perfusion during sepsis could explain the oxygen extraction defect of sepsis. The abnormal distribution of perfusion within organs during sepsis could be explained by endothelial injury, decreased erythrocyte and leukocyte deformability, microvascular obstruction, and changes in concentration of local and systemic vasoactive substances.

Impaired regulation of perfusion distribution within organs (such as the gut, heart, kidneys, and brain) may cause tissue hypoxia. Gut blood flow decreases dramatically in hemorrhagic or cardiogenic shock, and the decrease is out of proportion to the decrease in total cardiac output.[63–65] In the heart, there is redistribution of blood flow from the endocardium to the epicardium during hemorrhagic shock, which causes subendocardial patchy necrosis.[66,67] In the kidney there is redistribution of renal blood flow from outer to inner cortex and medulla in hypovolemic shock, which can cause ischemic damage.[68] Global cerebral perfusion is unchanged in hemorrhagic shock.[69–71]

Systemic inflammatory states impair the ability of the gut microcirculation to regulate perfused capillary density,[72] resulting in mismatch of oxygen supply to demand.[73] In particular, normal redistribution of blood flow to the metabolically active mucosa is impaired.[74]

Impaired Tissue Oxygen Extraction

Impaired tissue oxygen extraction could cause tissue hypoxia. Abnormal redistribution of perfusion within organs is one mechanism of impaired oxygen extraction. Maintenance of high perfused capillary density is important in regulating oxygen extraction because it keeps oxygen diffusion distances small.[75] Recently, perfused capillary density was demonstrated to be decreased in sepsis.[76] Low flow capillaries have high capillary oxygen extraction ratios; high flow capillaries have low capillary oxygen extraction ratios. Endothelial injury, microvascular obstruction, decreased blood cell deformability, and release of vasoactive mediators are all potential causes of increased heterogeneity of capillary transit times during sepsis.

Vascular reactivity to metabolic feedback could be disturbed in sepsis. The distribution of blood flow within organs is normally controlled by the sympathetic nervous system and by systemic and local vasoactive mediators.[77,78] Alpha receptor blockade impairs normal oxygen extraction capability of tissues, indicating that adrenergic alpha tone is important in the normal blood flow distribution during hemorrhagic shock. Thus vasodilators used in management of ARDS could interfere with regulation of blood flow within organs. For example, nitroprusside increases intrapulmonary shunt and can worsen arterial hypoxemia by interfering with hypoxic pulmonary vasoconstriction.

Increased Oxygen Demand

Tissue hypoxia can be caused by increased tissue oxygen demand if increased oxygen demand is not met by increased oxygen delivery. Examples of increased oxygen demand in the patients who have ARDS include fever, inadequate sedation, and increased respiratory muscle work.[43,44,79,80]

Sedation and paralysis of mechanically ventilated patients significantly decrease global oxygen consumption because of decreased respiratory muscle and possibly other skeletal muscle oxygen consumption.[81] Common therapeutic interventions such as sedation and physiotherapy may change oxygen uptake and increase the risk of imbalance between oxygen delivery and demand.[80–83] Finally, adrenergic agents can increase oxygen demand and oxygen consumption because of a thermogenic effect. Dobutamine may increase oxygen consumption in healthy volunteers up to 20%; however, the increase in oxygen demand caused by dobutamine may be less in critically ill patients.[84–86] If local blood flow does not increase enough to match increased oxygen demand induced by the drug, tissue hypoxia can develop. This is one possible mechanism to explain the development of gastric mucosal acidosis in response to adrenergic agents despite increased gut blood flow.[87,88]

Splanchnic oxygen demand is increased and may jeopardize splanchnic oxygenation in septic patients.[61,62,89,90] Endotoxin increases splanchnic oxygen consumption and splanchnic TNF release in healthy volunteers.[60] Although splanchnic blood flow distribution is similar in patients with trauma and patients who have sepsis, oxygen consumption of the splanchnic region of septic patients is significantly greater than splanchnic oxygen consumption in patients with trauma.[89]

Several studies found that survivors of critical illness have higher oxygen delivery and oxygen consumption compared to nonsurvivors.[91-93] However, these studies do not prove that the nonsurvivors were hypoxic because lower DO_2 and VO_2 alone do not indicate tissue hypoxia.

Pathologic Dependence of Oxygen Consumption on Oxygen Delivery

There is little evidence in studies of DO_2-VO_2 dependence to suggest an association between tissue hypoxia and multiple system organ failure because few studies of oxygen delivery and consumption examined MSOF.

There are a few studies of the relationship of oxygen delivery and consumption in response to acute interventions in patients with ARDS.[94-96] Prostaglandin E_1 increased oxygen delivery and consumption but did not affect survival in patients with ARDS.[94] Prostacyclin increased oxygen delivery in patients who had acute lung injury.[95] Oxygen consumption increased significantly only in nonsurvivors.

In a study of PEEP-induced changes of oxygen delivery and consumption, all patients who had low DO_2 at zero PEEP had dependence of oxygen consumption on oxygen delivery, developed MSOF, and died.[96] To summarize, there is little evidence in studies of DO_2-VO_2 dependence in ARDS to suggest an association between tissue hypoxia and multiple system organ failure.

Randomized Control Trials of Supranormal Oxygen Delivery: Effects on Multiple System Organ Failure

Randomized controlled clinical trials (RCTs) of supranormal oxygen delivery are another way to assess whether tissue hypoxia causes multiple system organ failure. Some randomized controlled trials of supernormal oxygen delivery examined the effects on development of MSOF. These studies found little evidence that supranormal DO_2 decreases the incidence of MSOF.

There are at least nine RCTs of supranormal oxygen delivery compared to normal oxygen delivery (Table 13.6).[97-104] In all of these studies, survival was the major endpoint. None of the RCTs rigorously evaluated the effects of supranormal oxygen delivery on multiple system organ failure. There are five RCTs of supranormal oxygen delivery in which single or multiple system organ failure was reported.[97-100,103,104] In three of these studies, some evidence indicated that supranormal DO_2 decreases MSOF.[97-100] Shoemaker and colleagues found that the average number of complications, including poorly defined single organ failures, was lower in surgical patients randomized to receive supranormal oxygen delivery compared to controls. Fleming and associates also found that the number of poorly defined single organ failures per patients was less in protocol patients than in controls in a study of trauma patients.[98]

Table 13.6. Randomized controlled trials of supranormal versus normal oxygen delivery

Author (ref.)	Year	Patients	No. of patients	Mortality (%) controls	Mortality (%) intervention	p-value
Shoemaker[97]	1988	Surgical	88	28	4	< 0.05
Bone[94]	1989	ARDS	100	48	60	NS
Fleming[98]	1992	Trauma	67	44	24	NS
Tuchschmidt[99]	1992	Septic shock	51	72	50	NS
Boyd[100]	1993	Surgical	107	22	6	< 0.05
Gutierrez[101]	1992	Critical, pHi normal	141	53	28	< 0.05
Gutierrez[101]	1992	Critical, pHi low	119	37	36	NS
Yu[102]	1993	Critical	67	34	34	NS
Hayes[103]	1994	Critical	109	34	54	< 0.05
Gattinoni[104]	1995	Critical	503	48	49	NS

Unfortunately, several recent RCTs of supranormal DO_2 do not report the effects of intervention of MSOF. Furthermore, several studies found no difference or even increased mortality and increased MSOF[103] associated with supranormal DO_2. Hence little evidence suggests that supranormal oxygen delivery decreases the incidence of MSOF.

Lactate

Increased arterial lactate levels may indicate anaerobic metabolism as a result of tissue hypoxia. Glycolysis occurs in the cytoplasm of virtually all cells. The end product of glycolysis is pyruvate. Pyruvate diffuses into mitochondria and is metabolized to carbon dioxide by the Krebs' cycle. Metabolism of glucose to pyruvate reduces the enzyme cofactor NAD^+ (nicotinamide adenine dinucleotide) to NADH. The electron transport chain oxidizes NADH to NAD^+ using molecular oxygen. Oxidative phyosphorylation produces adenosine triphosphate (ATP).[105] In steady state, pyruvate is in equilibrium with lactate and with the oxidized and reduced forms of the cofactor nicotinamide adenine dinucleotide (NAD^+ and NADH, respectively). During cellular anoxia, mitochondrial metabolism ceases and pyruvate is metabolized by lactic dehydrogenase (LDH) to lactate. Lactate diffuses out of cells and accumulates in extracellular fluid. Myocardium metabolizes lactate by oxidative metabolism. Liver and kidney convert lactate to glucose. However, when tissue hypoxia is severe, lactate production exceeds lactate utilization and therefore hyperlactatemia develops.[105]

Although the specific sources of excess lactate production in severe shock are not known, lactic acidosis usually indicates generalized tissue hypoxia.[106,107] Sources of excess lactate production during tissue hypoxia include lung, gut, muscle, and other organs. Interestingly, lung is a source of lactate production in patients who have

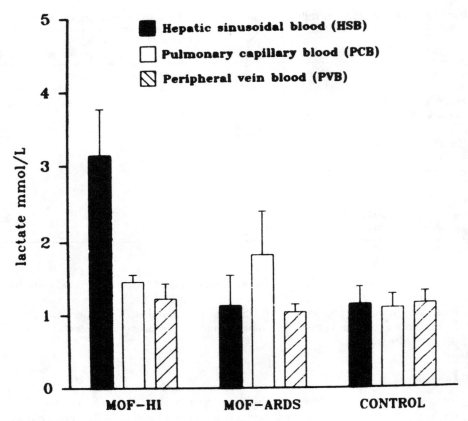

Figure 13.2. Mean ± SE serum levels of lactate from three different sites of blood sampling in the MOF groups and the control group. MOF-HI = multiple organ failure with hepatic involvement, MOF-ARDS = multiple organ failure with ARDS.[114] Lactate is highest in hepatic sinusoidal blood in patients who had MSOF with hepatic involvement.

ARDS. Normally lungs do not produce lactate.[108–111] The lungs of patients who have ARDS produce excess lactate compared to patients without ARDS,[112–114] and lactate release from the lungs increases with increasing severity of lung injury. Hepato-splanchnic bed was the main source of lactate of patients who have MSOF and hepatic dysfunction. In contrast, lungs were the main source of lactate in patients with MSOF who had ARDS[114] (Figure 13.2).

In general, there is a direct relationship between elevated lactate concentration and mortality of critically ill patients.[115] Furthermore, even in patients who have chronic liver disease there is a relationship between increased lactate and increased mortality.[116–118] Persistence of hyperlactatemia is also associated with increased mor-

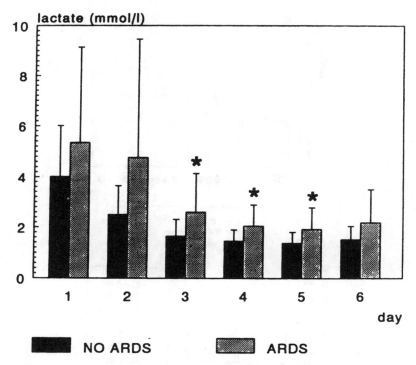

Figure 13.3. Mean lactate levels (+ SD) of 51 patients with multiple trauma divided into those with (n = 22) and without (n = 29) ARDS (* p < 0.05).[122] Lactate was higher in patients who had ARDS.

tality.[119–121] Also, lactate levels were moderately higher at the early phase post injury in multiple trauma patients who ultimately developed ARDS[122] (Figure 13.3). Studies of surgical and trauma patients, in general, find an association between increased lactate and development of MSOF.[122–127] Furthermore, initial and highest lactate levels and the duration of hyperlactatemia were significantly higher in trauma patients who developed organ failure compared to trauma patients who did not.[126]

Lactate levels, and especially the duration of hyperlactatemia, are also good predictors of MSOF in patients who have septic shock[127] (Figure 13.4). However, there are both hypoxic and nonhypoxic mechanisms of hyperlactatemia in septic shock, so the association of hyperlactatemia and MSOF in patients who have septic shock does not prove an hypoxic mechanism.

The association of hyperlactatemia and MSOF suggests an association between tissue hypoxia and MSOF in trauma patients and patients with hemorrhagic shock. However, in general, hyperlactatemia is only moderately predictive of MSOF in ARDS.

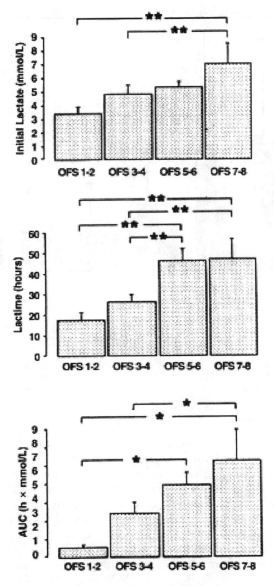

Figure 13.4. Initial blood lactate level, time during which blood lactate exceeded 2.0 mmol/L (lactime), and area under the curve (AUC) according to the organ failure score (OSF) (mean ± standard error of the mean). * p < 0.01. The area under the curve (AUC) for abnormal (above 2.0 mmol/L) lactate levels was calculated using initial and final lactate levels, and assuming a linear regression, according to this equation: AUC = 0.5 × lactime × (initial lactate + final lactate) – 2 × lactime. OFS = organ failure scoring.[127]

Gastric Tonometry

Monitoring splanchnic perfusion may be valuable in critically ill patients because the gut participates in the regulation of blood volume and systemic blood pressure, because in shock perfusion of vital organs such as brain and heart is maintained at the expense of gut, and because splanchnic hypoxia may be associated with the development of multiple system organ failure.[53–55,128–130]

The anatomy of gut mucosal blood flow and different metabolic requirements of the various layers of the gut make the surface of the mucosa very vulnerable to hypoperfusion. The parallel anatomy of the artery and vein in the intestinal villus allows countercurrent exchange of oxygen from the artery to the vein.[131] This results in lower tissue PO_2 at the villus tip. Furthermore, the high metabolic demand of the mucosa increases the risk of mucosal hypoxia during states of decreased oxygen delivery.[132]

There is an association between gastric mucosal acidosis, mortality, and MSOF. Several studies found an association between gastric mucosal acidosis and MSOF in critically ill adults. Gastric mucosal pH, measured within 24 hours after the onset of sepsis, was a better predictor of multiple organ dysfunction syndrome than oxygen-derived variables or lactate levels in septic patients.[133] Trauma patients who had pH_i < 7.25 at 24 hours after trauma were 4.5 times more likely to develop multiple system organ failure than patients who had pH_i > 7.25.[134] Gastric mucosal acidosis at the end of major surgery predicted postoperative multiple system organ failure.[135] Patients who had decreased pH_i at the time of ICU admission had more organ failure than patients who had normal (> 7.35) pH_i.[136] Thus these four studies suggest an association between gastric mucosal acidosis and MSOF.

In a large randomized controlled trial of therapy directed by gastric tonometry, Gutierrez and colleagues[101] found decreased mortality in patients managed by gastric tonometry if pH_i was normal at ICU admission. However, MSOF was not evaluated.

In summary, there is an association between gastric mucosal acidosis and multiple system organ failure. Also, no studies to date prove that gastric mucosal acidosis causes MSOF.

Potential Effects of Catecholamines and Other Interventions on Inflammation

Vasoactive adrenergic agents used to resuscitate patients who have ARDS have effects on inflammation that could influence the development of MSOF. The effects of catecholamines in clinical trials are usually attributed to effects on tissue oxygenation. Recent evidence suggests that catecholamines have effects on inflammation because catecholamines change levels of pro- and anti-inflammatory cytokines.

There are pro-inflamamtory cytokines, such as TNF and IL-6, and anti-inflammatory cytokines, such as IL-10.[137] Multiple system organ failure could be caused by

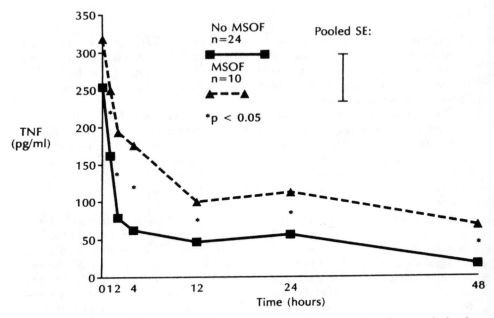

Figure 13.5. Figure 13.5. Mean TNF levels in septic shock patients who subsequently developed or did not develop MSOF. Note the persistent elevation in TNF levels in septic patients with MSOF.[139]

uncontrolled systemic inflammatory response and excessive cytokine action.[138] It has been suggested that if the balance between pro- and anti-inflammatory cytokines is altered, cytokines could cause organ injury both directly and indirectly.

In patients with sepsis, persistently high levels of tumor necrosis factor (TNF) and interleukin-6 (IL-6) are associated with multiple system organ failure and death[139] (Figure 13.5). In major surgery patients, multiple system organ failure is the most common cause of death.[100] Interestingly, elective and emergency surgery are associated with release of TNF and IL-6, and the greater the surgical trauma, the greater the release of TNF and IL-6.[140–142]

Catecholamines modulate cytokine production. Norepinephrine inhibits TNF-alpha production[143–145] by stimulation of beta-receptors. Adrenaline infusion prior to LPS challenge of human volunteers inhibited in vivo TNF appearance and increased IL-10 release, suggesting that adrenaline has anti-inflammatory effects (Figure 13.6).[146] Furthermore, low levels of IL-10 in bronchoalveolar lavage fluid of patients who have ARDS is associated with increased mortality.[147] Although dobutamine is probably the most widely used catecholamine in critical care, we are not aware of studies that have examined the effects of dobutamine on cytokine production.

Phosphodiesterase inhibitors also modify cytokine production in vitro and in

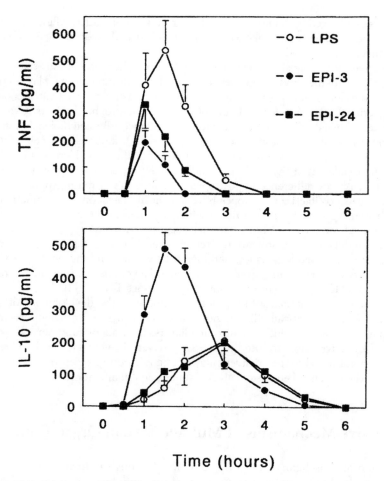

Figure 13.6. Mean (± SE) plasma concentrations of TNF (top) and IL-10 (bottom) after intravenous injection of LPS at t = 0. LPS, subjects injected with LPS only (n = 6); EPI-3, subjects infused with epinephrine (30 ng/kg per minute) from t = –3 to 6 hours (n = 5); EPI-24, subjects infused with epinephrine (30 ng/kg per minute) from –24 to 6 hours (n = 6). EPI-3 attenuated the LPS-induced increase in TNF levels and potentiated the rise in IL-10 levels (both p < 0.0005 vs. LPS only). EPI-24 only reduced TNF levels (p = 0.05 vs. LPS only), without any effect on IL-10 release.[146]

vivo. Pentoxyfylline inhibited TNF and IL-6 activity in a dose-related fashion in whole blood incubated with endotoxin.[148] In endotoxemic mice, both pentoxifylline and amrinone increased survival and decreased TNF production.[149,150] Human studies confirm the anti-inflammatory effects of phosphodiesterase inhibitors. In healthy volunteers challenged with endotoxin, a 4 hour infusion of pentoxifylline, started 30 minutes prior to endotoxin injection, totally blocked endotoxin-induced TNF but had no effect on IL-6 synthesis.[151]

Vasoactive drugs may also modify inflammation by other mechanisms than simply inhibition of cytokine production. Leukocyte-endothelial interactions play a critical role in the development of organ failure.[152] Leukocyte adherence to activated endothelium is a critical early step for initiation of release of neutrophil products. Cytokines stimulate endothelial cells to increase expression of surface adhesion molecules, such as E-selectin, intercellular adhesion molecule-1 (ICAM-1), and vascular cell adhesion molecule-1 (VCAM-1). Amrinone pretreatment significantly decreases cytokine-induced up-regulation of these adhesion molecules.[153] Pretreatment with dopexamine attenuates leukocyte adherence to postcapillary venules in rats during endotoxemia.[154] Therefore, it is possible that inotropes have beneficial effects on organ function and survival through some effects other than their effects on oxygen transport.

Very recent animal and clinical studies suggest that some types of mechanical ventilation induce lung inflammation. Tremblay and Slutsky compared the effects of low and high lung stretch using low and high tidal volume on lung cytokine levels in an animal model.[155] High lung stretch (i.e., large tidal volume) significantly increased production and levels of the pro-inflammatory cytokines TNF and IL-1.

To summarize, inflammatory mediators contribute to the development of organ failure and death in critically ill patients. Vasoactive drugs and other interventions have complex effects on inflammatory mediators. In trials of supranormal oxygen delivery, vasoactive drugs are used to increase oxygen delivery. Hence the potential effects of supranormal oxygen delivery may not be related to oxygen transport alone, but also to the beneficial effects of catecholamines on inflammation.

Alternative Mechanisms of Multiple System Organ Failure

Reperfusion after ischemia causes tissue injury. Although ischemia-induced tissue hypoxia can lead to irreversible tissue injury if the period of ischemia is sufficiently prolonged, frequently much of the tissue damage occurs after oxygenation is restored rather than during the period of ischemia. More specifically, ischemic tissues in a variety of organs are vulnerable to xanthine oxidase–mediated reperfusion injury.[156–158] Xanthine oxidase has been found in vascular endothelium as well as the gut epithelium. Under normal conditions, xanthine oxidase exists predominantly as xanthine dehydrogenase; however, with ischemia, xanthine dehydrogenase is converted to xanthine oxidase. As the same time, breakdown of ATP increases the level of purine metabolites hypoxanthine and xanthine. With reperfusion, oxygen becomes available and the xanthine oxidase–dependent oxidation of hypoxanthine and xanthine generates a burst of reactive oxygen metabolites (ROMs), such as hydroxyl radical ($\cdot$OH), that cause tissue injury.[156] Reperfusion injures cells directly.

Following reoxygenation, ROMs within cells may damage cell and organelle membranes, denature proteins, and disrupt the chromosomes. In addition, oxidants may escape from cells and injure adjacent cells as well as enter the circulation. This cellular damage may occur in all cells, but endothelial cells in the microvasculature appear to be especially affected; hence microcirculatory disruption is a prominent feature of severe reperfusion injury.[159] It is interesting to note that the crucial step, the conversion of xanthine dehydrogenase to xanthine oxidase, takes only 10 seconds in intestinal tissue, 8 minutes in cardiac muscle, and about 30 minutes in the liver, spleen, kidney, and lung.[160] This may explain the different relative susceptibility of these organs to ischemia-reperfusion-mediated tissue injury.

Serum lipofuscin is an indicator of toxic oxygen free radical damage and lipid peroxidation. Interestingly, increased concentrations of serum lipofuscin are predictive of development of ARDS and MSOF after major surgery and trauma.[161] Also, a recent clinical trial in ARDS showed shortened duration of lung injury in response to antioxidant therapy.[32] These findings support the role of toxic oxygen radicals and reperfusion injury in MSOF.

Reperfusion injury also stimulates inflammation. Polymorphonuclear leukocytes (PMNs) are required for the full expression of ischemia-reperfusion injury; oxidant injury appears to rapidly activate PMNs.[162,163] Macrophages are also stimulated by reperfusion. ROMs enhance pro-inflammatory cytokine production (i.e., TNF, IL-1, and IL-6). It is likely that these and other cytokines play an important role in amplifying the inflammatory response to ischemia and reperfusion. Among the many actions of the pro-inflammatory cytokines are direct cytotoxicity, PMN activation, and the stimulation of additional production of ROMs.[159]

A number of stimuli following shock and trauma may prime and activate leukocytes. These include ischemia, reactive oxygen metabolites, and cytokines.[164] Activated leukocytes can produce cellular injury by release of lysosomal enzymes and cytokines. Normally, circulating neutrophils do not adhere to vascular endothelium, and neutrophil adhesion to vascular endothelium is a key element in injury and inflammatory response.[165,166] When the endothelium is activated (e.g., by cytokines), neutrophils adhere to the endothelial surface.[165] Neutrophil adherence is facilitated by adhesion molecules expressed on neutrophils and endothelial cells.[165] The adherence of neutrophils to vascular endothelial surfaces creates a microenvironment in which activated neutrophils release products that cause endothelial damage leading to an increase in microvascular permeability and widespread edema. Excessive aggregation of neutrophils within the microvasculature can also lead to focal ischemia and organ dysfunction. It has been proposed that gut ischemia/reperfusion, secondary to splanchnic hypoperfusion, is responsible for creating the local inflammatory environment that primes circulating neutrophils to adhere to endothelial cell surfaces.[167]

Cytokines are another potential cause of MSOF, and an anticytokine hypothesis has dominated clinical trials in sepsis for several years. The hypothesis is that overproduction and persistently high levels of pro-inflammatory cytokines, such as interleukin-1 (IL-1), tumor necrosis factor (TNF), IL-6, and IL-8 cause multiple organ failure.[139,168] Cytokines increase the production of secondary mediators such as nitric oxide, arachidonic acid metabolites, bradykinin, and histamine. These secondary mediators activate neutrophils and endothelial cells to perpetuate tissue injury. However, cytokines are necessary for the immune response, and there are anti-inflammatory as well as pro-inflammatory cytokines. In addition, none of the attempts to modulate the biologic activity of cytokines with antibodies has been successful in improving outcome in several clinical trials.

To summarize, there are many potential causes for the development of multiple system organ failure. One event may activate several other pathways, which in turn may activate the release of mediators that cause MSOF.

Summary

We have reviewed the evidence for and against the hypothesis that occult tissue hypoxia causes multiple organ failure. We have reviewed several lines of evidence in attempting to link tissue hypoxia and multiple organ failure. The evidence includes the dependence of oxygen consumption on oxygen delivery; the value of hyperlactatemia and gastric tonometry in assessing tissue oxygenation; and the randomized controlled trials of supranormal oxygen delivery and the effects on the incidence of multiple organ failure. Despite our efforts, we were unable to show definitively that occult tissue hypoxia causes multiple organ failure. There are few animal models of multiple organ failure and virtually all have a nonshock mechanism.

The association between high lactate or gastric mucosal acidosis and development of multiple organ failure suggests but does not prove occult tissue hypoxia. It is most likely that the pathophysiology of multiple organ failure is multifactorial. The "two-hit" model of multiple organ failure is a relatively new approach to explain the pathophysiology of organ failure.[12] We suggest that occult tissue hypoxia may cause multiple organ failure by the two-hit hypothesis, although each of the two hits may be nonhypoxic.

We recommend potentially fertile areas for future investigation to test the hypothesis that occult tissue hypoxia causes multiple organ failure. It would be useful to reevaluate the timing of intervention and also the target patient population in randomized controlled trials of supranormal oxygen delivery. We believe that a preoperative strategy to optimize oxygen delivery in a homogeneous group of high-risk elective surgical patients requires further studies. Second, we suggest that the potential effect of splanchnic tissue hypoperfusion on outcome should be tested. If gastric tonometry is to be utilized, gastric-arterial CO_2 gradient, instead of gastric mucosal pH, should be used as the variable to trigger additional treatment. The additional treatment should also be directed by clear, reproducible algorithms. Finally, the two-hit model of multiple organ failure and the role of different "hits," such as tissue hypoxia, require further evaluation. Finally, we propose that the anti- and pro-inflammatory effects of catecholamines require further studies as an influence on MSOF.

References

1. Ferring M, Vincent J-L. Is outcome from ARDS related to the severity of respiratory failure? Eur Respir J 1997; 10:1297–1300.
2. Doyle RL, Szaflarski N, Modin GW, Wiener-Kronish JP, Matthay MA. Identification of patients with acute lung injury. Predictors of mortality. Am J Respir Crit Care Med 1995; 152:1818–1824.
3. Bone RC, Balk RA, Cerra FB, Dellinger RP, Fein AM, Knaus WA, Schein RM, Sibbald WJ. Definitions for sepsis and organ failure and guidelines for the use of innovative therapies in sepsis. Chest 1992; 101:1644–1655.
4. Fry DE, Pearlstein L, Fulton RL, Polk HC Jr. Multiple system organ failure: the role of uncontrolled infection. Arch Surg 1980; 115:136–140.
5. Knaus WA, Draper EA, Wagner DP, Zimmerman JE. Prognosis in acute organ-system failure. Ann Surg 1985; 202:685–693.
6. Marshall JC, Cook DJ, Christon NV, Bernard GR, Sprung CL, Sibbald WJ. Multiple organ dysfunction score: a reliable descriptor of a complex clinical outcome. Crit Care Med 1995; 23:1638–1652.
7. Hebert PC, Drummond AJ, Singer J, Bernard GR, Russell JA. A simple multiple system organ failure scoring system predicts mortality of patients who have sepsis syndrome. Chest 1993; 104:230–235.
8. Le Gall J-R, Klar J, Lemeshow S, Saulnier F, Alberti C, Artigas A, Teres D. The logistic organ dysfunction system. A new way to assess organ dysfunction in the intensive care unit. JAMA 1996; 276:802–810.
9. Vincent J-L, Moreno R, Takala J, Willatts S, De Mendonca A, Bruining H, Reinhart CK, Suter PM, Thijs LG. The SOFA (Sepsis-related Organ Failure Assessment) score to describe organ dysfunction/failure. Intensive Care Med 1996; 22:707–710.
10. Marshall JC, Sweeney D. Microbial infection and the septic response in critical surgical illness. Sepsis, not infection, determines outcome. Arch Surg 1990; 125:17–23.
11. Montgomery AB, Stager MA, Carrico CJ, Hudson LD. Causes of mortality in patients with the adult respiratory distress syndrome. Am Rev Respir Dis 1985; 132:485–489.
12. Deitch EA. Multiple organ failure: pathophysiology and potential future therapy. Ann Surg 1992; 216:117–134.
13. Tran DD, Groeneveld ABJ, van der Meulen J, Nauta JJP, van Schijndel RS, Thijs LG. Age, chronic disease, sepsis, organ system failure, and mortality in a medical intensive care unit. Crit Care Med 1990; 18:474–479.
14. Baue AE. Multiple, progressive, or sequential systems failure: a syndrome of the 1970's. Arch Surg 1975; 110:779–781.
15. Madoff RD, Sharpe SM, Fath JJ, Simmons RL, Cerra FB. Prolonged surgical intensive care. Arch Surg 1985; 120:698–702.
16. Rapoport J, Teres D, Lemeshow S, Avrunin JS, Haber R. Explaining variability of cost using a severity-of-illness measure for ICU patients. Med Care 1990; 28:338–348.
17. Oye RK, Bellamy PE. Patterns of resource consumption in medical intensive care. Chest 1991; 99:685–689.
18. Hudson LD. Multiple systems organ failure (MSOF): lessons learned from the adult respiratory distress syndrome (ARDS). Crit Care Clin 1989; 5:697–705.

19. Suchyta MR, Clemmer TP, Elliott CG, Orme JF, Weaver LK. The adult respiratory distress syndrome. A report of survival and modifying factors. Chest 1992; 101:1074–1079.

20. Bell RC, Coalson JJ, Smith JD, Johanson WG Jr. Multiple organ system failure and infection in adult respiratory distress syndrome. Ann Intern Med 1983; 99:293–298.

21. Anzueto A, Baughman RP, Guntupalli KK, Weg JG, Wiedemann HP, Raventos AA, Lemaire F, Long W, Zaccardelli DS, Pattishall EN. Aerolized surfactant in adults with sepsis-induced acute respiratory distress syndrome. N Engl J Med 1996; 334:1417–1421.

22. Russell JA, Ronco JJ, Lockhat D, Belzberg A, Kiess M, Dodek PM. Oxygen delivery and consumption and ventricular preload are greater in survivors than in nonsurvivors of the adult respiratory distress syndrome. Am Rev Respir Dis 1990; 141:659–665.

23. DiRusso SM, Nelson LD, Safcsak K, Miller RS. Survival in patients with severe adult respiratory distress syndrome treated with high-level positive end-expiratory pressure. Crit Care Med 1995; 23:1485–1496.

24. Dorinsky PM, Gadek JE. Mechanisms of multiple nonpulmonary organ failure in ARDS. Chest 1989; 96:885–892.

25. Gregory TJ, Steinberg KP, Spragg R, Gadek JE, Hyers TM, Longmore WL, Moxley MA, Cai G-Z, Hite RD, Smith RM, Hudson LD, Crim C, Newton PP, Mitchell BR, Gold AL. Bovine surfactant therapy for patients with acute respiratory distress syndrome. Am J Respir Crit Care Med 1997; 155:1309–1315.

26. Gattinoni L, Bombino M, Pelosi P, Lissoni A, Pesenti A, Fumagalli R, Tagliabue M. Lung structure and function in different stages of severe adult respiratory distress syndrome. JAMA 1994; 271:1772–1779.

27. Knaus WA, Sun X, Hakim RB, Wagner DP. Evaluation of definitions for adult respiratory distress syndrome. Am J Respir Crit Care Med 1994; 150:311–317.

28. Amato MBP, Barbas CSV, Medeiros DM, Magaldi RB, de Paula Pinto Schettino G, Lorenzi-Filho G, Takagaki TY, Carvalho CRR. Effect of a protective-ventilation strategy on mortality in the acute respiratory distress syndrome. N Engl J Med 1998; 338:347–354.

29. Suchyta MR, Clemmer TP, Ormeo JF, Morris AH, Elliott CG. Increased survival of ARDS patients with severe hypoxemia (ECMO criteria). Chest 1991; 99:951–955.

30. Morris AH, Wallace CJ, Menlove RL, Clemmer TP, Orme JF Jr, Weaver LK, Dean NC, Thomas F, East TD, Pace NL, Suchyta MR, Beck E, Bombino M, Sittig DF, Böhm S, Hoffmann B, Becks H, Butler S, Pearl J, Rasmusson B. Randomized clinical trial of pressure-controlled inverse ratio ventilation and extracorporeal CO_2 removal for adult respiratory distress syndrome. Am J Respir Crit Care Med 1994; 149:295–305.

31. Dellinger RP, Zimmerman JL, Taylor RW, Straube RC, Hauser DL, Criner GJ, Davis K Jr, Hyers TM, Papadakos P. Effects of inhaled nitric oxide in patients with acute respiratory distress syndrome: results of a randomized phase II trial. Crit Care Med 1998; 28:15–23.

32. Bernard GR, Wheeler AP, Arons MM, Morris PE, Paz HL, Russell JA, Wright PE. A trial of antioxidants N-acetylcysteine and Procysteine in ARDS. Chest 1997; 112:164–172.

33. Gutierrez G, Lund N, Bryan-Brown CW. Cellular oxygen utilization during multiple organ failure. Crit Care Clin 1989; 5(2):271–287.

34. Finch CA, Lenfant C. Oxygen transport in man. N Engl J Med 1972; 286:407–415.

35. Weiskopf RB, Viele MK, Feiner J, Kelley S, Lieberman J, Noorani M, Leung JM, Fisker DM, Murray WR, Toy P, Moore MA. Human cardiovascular and metabolic response to acute severe isovolemic anemia. JAMA 1998; 279:217–221.

36. Hebert PC, Wells G, Marshall J, Martin C, Tweeddale M, Pagliarello G, Blajchman M. Transfusion requirements in critical care: a pilot study. JAMA 1995; 273:1439–1444.

37. Levine E, Rosen A, Sehgal L, Gould S, Sehgal H, Moss G. Physiologic effects of acute anemia: implication for a reduced transfusion trigger. Transfusion 1992; 30:11–16.
38. Tremper KK, Barker SJ. Blood-gas analysis. In Principles of critical care, eds JB Hall, GA Schmidt, LDH Wood, McGraw-Hill, New York, 1992, pp. 181–196.
39. Hebert PC, Wells G, Tweeddale M, Martin C, Marshall J, Pham BA, Blajchman M, Schweitzer I, Pagliarello G. Does transfusion practice affect mortality in critically ill patients? Am J Respir Crit Care Med 1997; 155:1618–1623.
40. Ronco JJ, Phang PT, Walley KR, Wiggs B, Fenwick JC, Russell JA. Oxygen consumption is independent of changes in oxygen delivery in severe adult respiratory distress syndrome. Am Rev Respir Dis 1991; 143:1267–1273.
41. Marik PE, Sibbald WJ. Effect of stored-blood transfusion on oxygen delivery in patients with sepsis. JAMA 1993; 269:3024–3029.
42. Cherniac RM. The oxygen consumption and efficiency of the respiratory muscles in health and emphysema. J Clin Invest 1959; 38:494–499.
43. Field S, Kelly SM, Macklem PT. The oxygen cost of breathing in patients with cardiorespiratory disease. Am Rev Resp Dis 1982; 126:9–13.
44. Viires N, Sillye G, Aubier M, Rassidakis A, Roussos C. Regional blood flow distribution in dog during induced hypotension and low cardiac output. Spontaneous breathing versus artificial ventilation. J Clin Invest 1982; 72:935–947.
45. Mohsenifar Z, Hay A, Hay J, Lewis MI, Koerner SK. Gastric intramucosal pH as a predictor of success or failure in weaning patients from mechanical ventilation. Ann Intern Med 1993; 119:794–798.
46. Suter PM, Fairley HB, Isenberg MD. Optimum end-expiratory airway pressure in patients with acute pulmonary failure. N Engl J Med 1975; 292:284–288.
47. Manny J, Justice R, Hetchman HB. Abnormalities in organ blood flow and its distribution during positive end-expiratory pressure. Surgery 1979; 85:425–432.
48. Matuschak GM, Pinsky MR, Rogers RM. Effects of positive end-expiratory pressure on hepatic blood flow and performance. J Appl Physiol 1987; 62:1377–1383.
49. Berstein AD, Gnidec AA, Rutledge FS, Sibbald NJ. Hyperdynamic sepsis modifies a PEEP-mediated redistribution in organ blood flows. Am Rev Respir Dis 1990; 141:1198–1208.
50. Geiger K, Georgieff M, Lutz H. Side effects of positive pressure ventilation on hepatic function and splanchnic circulation. Int J Clin Monit Comput 1986; 69:103–106.
51. Arvidsson D, Almquist P, Haglund U. Effects of positive end-expiratory pressure on splanchnic circulation and function in experimental peritonitis. Arch Surg 1991; 126:631–636.
52. Fujita Y, Sakai T, Ohsumi A, Takaori M. Effects of hypocapnia and hypercapnia on splanchnic circulation and hepatic function in the beagle. Anesth Analg 1989; 69:152–157.
53. Rowell LB, Brengelman GL, Blackmon JR, Twiss RD, Kusumi F. Splanchnic blood flow and metabolism in heat-stressed man. Appl Physiol 1968; 24:475–484.
54. Price HL, Deutsch S, Marshall BE, Stephen GW, Behar MG, Neufeld GR. Hemodynamic and metabolic effects of hemorrhage in man with particular reference to the splanchnic circulation. Circ Res 1966; 18:469–474.
55. Edouard AR, Degremont A-C, Duranteau J, Pussard E, Berdeaux A, Samii K. Heterogeneous regional vascular responses to simulated transient hypovolemia in man. Intensive Care Med 1994; 20:414–420.

56. Duranteau J, Sitbon P, Vicaut E, Descorps-Declere A, Vugue B, Samii K. Assessment of gastric mucosal perfusion during simulated hypovolemia in healthy volunteers. Am J Respir Crit Care Med 1996; 154:1653–1657.

57. Uusaro A, Ruokonen E, Takala J. Estimation of splanchnic blood flow by the Fick principle in man and problems in the use of indocyanine green. Cardiovasc Res 1995; 30:106–112.

58. Lang CH, Bagby GJ, Ferguson JL, Spitzer JJ. Cardiac output and redistribution of organ blood flow in hypermetabolic sepsis. Am J Physiol 1984; 246:R331–R337.

59. Xu D, Qi L, Guillory D, Cruz N, Berg R, Deitch EA. Mechanisms of endotoxin-induced intestinal injury in a hyperdynamic model of sepsis. J Trauma 1993; 34:676–683.

60. Fong Y, Marano MA, Moldaver LL, Wei H, Calvano SE, Kenney JS, Allison AC, Cerami A, Shires GT, Lowry SF. The acute splanchnic and peripheral tissue metabolic response to endotoxin in humans. J Clin Invest 1990; 85:1896–1904.

61. Dahn MS, Lange P, Wilson RF, Jacobs LA, Mitchell RA. Hepatic blood flow and splanchnic oxygen consumption measurements in clinical sepsis. Surgery 1990; 107:295–301.

62. Ruokonen E, Takala J, Kari A, Saxen H, Mertsola J, Hansen EJ. Regional blood flow and oxygen transport in septic shock. Crit Care Med 1993; 21:1296–1303.

63. Bailey RW, Morris JB, Hamilton SR, Bulkley GB. The pathogenesis of non-occlusive ischaemic colitis. Ann Surg 1986; 203:590–599.

64. McNeill JR, Stark RD, Greenway CV. Intestinal vasoconstriction after hemorrhage: roles of vasopressin and angiotensin. Am J Physiol 1970; 219:1342–1347.

65. Carter EA, Tompkins RG, Yarmush ML, Walker WA, Burke JF. Redistribution of blood flow after thermal injury and hemorrhagic shock. J Appl Physiol 1988; 65:1782–1788.

66. Carlton EL, Selinger SL, Utley J, Hoffman JIE. Intramyocardial distribution of blood flow in hemorrhagic shock in anesthetized dogs. Am J Physiol 1976; 230:41–49.

67. Archie JP, Mertz WR. Myocardial oxygen delivery after experimental shock. Ann Surg 1978; 187:205–210.

68. Ratcliffe PJ, Moonen CTW, Holloway PA, Ledingham JG, Radda GK. Acute renal failure in hemorrhagic hypotension: cellular energetics and renal function. Kidney Int 1986; 30:355–360.

69. Wyler F, Neutze JM, Rudolp AM. Effects of endotoxin on distribution of cardiac output in unanesthetized rabbits. Am J Physiol 1970; 219:246–251.

70. Kreimeier U, Brückner WB, Niemczyk S, Messmer K. Hyperosmotic saline dextran for resuscitation from traumatic-hemorrhagic hypotension: effect on regional blood flow. Circ Shock 1990; 32:83–99.

71. Miller CF, Breslow MJ, Shapiro RM, Traystman RF. Role of hypotension in decreasing cerebral blood flow in porcine endotoxemia. Am J Physiol 1987; 253:H956–H964.

72. Drazenovic R, Samsel RW, Wylam ME, Doerschuk CM, Schumacker PT. Regulation of perfused capillary density in canine intestinal mucosa during endotoxemia. J Appl Physiol 1992; 72:259–265.

73. Humer MF, Phang PT, Friesen BP, Allard MF, Goddard CM, Walley KR. Heterogeneity of gut capillary transit times and impaired gut oxygen extraction in endotoxemic pigs. J Appl Physiol 1996; 81(2):895–904.

74. Connolly HV, Maginniss LA, Schumacker PT. Transit time heterogeneity in canine small intestine: significance for oxygen transport. J Clin Invest 1997; 99:228–238.

75. Tenney SM. A theoretical analysis of the relationship between venous blood and mean tissue oxygen pressures. Respir Physiol 1974; 20:283–296.

76. Lam C, Tyml K, Martin C, Sibbald W. Microvascular perfusion is impaired in a rat model of normotensive sepsis. J Clin Invest 1994; 94:2077–2083.

77. Moncada S, Palmer RM, Higgs EA. Nitric oxide: physiology, pathophysiology, and pharmacology. Pharmacol Rev 1991; 43:109–142.

78. Cohen RA, Shepherd JT, Vanhoutte PM. Inhibitory role of the endothelium in the response of isolated coronary arteries to platelets. Science 1983; 221:273–274.

79. Manthous CA, Hall JB, Olson D, Singh M, Chatila W, Pohlman A, Kushner R, Schmidt GA, Wood LDG. Effect of cooling on oxygen consumption in febrile critically ill patients. Am J Respir Crit Care Med 1995; 151:10–14.

80. Boyd O, Grounds M, Bennett D. The dependency of oxygen consumption on oxygen delivery in critically ill postoperative patients is mimicked by variations in sedation. Chest 1992; 101:1619–1624.

81. Manthous CA, Hall JB, Kushner R, Schmidt GA, Russo G, Wood LDG. The effect of mechanical ventilation on oxygen consumption in critically ill patients. Am J Respir Crit Care Med 1995; 151:210–214.

82. Weissman C, Kemper M. The oxygen uptake-oxygen delivery relationship during ICU interventions. Chest 1991; 99:430–435.

83. Weissman C, Kemper M, Damask MC, Askanazi J, Hyman AI, Kinney JM. Effect of routine intensive care interactions on metabolic rate. Chest 1984; 86:815–818.

84. Bhatt S, Hutchinson R, Tomlinson B, Oh T, Mak M. Effects of dobutamine on oxygen supply and uptake in healthy volunteers. Br J Anaesth 1992; 69:298–303.

85. Green C, Frazer R, Underhill S, Maycock P, Fairhurst J, Campbell I. Metabolic effects of dobutamine in normal man. Clin Sci 1992; 82:77–83.

86. Uusaro A, Hartikainen J, Parviainen M, Takala J. Metabolic stress modifies the thermogenic effect of dobutamine in man. Crit Care Med 1995; 23:674–680.

87. Uusaro A, Ruokonen E, Takala J. Gastric mucosal pH does not reflect changes in splanchnic blood flow after cardiac surgery. Br J Anaesth 1995; 74:149–154.

88. Parviainen I, Ruokonen E, Takala J. Dobutamine-induced dissociation between changes in splanchnic blood flow and gastric intramucosal pH after cardiac surgery. Br J Anaesth 1995; 74:277–282.

89. Dahn MS, Lange P, Lobdell K, Hans B, Jacobs LA, Mitchell RA. Splanchnic and total body oxygen consumption differences in septic and injured patients. Surgery 1987; 101:69–80.

90. Wilmore DW, Goodwin CW, Aulick LH, Powanda MC, Mason AD, Pruitt BA Jr. Effect of injury and infection on visceral metabolism and circulation. Ann Surg 1980; 192:491–500.

91. Shoemaker WC, Appel PL, Kram HB. Tissue oxygen debt as a determinant of lethal and nonlethal postoperative organ failure. Crit Care Med 1988; 16:1117–1120.

92. Shoemaker WC, Appel PL, Kram HB. Role of oxygen debt in the development of organ failure, sepsis, and death in high-risk surgical patients. Chest 1992; 102:208–215.

93. Russell JA, Ronco JJ, Lockhat D, Belzberg A, Kiess M, Dodek PM. Oxygen delivery and consumption and ventricular preload are greater in survivors than in nonsurvivors of the adult respiratory distress syndrome. Am Rev Respir Dis 1990; 141:659–665.

94. Bone RC, Slotman G, Maunder R, Silverman H, Hyers TM, Kerstein MD, Ursprung JJ. Randomized double-blind, multicenter study of prostaglandin E$_1$ in patients with the adult respiratory distress syndrome. Chest 1989; 96:114–119.

95. Bihari D, Smithies M, Gimson A, Tinker J. The effects of vasodilation with prostacyclin on oxygen delivery and uptake in critically ill patients. N Eng J Med 1987; 317:397–403.

96. Spec-Marn A, Tos L, Kremzar B, Milic-Emili J, Ranieri VM. Oxygen delivery-consumption relationship in adult respiratory distress syndrome patients: the effects of sepsis. J Crit Care 1993; 8:43–50.

97. Shoemaker WC, Appel PL, Kram HB, Waxman K, Lee TS. Prospective trial of supranormal values of survivors as therapeutic goals in high-risk surgical patients. Chest 1988; 94:1176–1186.

98. Fleming A, Bishop M, Shoemaker W, Appel P, Sufficool W, Kuvhenguwha A, Kennedy F. Prospective trial of supranormal values as goals of resuscitation in severe trauma. Arch Surg 1992; 127:1175–1181.

99. Tuchschmidt J, Fried J, Astiz M, Rackow E. Elevation of cardiac output and oxygen delivery improves outcome in septic shock. Chest 1992; 102:216–220.

100. Boyd O, Grounds RM, Bennett ED. A randomized clinical trial of the effect of deliberate perioperative increase of oxygen delivery on mortality in high-risk surgical patients. JAMA 1993; 270:2699–2707.

101. Gutierrez G, Palizas F, Doglio G, Wainsztein N, Gallesio A, Pacin J, Dubin A, Schiavi E, Jorge M, Pusajo J, Klein F, San Roman E, Dorfman B, Shottlender J, Giniger R. Gastric intramucosal pH as a therapeutic index of tissue oxygenation in critically ill patients. Lancet 1992; 339:195–199.

102. Yu M, Levy MM, Smith P, Lisa A. Effect of maximizing oxygen delivery on morbidity and mortality rates in critically ill patients: a prospective, randomized, controlled study. Crit Care Med 1993; 21:830–838.

103. Hayes MA, Timmins AC, Yau EHS, Palazzo M, Hinds CJ, Watson D. Elevation of systemic oxygen delivery in the treatment of critically ill patients. N Engl J Med 1994; 330:1717–1722.

104. Gattinoni L, Brazzi L, Pelosi P, Latini R, Tognoni G, Pesenti A, Fumagalli R. A trial of goal-oriented hemodynamic therapy in critically ill patients. N Engl J Med 1995; 333:1025–1032.

105. Kruse JA, Carlson RW. Lactate metabolism. Crit Care Clin 1987; 5:725–746.

106. Arieff AI, Graf L. Pathophysiology of type A hypoxic lactic acidosis in dogs. Am J Physiol 1987; 253:271–276.

107. Weil MH, Afifi AA. Experimental and clinical studies on lactate and pyruvate as indicators of the severity of acute circulatory failure. Circulation 1970; 41:989–994.

108. Strauss B, Caldwell PRB, Fritss HW Jr. Observations on a model of proliferative lung disease: I. Transpulmonary arteriovenous differences in lactate, pyruvate and glucose. J Clin Invest 1970; 49:1305–1310.

109. Sayeed MM. Pulmonary cellular dysfunction in endotoxin shock: metabolic and transport derangements. Circ Shock 1982; 9:335–355.

110. Mitchel AM, Cournaud A. The fate of circulating lactic acid in the human lung. J Clin Invest 1955; 34:471–476.

111. Harris P, Bailey T, Bateman M. Lactate, pyruvate, glucose and free fatty acid in mixed venous and arterial blood. J Appl Physiol 1963; 18:933–936.

112. Brown SD, Clark C, Gutierrez G. Pulmonary lactate release in patients with sepsis and the adult respiratory distress syndrome. J Crit Care 1996; 11:2–8.

113. Kellum JA, Kramer DJ, Lee K, Mankad S, Bellomo R, Pinsky MR. Release of lactate by the lung in acute lung injury. Chest 1997; 111:1301–1305.

114. Douzinas EE, Tsidemiadou PD, Pitaridis MT, Andrianakis I, Bobota-Chloraki A, Kat-

souyanni K, Sfyras D, Malagari K, Roussos C. The regional production of cytokines and lactate in sepsis-related multiple organ failure. Am J Respir Crit Care Med 1997; 155:53–59.

115. Broder G, Weil MH. Excess lactate: an index of reversibility of shock in human patients. Science 1964; 143:1457–1459.

116. Vitek V, Cowley RA. Blood lactate in the prognosis of various forms of shock. Ann Surg 1971; 173:308–313.

117. Bakker J, Coffernils M, Leon M, Gris P, Vincent JL. Blood lactate levels are superior to oxygen-derived variables in predicting outcome in human septic shock. Chest 1991; 99:956–962.

118. Kruse JA, Zaidi SAJ, Carlson R. Significance of blood lactate levels in critically ill patients with liver disease. Am J Med 1987; 83:77–82.

119. Vincent JL, Dufaye P, Berre J, Leeman M, Degante SP, Kahn RJ. Serial lactate determinations during circulatory shock. Crit Care Med 1983; 11:449–451.

120. Falk JL, Rackow EC, Laevy J, Astiz ME, Weil MH. Delayed lactate clearance in patients surviving circulatory shock. Acute Care 1985; 11:212–215.

121. Parker MM, Shelhamer JH, Natanson C, Alling DW, Parillo JE. Serial cardiovascular variables in survivors and nonsurvivors of human septic shock: heart rate as an early predictor of prognosis. Crit Care Med 1987; 15:923–929.

122. Roumen RMH, Redl H, Schlag G, Sandtner W, Koller W, Goris RJA. Scoring systems and blood lactate concentrations in relation to the development of adult respiratory distress syndrome and multiple organ failure in severely traumatized patients. J Trauma 1993; 35:349–355.

123. Sauaia A, Moore EA, Moore EE, Haenel JB, Read RA, Lezotte DC. Early predictors of postinjury multiple organ failure. Arch Surg 1994; 129:39–45.

124. Moore FA, Haenel JB, Moore EE, Whitehill TA. Incommensurate oxygen consumption in response to maximal oxygen availability predicts postinjury multiple organ failure. J Trauma 1992; 33:58–65.

125. Cerra FB, Negro F, Abrams J. APACHE II score does not predict multiple organ failure or mortality in postoperative surgical patients. Arch Surg 1990; 125:519–522.

126. Manikis P, Jankowski S, Zhang H, Kahn RJ, Vincent JL. Correlation of serial blood lactate levels to organ failure and mortality after trauma. Am J Emerg Med 1995; 13:619–622.

127. Bakker J, Gris P, Coffernils M, Kahn RJ, Vincent JL. Serial blood lactate levels can predict the development of multiple organ failure following septic shock. Am J Surg 1996; 171:221–226.

128. Bulkley GB, Oshima A, Bailey RW. Pathophysiology of hepatic ischemia in cardiogenic shock. Am J Surg 1986; 151:87–97.

129. Arvidsson D, Rasmunssen I, Almquist P, Niklansson F, Haglund U. Splanchnic oxygen consumption in septic and hemorrhagic shock. Surgery 1991; 109:190–197.

130. Meakins JL, Marshall W. The gastrointestinal tract: the "motor" of MOF. Arch Surg 1986; 121:197–201.

131. Lundgren O, Haglund U. The pathophysiology of the countercurrent exchanger. Life Sciences 1978; 23:1411–1422.

132. Bohlen HG. Intestinal tissue PO_2 and microvascular responses during glucose exposure. Am J Physiol 1980; 238:H164–H171.

133. Marik PE. Gastric intramucosal pH. A better predictor of multiorgan dysfunction and death than oxygen derived variables in patients with sepsis. Chest 1993; 104:225–229.

134. Miller PR, Chang MC, Meredith JW. Comparison of pH$_i$ and mucosal-arterial CO_2 gap as predictors of outcome in trauma patients. Chest 1996; 110(4):138S.

135. Mythen MG, Webb AR. Intra-operative gut mucosal hypoperfusion is associated with increased post-operative complications and cost. Intensive Care Med 1994; 20:99–104.

136. Doglio GR, Pusajo JF, Egurrola MA, Bonfigli GC, Parra C, Vetere L, Hernandez MS, Fernandez S, Palizas F, Gutierrez G. Gastric mucosal pH as a prognostic index of mortality in critically ill patients. Crit Care Med 1991; 19:1037–1040.

137. Bone RC. Toward a theory regarding the pathogenesis of the systemic inflammatory response syndrome: what we do and do not know about cytokine regulation. Crit Care Med 1996; 24:163–172.

138. Beal AL, Cerra FB. Multiple organ failure syndrome in the 1990s. Systemic inflammatory response and organ dysfunction. JAMA 1994; 271:226–233.

139. Pinsky MR, Vincent J-L, Deviere J, Alegre M, Kahn RJ, Dupont E. Serum cytokine levels in human septic shock. Relation to multiple-system organ failure and mortality. Chest 1993; 103:565–575.

140. Cruickshank AM, Fraser WD, Burns HJG, van Damme J, Shenkin A. Response of serum interleukin-6 in patients undergoing elective surgery of varying severity. Clin Sci 1990; 79:161–165.

141. Tang GJ, Kuo CD, Yen TC, Kuo HS, Yien HW, Lee TY. Perioperative plasma concentrations of tumor necrosis factor-alpha and interleukin-6 in infected patients. Crit Care Med 1996; 24:423–428.

142. Kragsbjerg P, Holmberg H, Vikerfors T. Serum concentrations of interleukin-6, tumour necrosis factor-alpha, and C-reactive protein in patients undergoing major operations. Eur J Surg 1995; 161:17–22.

143. van der Poll T, Jansen J, Endert E, Sauerwein HP, van Deventer SJH. Noradrenaline inhibits lipopolysaccharide-induced tumor necrosis factor and interleukin-6 production in human whole blood. Infect Immun 1994; 62:2046–2050.

144. Hu X, Goldmuntz EA, Brosnan CF. The effect of norepinephrine on endotoxin-mediated macrophage activation. J Neuroimmunol 1991; 31:35–42.

145. Severn A, Rapson NT, Hunter CA. Regulation of tumor necrosis factor production by adrenaline and β-adrenergic agonists. J Immunol 1992; 148:3441–3445.

146. van der Poll T, Coyle SM, Barbosa K, Braxton CC, Lowry SF. Epinephrine inhibits tumor necrosis factor-α and potentiates interleukin-10 production during human endotoxemia. J Clin Invest 1996; 97:713–719.

147. Donnelly SC, Strieter RM, Reid P, Kunkel SL, Burdick MD, Armstrong I, Mackenzie A, Haslett C. The association between mortality rates and decreased concentrations of interleukin-10 and interleukin-1 receptor antagonist in the lung fluid of patients with the adult respiratory distress syndrome. Ann Intern Med 1996; 125:191–196.

148. Barton MH, Moore JN. Pentoxifylline inhibits mediator synthesis in an equine in vitro whole blood model of endotoxemia. Circ Shock 1994; 44:216–220.

149. Schade UF. Pentoxifylline increases survival in murine endotoxin shock and decreases formation of tumor necrosis factor. Circ Shock 1990; 31:171–181.

150. Giroir BP, Beutler B. Effect of amrinone on tumor necrosis factor production in endotoxic shock. Circ Shock 1992; 36:200–207.

151. Zabel P, Wolter DT, Schonharting MM, Schade UF. Oxpentifylline in endotoxemia. Lancet 1989; 2:1474–1478.

152. Adams DH, Nash GB. Disturbance of leucocyte circulation and adhesion to the endothelium as factors in circulatory pathology. Br J Anaesth 1996; 77:17–31.

153. Fortenberry JD, Huber AR, Owens ML. Inotropes inhibit endothelial cell surface adhesion molecules induced by interleukin-1β. Crit Care Med 1997; 25:303–308.

154. Schmidt W, Schmidt H, Hacker A, Gebhard M-M, Martin E. Influence of dopexamine on leukocyte adherence and vascular permeability in postcapillary venules during endotoxemia. Crit Care Med 1997; 25(1 Suppl):A42.

155. Tremblay L, Valenza F, Ribeiro SP, Li J, Slutsky AS. Injurious ventilatory strategies increase cytokines and c-fos m-RNA expression in an isolated rat lung model. J Clin Invest 1997; 99:944–952.

156. Moore FA, Moore EE. Evolving concepts in the pathogenesis of postinjury multiple organ failure. Surg Clin North Am 1995; 75:257–277.

157. Nielsen VG, Tan S, Weinbroum A, McCammon AT, Samuelson PN, Gelman S, Parks DA. Lung injury after hepatoenteric ischemia-reperfusion: role of xanthine oxidase. Am J Respir Crit Care Med 1996; 154:1364–1369.

158. Nielsen VG, Tan S, Baird MS, McCammon AT, Parks DA. Gastric intramucosal pH and multiple organ injury: impact of ischemia-reperfusion and xanthine oxidase. Crit Care Med 1996; 24:1339–1344.

159. Waxman K. Shock: ischemia, reperfusion, and inflammation. New Horiz 1996; 4:153–160.

160. McCord JM. Oxygen-derived free radicals in post-ischemic tissue injury. N Engl J Med 1985; 312:159–163.

161. Roumen RMH, Hendriks TH, de Man RM, Goris RJA. Serum lipofuscin as a prognostic indicator of adult respiratory distress syndrome and multiple organ failure. Br J Surg 1994; 81:1300–1305.

162. Goldman G, Welbourn R, Klausner JM, Kobzik L, Valeri CR, Shepro D, Hechtman HB. Mast cells and leukotrienes mediate neutrophil sequestration and lung edema after remote ischemia in rodents. Surgery 1992; 112:578–586.

163. Punch J, Rees R, Cashmer B, Oldham K, Wilkins E, Smith DJ Jr. Acute lung injury following reperfusion after ischemia in the hind limb of rats. J Trauma 1991; 31:760–765.

164. Partnick DA, Moore FA, Moore EE, Barnett CC Jr, Silliman CC. Neutrophil priming and activation in the pathogenesis of postinjury multiple organ failure. New Horiz 1996; 4:194–210.

165. Pastores S, Katz DP, Kvetan V. Splanchnic ischemia and gut mucosal injury in sepsis and the multiple organ dysfunction syndrome. Am J Gastroenterol 1996; 91:1697–1710.

166. Cipolle MD, Pasquale MD, Cerra FB. Secondary organ dysfunction. From clinical perspectives to molecular mediators. Crit Care Clin 1993; 9:261–298.

167. Moore EE, Moore FA, Franciose RJ, Kim FJ, Biffl WL, Banerjee A. The postischemic gut serves as a priming bed for circulating neutrophils that provoke multiple organ failure. J Trauma 1994; 37:881–887.

168. Livingston DH, Mosenthal AC, Deitch EA. Sepsis and multiple organ dysfunction syndrome: a clinical-mechanistic overview. New Horiz 1995; 3:257–266.

14

Outcome and Long-Term Care of ARDS

Richard K. Albert

Introduction

A variety of treatments have been tried in patients with acute respiratory distress syndrome (ARDS) in an attempt to prevent, reverse, or diminish the inflammatory response that occurs in this setting. Although preliminary data with more recently studied interventions such as ketoconazole, surfactant replacement, and partial liquid ventilation seem promising,[1–5] no approaches have yet been shown to alter survival, shorten the duration of ventilation or hospitalization, or reduce the frequency of ARDS-associated morbidity.

In lieu of data indicating a beneficial effect with any specific therapy, treatment of ARDS has focused on adjusting the fraction of inspired oxygen (FiO_2) and positive end-expiratory pressure (PEEP) so as to reduce the likelihood of oxygen toxicity and/or barotrauma (recently, and appropriately renamed volutrauma[6]). More recent observations indicating that much of the lung in patients with ARDS is not ventilated,[7] along with the rediscovery that ventilation with high volumes actually *causes* lung injury,[8–10] has led to the development of new ventilatory strategies designed to minimize this potential problem.[11]

Although the more recent changes in supportive therapy of ARDS may not have been employed sufficiently long for differences in morbidity and/or mortality to become apparent, until just recently there was little evidence suggesting that the course of ARDS had been altered by any of these interventions. This chapter summarizes published information pertaining to the survival of patients with ARDS and how the episode of acute lung injury affects symptoms, roentgenographs, and pulmonary function. Aspects of appropriate management of patients after they are discharged from the ICU and from the hospital are also reviewed.

James A. Russell and Keith R. Walley, eds. *Acute Respiratory Distress Syndrome*. Printed in the United States of America. Copyright © 1999. Cambridge University Press. All rights reserved.

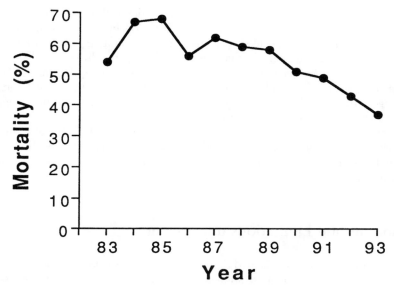

Figure 14.1. Improved survival of patients with acute respiratory distress syndrome: 1983–1993. (Modified from Milberg JA, Davis DR, Steinberg KP, Hudson LD. Improved survival of patients with acute respiratory distress syndrome (ARDS): 1983–1993. JAMA 1995; 273:306–309.)

Survival

The mortality of ARDS has generally exceeded 50% since the condition was recognized in 1967.[12–14] One difficulty in quantifying survival is that a variety of factors has been found to influence mortality in these patients. Accordingly, the demographics and various conditions resulting in ARDS in the specific population being studied influence the results observed, as may potential differences in management. Milberg and colleagues[15] noted that mortality at a single institution (with a consistent definition of ARDS) had improved from 55% to 65% in the 1980s to a low of 37% in 1993 (Figure 14.1). This observation supports the results from less well-designed studies by other investigators.[16–18] Interestingly, Milberg et al.[15] found that adjusting for age, ARDS risk factor, and degree of injury and/or severity of illness (i.e., factors previously shown to affect mortality) had a remarkably small effect on the results observed. It was not possible for the authors to evaluate the cause of this apparent change, but a number of potential explanations were suggested including (1) that patients entering their study had become less ill or less severely injured in more recent years; (2) that supportive care of the critically ill had improved; and/or (3) that newer modes of ventilation or pharmacologic interventions had been beneficial.[15] A considerable number of laboratory studies utilizing a variety of animal models of acute lung injury (but with *no* confirmation in studies of humans with ARDS) suggest that the most likely explanation for this finding pertains to improvements in supportive care; namely, that physicians have generally become less aggressive with PEEP and/or hemodynamic interventions aimed at "optimizing" or "maximizing" oxygen delivery, and more content with simply adjusting ventilatory, gas exchange, and hemodynamic variables to levels that provide adequate support, thereby avoiding iatrogenic complications.

Regardless of the explanation, the observation that ARDS mortality may be improving over time means all future studies designed to investigate new therapeutic interventions in this patient population must at least include a control group that is concurrently observed.

Symptoms and Limitations in Survivors

A number of early reports indicated that the majority of ARDS survivors were symptom free.[12,19–25] In most of these studies, however, symptoms were not aggressively sought, and in some, the results were likely biased by the fact that patients with mild illness were included. For example, no respiratory symptoms were found in a series reported by Douglas and colleagues[20] in which ARDS survival was 80% and in a study by Yahav and colleagues[22] in which only 66% required mechanical ventilation, and many of those did not require PEEP to maintain oxygenation.

Data from more recent studies with more rigorously defined populations that included more severely affected patients suggest that up to 66% will have some respiratory symptoms following recovery[26,27] (although these studies may overestimate this risk as a result of a high frequency of smoking prior to the ARDS episode).

The most systematic evaluation of symptoms following ARDS was done by Ghio and associates,[28] who found cough, sputum production, and/or dyspnea in 21 of 25 patients (84%) studied between 0.3 and 7.5 years after their episode. Although there was a tendency for improvement to occur over time, more than one-half of those questioned more than a year following their episode continued to be symptomatic. Smoking status had no association with symptoms, although 29% of the those studied were smokers. Fewer than half of those with pulmonary symptoms had abnormal pulmonary function tests, and those with abnormal tests were no more likely to be symptomatic than those having normal tests.

McHugh and colleagues[29] have provided another way of evaluating the importance of post-ARDS respiratory symptoms by following self-perceived health assessments in 52 patients discharged after an episode of ARDS that required intubation and mechanical ventilation. Health was assessed using the Sickness Impact Profile ("normal" scores obtained from a healthy population = < 5). Median scores post-ARDS decreased from 33 within 2 weeks of extubation to 12 at 3 months, and further decreased to 7 at 1 year (ranges or data indicating the number of patients with normal vs. abnormal scores at the three time points were not included). Despite the 1 year values slightly exceeding the average score of normal subjects, complaints were more frequently associated with general health than with lung problems specifically.

Roentgenographic Changes in Survivors

Although the availability of information pertaining to the roentgenographic course of patients with ARDS following hospital discharge is limited, chest x-rays of patients who survive without complications are generally thought to return to normal.[30] Anecdotal cases of diffuse interstitial fibrosis and cyst formation (possibly as a result of ventilator-induced lung injury) have been reported,[31–33] and these changes have been likened to those found in the bronchopulmonary dysplasia that occurs as a consequence of the infant respiratory distress syndrome and/or its treatment.[33] Occasionally these patients are so severely compromised that lung transplantation is considered.

Pulmonary Function Test Abnormalities

Spirometry

Mild to moderate reductions in the forced expiratory volume in 1 second (FEV_1) (i.e., 50% to 75% predicted) are commonly seen early in the post-ARDS period.[26] The forced vital capacity (FVC) is generally reduced to a similar extent resulting in a normal FEV_1/FVC, thereby suggesting a restrictive defect (see discussion of lung volumes later). On occasion the reductions are severe (e.g., FEV_1's of 20% to 25% predicted). These abnormalities tend to improve over time to the extent that normal or near normal values are generally seen by 1 year in those who initially have mild to moderate reductions. Those with severe reductions improve much less and much less commonly.

A subset of ARDS survivors ranging from 14% to 50% of the various reported series[20,26–28] are left with at least mild airflow limitation (i.e., $FEV_1/FVC < 65\%$, forced expiratory flow from 25% to 75% of the VC, < 50% predicted) even in the absence of a smoking history prior to the ARDS episode.[24]

Airway Resistance

Increased airway resistance is characteristic of acute ARDS,[34–37] but the abnormality improves with resolution[25] presumably as a result of the improvement in the airway inflammation[34] and/or the increase in total lung capacity (TLC) that occurs as ARDS resolves.[37]

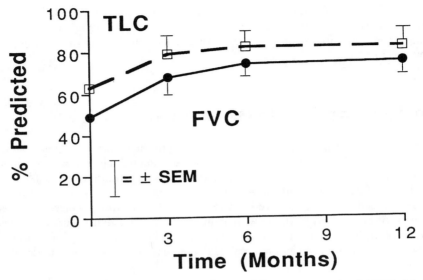

Figure 14.2. Improvement in lung volumes over time following an episode of ARDS. (Modified from McHugh LG, Milberg JA, Whitcomb ME, Schoene RB, Maunder RJ, Hudson LD. Recovery of function in survivors of the acute respiratory distress syndrome. Am J Respir Crit Care Med 1995; 150:90–94.)

Airway Hyperreactivity

Bronchial hyperreactivity in response to methacholine and/or exercise has been observed in 3 of 9 patients as long as 1 year following their episode of ARDS.[38] Neither the frequency with which this abnormality occurs nor its associated or predisposing factors are known at this time.

Lung Volumes

Lung volumes are reduced in most patients when measured within 2 weeks of extubation and/or at discharge following an episode of ARDS, but these abnormalities improve during the first 3 to 6 months of recovery[21,22,25,26,29,39] (Figure 14.2). Those with more severe ARDS and those with more severe restriction at the time of discharge improve less.[26,29]

A small subset of patients have a chronically elevated residual volume with a normal or mildly reduced TLC and no evidence of airflow limitation,[19–21, 40] perhaps as a manifestation of small airway injury that occurs during the acute phase of the syndrome.

Dead Space

Dead space ventilation (V_D/V_T) is generally increased early in the recovery phase of ARDS and improves over time in many, but not all of the affected patients.[21,24,40,41] The normal exercise-associated *fall* in V_D/V_T occurs to a lesser extent in these patients.

Diffusing Capacity

From 75% to 100% of ARDS survivors have a reduced diffusion capacity (DL_{CO}), making it the most common pulmonary function test abnormality seen in these patients.[26,28,29] Although some of these patients improve during the first year, 40% to 80% of those studied continue to have mild reductions that persist even after 1 year.[21,24,26–29,39,40] As with lung volumes, those with the most severely reduced DL_{CO}s tend to have the least improvement.[26]

Failure of the DL_{CO} to return to normal in most ARDS survivors contrasts with the improvements in spirometry and lung volumes that generally occur in these patients. Low DL_{CO}s, together with persistent abnormalities in V_D/V_T, suggest that the pulmonary vasculature may have been destroyed or obstructed by the acute injury, by the inflammatory response, and/or by the repair mechanism associated with the episode of ARDS. Many histologic studies demonstrate a loss and/or thrombosis of the pulmonary microcirculation in the acute phase of ARDS.[42]

Arterial Blood Gases

Elliott and colleagues[24,25] found in 11 of 13 (85%) ARDS survivors an alveolar-to-arterial oxygen difference ($A\text{-}aDO_2$) that was normal at rest (measured 1 month after the episode of ARDS), but elevated with exercise. This gas exchange abnormality can occur in the setting of normal spirometry and lung volumes.[41]

Given that most survivors have a normal $A\text{-}aDO_2$ at rest, it is not surprising to find that shunt fraction is generally normal or only minimally abnormal.[20,21,40]

Medical Management of Patients after Discharge

Management should be tailored to the severity of the patient's respiratory symptoms. In many instances no pulmonary-specific follow-up or management will be necessary. At the other extreme are a few patients with irreversible pulmonary disease (obstruction and/or restriction) of a severity that prompts evaluation for lung transplantation. Because the long-term symptoms and physiology may be so variable, nothing can be recommended on a routine basis.

Similarly, because of the numerous types of post-ARDS problems that may occur, patients complaining of dyspnea, cough, or any other respiratory symptoms require a thorough history and physical examination along with roentgenographic, pulmonary physiologic, and potentially a bronchoscopic evaluation.

History

Although respiratory complaints are likely to be related to the episode of ARDS, other causes should be sought as directed by the patient's age, chronic medical or surgical problems, medications, smoking history, and family history. Given that pulmonary function returns to normal or close to normal in the large majority of ARDS survivors, it is important to seek other, nonpulmonary explanations for respiratory complaints.

Most, but not all, studies indicate that the likelihood of developing chronic respiratory symptoms following an episode of ARDS is related to the degree of abnormality in thoracic compliance, pulmonary artery pressure, and shunt fraction measured during the first days of ARDS, the duration of mechanical ventilation, and the need for higher levels of PEEP.[28,37] Accordingly, reviewing the patient's hospital course may allow estimation of the likelihood that post-ARDS respiratory symptoms are indeed the result of the ARDS episode. Other variables associated with an increased incidence of postoperative pulmonary problems include increases in pulmonary vascular resistance, pulmonary arterial pressures, and A-aDO$_2$ measured during the first week of the episode of ARDS.[26] The presence of barotrauma and the need for an FiO$_2$ > 0.6 for longer than 24 hours have both been associated with a reduced DL$_{CO}$ measured 1 year later.[39] Unfortunately, two other small studies confuse the issue because they found no correlation between abnormalities in pulmonary function and the severity of ARDS, the duration of mechanical ventilation,[22] the duration of PEEP therapy, or the initial arterial oxygen tension.[40] Despite these contradictions, the majority of the data support the association between the presence of chronic pulmonary dysfunction and the severity of the ARDS episode.

The etiology of the episode of ARDS may be associated with the development of chronic pulmonary dysfunction, although there are conflicting data. Some studies indicate that the ARDS resulting from viral pneumonia or from gram-negative pneumonia is more likely to result in pulmonary fibrosis and dysfunction;[31,32] others suggest no association between the presumed cause of ARDS and the long-term prognosis.[26,28]

Having a history of smoking does not seem to predispose ARDS survivors to more severe ARDS or to more abnormal pulmonary function after recovery.[26,39] This is an interesting observation in lieu of the increased number of neutrophils found in bronchoalveolar lavage of asymptomatic smokers and the hypothesis that the lung damage resulting in ARDS is neutrophil mediated.

Some aspects of the "supportive" care of patients with ARDS (i.e., excessive tidal volume, excessive or insufficient levels of PEEP, high FiO$_2$) may also predispose to long-term pulmonary compromise.[8,10] Reviewing the type of ventilatory support used during the acute phase of ARDS may assist in assessing the likelihood of ARDS-induced chronic lung injury.

Physical Examination

Although chest roentgenograms and pulmonary function tests are more sensitive screening tests for pleural and parenchymal lung disease, as well as for airflow limitation or restrictive lung disease, the physical examination can suggest interstitial fibrosis, a paralyzed hemidiaphragm, or cardiac, liver, or other disease that may possibly be responsible for the specific respiratory symptom being evaluated.

Pulmonary Function Testing

In absence of findings pointing to a nonpulmonary cause of respiratory symptoms, spirometry should be measured along with lung volumes (ideally by plethysmography) and a DL_{CO}. Flow volume loops should also be routinely obtained to evaluate the possibility of laryngotracheal stenosis, a well-recognized consequence of prolonged intubation[43] and/or vocal cord dysfunction. ABGs should be obtained in every patient, regardless of the results of screening pulmonary function tests because the A-aDO$_2$ may be increased despite normal airflow and lung volumes. If resting ABGs are normal and respiratory symptoms remain unexplained, an ABG during exercise is indicated.

The results of these studies may be interpreted only in lieu of the natural history of the pulmonary abnormalities that result from ARDS as discussed earlier. The implications of reductions in airflow, lung volumes, and/or DL_{CO} depend on how long after the episode of ARDS the abnormality is noted. Improvements would be expected if the abnormalities were found within a few months of discharge, but would be much less likely to occur if noted 6 to 12 months hence.

Bronchoscopy

Because the sensitivity of the flow-volume loop for upper airway abnormalities is not known, it may also be reasonable for patients with complaints of dyspnea to undergo laryngoscopy and/or bronchoscopy.

Summary

Although many patients report dyspnea following ARDS, the symptom does not correlate with PFT abnormalities. Most ARDS survivors have persistent, mild reductions of DL_{CO} even as long as a year following their episode of ARDS. The lung volumes and flows return to normal in the large majority, although a subset including those with the most severe ARDS have persistent impairment. Both obstructive and restrictive patterns may be seen. This subgroup may be predicted with reasonable accuracy by reviewing the degree of acute lung injury at the time of ARDS as assessed by the FiO$_2$, PEEP level used, and/or the gas exchange abnormality seen in the first few days of the episode.

In the first year after ARDS most physiologic abnormalities improve, with the greatest degree of improvement occurring in the first 3 months. If deficits persist at 1 year, further improvement is unlikely.

References

1. Yu M, Tomasa G. A double-blind, prospective, randomized trial of ketoconazole, a thromboxane synthesis inhibitor, in the prophylaxis of the adult respiratory distress syndrome. Crit Care Med 1993; 21:1635–1642.
2. Weg JG, Balk RA, Tharatt RS, Jenkinson SG, Shah JB, Zaccardelli D, Horton J, Pattishall EN. Safety and potential efficacy of an aerosolized surfactant in human sepsis-induced adult respiratory distress syndrome. JAMA 1994; 272:12599–12660.
3. Haslam PL, Hughes DA, MacNaughton PD, Baker CS, Evans TW. Surfactant replacement therapy in late-stage adult respiratory distress syndrome. Lancet 1994; 343: 1009–1011.
4. Spragg RG, Gilliard N, Richman P, Smith RM, Hite RD, Pappert D, Robertson B, Curstedt T, Strayer D. Acute effects of a single dose of porcine surfactant on patients with the adult respiratory distress syndrome. Chest 1994; 105:195–202.
5. Hirschl RB, Pranikoff T, Wise C, Overbeck MC, Gauger P, Schreiner RJ, Dechert R, Bartlett RH. Initial experience with partial liquid ventilation in adult patients with the acute respiratory distress syndrome. JAMA 1995; 275:383–389.
6. Dreyfuss D, Saumon G. Barotrauma is volutrauma, but which volume is the one responsible? Intensive Care Med 1992; 18:139–141.
7. Gattinoni L, Mascheroni D, Torresin A, Marcolin R, Fumagalli R, Vesconi S, Rossi GP, Rossi F, Baglioni S, Bassi F, Nastri G, Pesenti A. Morphological response to positive end expiratory pressure in acute respiratory failure. Computerized tomography study. Intensive Care Med 1986; 12:137–142.
8. Webb H, Tierney D. Experimental pulmonary edema due to intermittent positive pressure ventilation with high inflation pressures: protection by positive end-expiratory pressure. Am Rev Respir Dis 1974; 110:556–565.
9. Hernandez L, Peevy K, Moise A, Parker J. Chest wall restriction limits high airway pressure induced lung injury in young rabbits. J Appl Physiol 1989; 66:2364–2368.
10. Dreyfuss D, Basset G, Soler P, Saumon G. Intermittent positive-pressure hyperventilation with high inflation pressures produces pulmonary microvascular injury in rats. Am Rev Respir Dis 1985; 132:880–884.
11. Slutsky AS. Mechanical ventilation. American College of Chest Physicians' Consensus Conference. Chest 1993; 104:1833–1859.
12. Ashbaugh DG, Bigelow DB, Petty TL, Levine BE. Acute respiratory distress in adults. Lancet 1967; 2:319–323.
13. Fowler A, Hamman R, Zerbe G, Benson K, Hyers T. Adult respiratory distress syndrome. Prognosis after onset. Am Rev Respir Dis 1985; 132:472–478.
14. Sloane P, Gee M, Gottlieb Albertine K, Peters S, Burns J, et al. A multicenter registry of patients with acute respiratory distress syndrome. Am Rev Respir Dis 1992; 146:419–426.

15. Milberg JA, Davis DR, Steinberg KP, Hudson LD. Improved survival of patients with acute respiratory distress syndrome (ARDS): 1983–1993. JAMA 1995; 273:306–309.

16. Morris AH, Wallace CJ, Menlow RL, et al. Randomized clinical trial of pressure-controlled inverse ratio ventilation and extracorporeal CO_2 removal for adult respiratory distress syndrome. Am J Respir Crit Care Med 1994; 149:295–305.

17. Zapol WM, Frikker MJ, Lynch K, Pontoppidan H, Wilson RS. The adult respiratory distress syndrome at Massachusetts General Hospital: etiology, progression and survival rates 1978–88. In Acute respiratory failure, eds WM Zapol, F Lemaire. New York, Marcel Dekker, 1990, 367–380.

18. Suchya MR, Clemmer TP, Orme JF, Morris AH, Elliot CG. Increased survival of ARDS patients with severe hypoxemia (ECMO criteria). Chest 1991; 99:951–955.

19. Yernault J, Englert M, Sergysels R, DeCoster A. Pulmonary mechanics and diffusion after "shock lung." Thorax 1975; 30:252–257.

20. Douglas M, Downs J. Pulmonary function following severe acute respiratory failure and high levels of positive end-expiratory pressure. Chest 1977; 71:18–23.

21. Rotman H, Lavelle T, Dimcheff D, VandenBelt R, Weg J. Long-term physiologic consequences of the adult respiratory distress syndrome. Chest 1977; 71:190–192.

22. Yahav J, Lieberman P, Mollo M. Pulmonary function following the adult respiratory distress syndrome. Chest 1978; 74:247–250.

23. Kahn F, Parekh A. Reversible platypnea and orthodeoxia following recovery from adult respiratory distress syndrome. Chest 1979; 75:526–528.

24. Elliott G, Morris A, Cengiz M. Pulmonary function and exercise gas exchange in survivors of adult respiratory distress syndrome. Am Rev Respir Dis 1981; 123:492–495.

25. Alberts W, Priest G, Moser K. The outlook for survivors of ARDS. Chest 1983; 84:272–274.

26. Peters J, Bell R, Prihoda T, Harris G, Andrews C, Johanson W. Clinical determinants of abnormalities in pulmonary functions in survivors of the adult respiratory distress syndrome. Am Rev Respir Dis 1989; 139:1163–1168.

27. Lakshminarayan S, Stanford R, Petty T. Prognosis after recovery from adult respiratory distress syndrome. Am Rev Respir Dis 1976; 113:7–16.

28. Ghio A, Elliot C, Crapo R, Berlin S, Jensen R. Impairment after adult respiratory distress syndrome. An evaluation based on American Thoracic Society recommendations. Am Rev Respir Dis 1989; 94:526–530.

29. McHugh LG, Milberg JA, Whitcomb ME, Schoene RB, Maunder RJ, Hudson LD. Recovery of function in survivors of the acute respiratory distress syndrome. Am J Respir Crit Care Med 1995; 150:90–94.

30. Johnson TH, Altman AR, McCaffree RD. Radiologic considerations in the adult respiratory distress syndrome treated with positive end-expiratory pressure (PEEP). Clin Chest Med 1982; 3:89–100.

31. Winterbauer R, Ludwig W, Hammar S. Clinical course, management and long term sequelae of respiratory failure due to influenza viral pneumonia. Johns Hopkins Med J 1977; 141:148–155.

32. Pearson R, Hall W, Menegris M, Douglas R. Diffuse pneumonitis due to adenovirus type 21 in a civilian. Chest 1980; 78:107–109.

33. Churg A, Golden J, Fligiel S, Hogg J. Case reports: bronchopulmonary dysplasia in the adult. Am Rev Respir Dis 1983; 127:117–120.

34. Wright P, Bernard G. The role of airflow resistance in patients with adult respiratory distress syndrome. Am Rev Respir Dis 1989; 139:1169–1174.

35. Eissa N, Ranieri V, Corbeil C, Chasse M, Broidy J, Milic-Emili J. Effects of positive end-expiratory pressure, lung volume and inspiratory flow on interrupter resistance in patients with ARDS. Am Rev Respir Dis 1991; 144:538–543.

36. Presenti A, Pilosi P, Rossi N, Virtuani A, Brazzi L, Rossi A. The effect of positive end-expiratory pressure on respiratory resistance in patients with the adult respiratory distress syndrome and in normal anesthetized subjects. Am Rev Respir Dis 1991; 144:101–107.

37. Tantucci C, Corbeil C, Chasse M, Rabatto F, Nava S, Braidy J, et al. Flow and volume dependence of respiratory system flow resistance in patients with adult respiratory distress syndrome. Am Rev Respir Dis 1992; 145:355–360.

38. Simpson D, Goodman M, Spector S, Pettry T. Long-term follow-up and bronchial reactivity testing in survivors of the adult respiratory distress syndrome. Am Rev Respir Dis 1978; 117:449–454.

39. Elliott G, Rasmusson B, Crapo R, Morris A, Jensen R. Prediction of pulmonary function abnormalities after adult respiratory distress syndrome (ARDS). Am Rev Respir Dis 1987; 135:634–638.

40. Klein J, van Haeringen J, Sluiter H, Holloway R, Peset R. Pulmonary function after recovery from the adult respiratory distress syndrome. Chest 1976; 69:608–611.

41. Buchser E, Leuenberger P, Chiolero R, Perret C, Freeman J. Reduced pulmonary capillary blood volume as a long-term sequel of ARDS. Chest 1985; 87:608–611.

42. Bachofen M, Weibel E. Alterations of the gas exchange apparatus in adult respiratory insufficiency associated with septicemia. Am Rev Respir Dis 1977; 116:589–616.

43. Elliott C, Rasmussen B, Crapo R. Upper airway obstruction following adult respiratory distress syndrome. Chest 1988; 94:526–530.

Index

Abdominal examination, 15
Abdominal trauma, 203–4
Accessory muscles, and diaphragmatic weakness, 185
Acetaminophen, 154, 242
Acetazolamide, 93
Acidosis. *See* Metabolic acidosis; Respiratory acidosis
Acinetobacter spp., 252, 268t
ACTH stimulation test, 113
Acute lung injury (ALI)
  diagnosis of, 8
  fibrosing alveolitis and, 282–90
  growth factors, 290–4
  mediators of, 11
  quality of life for survivors of, 41
  removal of excess fluid and protein, 276–81
  standardized scoring systems for, 29
Acute respiratory distress syndrome (ARDS)
  approach to clinical management of, 1–2
  cardiovascular system and, 10–11, 12, 15, 108–20, 212–13, 211t, 107
  chest radiology and diagnosis of, 16–23
  clinical evaluation of patients, 11–16
  definition of, 1, 6–8, 30t
  epidemiology and risk factors for, 8–9, 29, 31–41, 305–9
  history of, 8
  idiopathic, 60

importance of in critical care medicine, 1
mediators of injury, 11
outcome of, 335–41
pathology and pathophysiology of, 9–11, 48–54, 57–8, 68–9
survivors of, 1, 11, 40–1, 336–41
Adenosine triphosphate (ATP), 310
Adrenaline
  anti–inflammatory effects of, 320
  lactate levels and, 129, 130
  venous return and, 113, 114–15
Adrenocortical insufficiency, 228
Adult respiratory distress syndrome, 8
Advanced Trauma Life Support (ATLS), 11, 197–9
Age, and mortality from ARDS, 39
Airflow, and inverse ratio ventilation, 147f
Airway, breathing, and circulation (ABC) approach, 14, 213
Airway, survivors of ARDS and hyperreactivity of, 338
Airway management
  chest tubes and, 190–1
  endotracheal intubation and, 183–4, 186–9
  hypoventilation and, 94t, 95–6
  inhaled bronchodilators and, 191
  mask CPAP and, 185

mechanical ventilation and, 184–5, 190
for prevention of nosocomial pneumonia, 268–9
total patient care and, 183–91
tracheostomy and, 189–90
Airway obstruction, 94t, 95, 191
Airway pressure
  hypercapnia and, 156
  inverse-ratio ventilation and, 147f
  lung compliance and, 99
  PEEP and increase in, 90
  respiratory mechanics and, 98, 159
  venous return, 151
Airway pressure-release ventilation (APRV), 148, 149f
Airway resistance
  measurement of at bedside, 100
  mechanical ventilation, 151
  survivors of ARDS and, 337
Albumin, 280
Alpha-1-antiprotease, 244
Alpha adrenergic agents, 121, 216
Alveolar-arterial oxygen partial pressure difference (AaDO$_2$), 88
Alveolar-capillary membrane, and gas transport, 81
Alveolar ducts, 50f, 51f
Alveolar fluid
  acute lung injury and removal of excess, 276–81
  pathophysiology of ARDS and, 10
Alveolar hypoventilation, 104

Alveolar macrophage, and inter-
    leukin-8, 68
Alveolar overdistension, and
    mechanical ventilation, 141
Alveolar oxygen pressure, 82
American College of Chest Physi-
    cians, 206
American College of Surgeons,
    197
American Thoracic Society
    (ATS), 8, 22, 23t, 29
Aminoglycosides, 216, 264, 265
Amiodarone, 58, 59f
Ampicillin, 209t
AMPLE history, 12
Amrinone, 123t, 322
Amyotrophic lateral sclerosis,
    94t, 95
Analgesics, and oxygen satura-
    tion, 152
Anatomy, and primary survey of
    ARDS patient, 12
Anemia
    as complication of ARDS, 219,
        220
    multiple system organ failure
        and, 310–11
    oxygen delivery and, 120–1
Anesthesia, topical, 188
Animal models
    for gut-liver-lung connection
        and sepsis, 72
    for inflammation and lung
        injury, 74–6
Antacids, 270
Anteromedial pneumothoraces, 20
Antibiotics
    nosocomial pneumonia and,
        212, 263–6, 267t, 268t
    prophylactic, 271–2
    sepsis and, 208, 209t
Antibody-coated bacteria, 259
Anti-cytokine agents, 239–41
Anti-endotoxin immunotherapy,
    238–9
Anti–inflammatory mediators,
    66–7
Antioxidants, 241–2, 293
Antiproteases, 244
Antipyretics, 152
Anti-TNF antibodies, 240
Anxiety, and weaning from
    mechanical ventilation, 167
Aortic stenosis, 119
APACHE II scores, 36, 39, 131
Apoptosis, 288, 290
ARDS. See Acute respiratory dis-
    tress syndrome
Arrhythmias, 190, 213

Arterial blood gases (ABG),
    86–7, 169, 339
Arterial circulation, and systemic
    vascular resistance, 113
Arterial hypoxemia, 82–7, 127–8.
    See also Hypoxemia
Aspiration, of gastric contents
    clinical evaluation of ARDS
        patient and, 14, 15
    head injury and, 200–1
    intubation and, 188–9
    nosocomial pneumonia and,
        253, 255–6, 258–9, 269
    pathology of ARDS and, 57
    as risk factor for ARDS, 36–7,
        39
Assist-control (AC) ventilation,
    144, 145, 146f
Asthma, 94t, 95, 96
Auscultation, of chest, 12
Auto PEEP. See also Intrinsic
    PEEP
    hypercapnia, 155
    mechanical ventilation, 145–7,
        148, 151
Aztreonam, 265, 267t

Bacteria
    pneumonia, 36, 60, 235
    sepsis and, 206, 208
Barbiturates, and intubation, 141
Barotrauma
    chest radiograph and, 19
    chest tubes and, 190–1
    intrinsic PEEP and, 101, 152
    mechanical ventilation and,
        145, 146–7, 148, 151, 156–8
    morbidity from ARDS, 40
    pneumoperitoneum and,
        214–16
    as respiratory complication of
        ARDS, 210–11
Basic fibrotic growth factor
    (bFGF), 291t, 294
Benzodiazepines
    hypoventilation and, 93
    intubation and, 141
    sedation and, 194
Beta adrenergic agents, 121, 276
Beta-lactam antibiotics, 264, 265
Beta$_2$-selective agents, 191
Bicarbonates, 126, 129, 156
Bilateral chest tubes, 157
Bilateral phrenic nerve injury,
    94t, 95
Biphasic positive airway pressure
    (BIPAP), 148, 149f
Blind intubation, 187
Blood plasma, and fibronectin, 284

Blood pressure, 121–2. See also
    Hypertension; Hypotension
Blood transfusions
    benefits of to ARDS patients,
        220
    cardiovascular management
        and, 128–9
    multiple as risk factor for
        ARDS, 36, 37t, 38, 39
    oxygenation of venous blood
        and, 152
Blunt chest trauma, 16
Botulism, 94t, 95
Bowel ileus, 213
Brain, and multiple system organ
    failure, 211t
Brain injury, 200
Breathing, weaning trials and
    increased work of, 167–8
Bronchial hyperreactivity, 338
Bronchiolitis, 58
Bronchiolitis obliterans and orga-
    nizing pneumonia (BOOP),
    60
Bronchoalveolar lavage (BAL)
    interleukin-8 and, 68–9
    nosocomial pneumonia and,
        259, 260–1
Bronchodilators, 173, 191
Bronchopulmonary dysplasia
    (BPD), 52, 54, 56f, 57f
Bronchoscopy, 259–61, 341
Burns, assessment of and patient
    care, 204–5

Capnograph, 97
Carbapenem, 265
Carbohydrates, and enteral nutri-
    tion, 192
Carbon dioxide
    alveolar-capillary membrane
        and elimination of, 81
    alveolar ventilation and, 92
    dead space and, 154
    gastric mucosal, 130–2
    hypoventilation and, 94t
    measures of production, 97
    pulmonary wedge pressure and
        elimination of, 126
    respiratory muscle pump load
        and, 167
    sodium bicarbonate and, 156
Cardiac function curves, 108,
    115–16
Cardiac index, 121, 122
Cardiac ischemia, 156
Cardiac output
    carbon dioxide and, 93
    hypotension, 158

maintenance of adequate in ARDS patients, 120–5
in survivors of ARDS, 11
venous return and, 113–17
Cardiac tamponade, 201, 202
Cardiogenic failure, 17–18
Cardiogenic pulmonary edema, 13–14, 17–18
Cardiogenic shock, 127
Cardiopulmonary arrest, 184
Cardiopulmonary bypass, 37t, 164
Cardiovascular failure, and organ system failure scoring system (OSF), 306t
Cardiovascular management, for ARDS patients
principles of, 120–9
tools and tests for, 129–32
Cardiovascular system. *See also* Congestive heart failure; Coronary artery disease
clinical evaluation of ARDS patient, 12, 15
complications of ARDS and, 212–13
pathophysiology of ARDS and, 10–11, 108–20
prevention and treatment of multiple system organ failure, 211t
Case-control studies, of ARDS, 31, 32t
Case-fatality rates, from ARDS, 39–40
Case series studies, of ARDS, 31, 32t
Catecholamines
multiple system organ failure and, 319–22
venous return and, 116
Catheters and catheterization
chest radiograph and venous, 18
pulmonary artery and, 18, 130, 223
suctioning cathers, 269
Causality, and association between risk factors and ARDS, 33
C-C chemokine family, 69–70
Cecal ligation/puncture model (CLP), 75–6
Cefoperazone, 265
Cefotaxime, 265, 267t, 272
Ceftazidime, 209t, 265, 267t
Ceftriaxone, 209t, 265, 267t
Cefuroxime, 265
Cell-to-cell communication, and inflammation, 72–3

Cell death, and acute lung injury, 288, 290
Centers for Disease Control, 256–7
Central cyanosis, 185
Central hypoventilation, 93
Central nervous system. *See also* Neurologic system
complications of ARDS and, 218
dysfunction of and mortality for ARDS, 16
hypoventilation and, 93, 94t
Cephalosporins, 265
Cerebral infarction, 218–19
Cerebral perfusion pressure, 200
Cervical spine injury, 94t, 95, 201. *See also* Spine injury
Chemical and drug ingestion, 58
Chemokines, 67–71
Chemotherapeutic toxicity, and pneumocytes, 52
Chest radiology
complications of ARDS and, 19–21
Computerized tomography scanning of thorax, 22
diagnosis of ARDS, 16–17
differential diagnosis of ARDS, 17–18
endotracheal intubation and, 18, 187
lung contusion and, 203
lung injury score and, 7t
pneumonia and, 261
Chest trauma
assessment and patient care, 201–3
blunt force and, 16
chest tubes, 191
Chest tubes, 157–8, 190–1
Chest wall, and hypoventilation, 94t, 95
Chloramphenicol, 209t
Chronic obstructive pulmonary disorder (COPD), 102, 119, 140, 168
Cilastin, 265
Ciprofloxacin, 209t
Circumferential chest burns, 205
Clinical evaluation, of patients with ARDS
airway management and, 183–91
complications of ARDS and, 210–28
gastrointestinal assessment and care, 191–2, 193f
medical history and, 13–14

neurologic assessment and care, 194–5, 196f
oxygenation and, 86–7
physical examination and, 14–16
primary survey and resuscitation, 11–13
secondary survey and, 13
sepsis syndrome and, 205–10
trauma assessment and care, 197–205
Cloxacillin, 209t
Coagulation, of blood
complications of ARDS and, 219–20
multiple system organ failure and, 211t
Cohort study, 31
Collagens, 285, 288
Colloid solutions, and fluid resuscitation, 126–7
Coma, and central nervous system, 218–19. *See also* Consciousness
Complications, of ARDS
chest radiograph and, 19–21
laboratory assessment for, 22–23
therapy for, 210–28
Complications, of endotracheal intubation, 188, 189t
Complications, of mechanical ventilation, 156–8
Complications, of tracheostomy, 189–90
Computerized tomography (CT) scanning
abdominal trauma and, 203–4
of thorax, 22
Confounding conditions or therapies, 33, 38
Congestive heart failure, 15, 94t, 95
Connective tissue activating protein-111, 67–8
Consciousness, levels of, 14, 184. *See also* Coma
Continuous lateral rotational therapy, 268
Continuous oximetry, 86
Continuous positive airway pressure (CPAP), 174, 185
Continuous renal replacement therapy, 217–18
Continuous venovenous therapy, 218
Cooling, of patient. *See also* Temperature, body
carbon dioxide production and, 154

Cooling (*Continued*)
 oxygenation of venous blood
   and, 152
Coronary artery disease, 156
Corticosteroids
 adrenocortical insufficiency
   and, 228
 immunosuppression and, 256
 as innovative therapy in early
   stages of ARDS, 235–8
 myopathy and neuromuscular
   blocking agents, 195, 219
 sepsis and, 208
Cough reflex, and intubation, 184
Crash induction, intubation by,
   186
Critical care medicine, and
   ARDS, 1
Critical illness polyneuropathy, 219
CROP index, 171–3
Crystalloid solutions, and fluid
   resuscitation, 126–7
C-X-C chemokines, 67–9
Cyclooxygenase inhibitors, 239
Cyclosporin A, 75
Cysteine, 242
Cytokines
 animal models of inflammation
   and lung injury, 74–6
 anticytokine agents, 239–41
 catecholamines and production of, 320
 cell-to-cell communication
   during inflammation, 72–3
 chemokines and, 67–71
 gut-liver-lung connection and
   sepsis, 71–2
 initiation and maintenance of
   systemic inflammation, 65–6
 as mediators of injury in
   ARDS, 11, 66–7
 multiple system organ failure,
   323–4
 PEEP and, 125
 sepsis syndrome and, 206–8

Dead space, of upper airways
 carbon dixoide production and,
   97
 hypercapnia and, 154–5
 survivors of ARDS and, 339
 total tidal volume and, 92
 weaning from mechanical ventilation and, 167
Death. *See also* Mortality
 causes of in ARDS patients, 9,
   309t
 multiple system organ failure as
   predictor of, 304

multiple trauma and, 197
Decision-making algorithms, 221
Decubitus chest radiograph, 20–21
Deep venous thrombosis (DVT),
   221, 222, 223
Dermatology, and complications
   of ARDS, 218
Diagnosis, of ARDS. *See also*
   Differential diagnosis
 chest radiology and, 16–17
 laboratory assessment and,
   22–23
 of nosocomial pneumonia,
   256–63
Dialysis, indications for, 217
Diaphragmatic fatigue, and weaning from mechanical ventilation, 167
Diarrhea, and enteral nutrition,
   192
Diastolic filling, and right heart
   failure, 112–13
Diastolic ventricular dysfunction,
   212
Diazepam, 188, 194
Differential diagnosis, of ARDS
 chest radiographs and steps in,
   17–18
 gas exchange and, 158
 medical history of patient and,
   13–14
 pathology and, 58, 60
Differential misclassification, 29
Diffuse alveolar damage (DAD),
   9, 48
Diffusing capacity, 339
Direct pulmonary insults, 16
Discharge, medical management
   of ARDS survivors after,
   339–41
Disseminated intravascular coagulation (DIC), 37, 39
Diuretics, 93
Dobutamine, 122, 123t, 313
Dopamine
 hemodynamic function and,
   116, 122, 123t
 hypotension after intubation
   and, 189
Dopexamine, 122, 322
Dose-response relationship, and
   inhalation of nitric oxide, 154
Drowning. *See* Near-drowning
Drug-induced disorders, and res-
   piratory muscle dysfunction,
   166
Drug-related adverse events, 243.
   See also Side effects
Drugs. *See also* Antibiotics; Innov-

ative therapy; Neuromuscular
   blocking agents; Vasopressors
   and inotropes; specific medications
 arrhythmias and, 213
 CNS depressants and hypoventilation, 93
 interstitial nephritis and, 216
 intubation and, 141, 187–8
 oxygen saturation levels and,
   152
 rashes and, 218
 wheezing and, 191
Dynamic hyperinflation, 101,
   164–5, 166f

E5 (murine antibody), 238–9
Echocardiography, 222
Edema, and pulmonary wedge
   pressure, 125–6. *See also*
   Pulmonary edema
Eicosanoids, 239, 242–3
Elastase, 256
Electrolyte abnormalities, and
   hypoventilation, 94t, 95
ELR motif, 68, 69t
Emergency management, of multiple trauma, 197–8
Emergent intubation, 184
Emphysema, 94t, 95
Empiric antimicrobial therapy,
   265–6
End-diastolic pressure
 cardiac output and, 109f, 111f,
   115f
 venous return and, 114f
Endocrine system
 complications of ARDS and,
   228
 respiratory muscle pump failure
   and disturbances of, 165–6
Endothelium, and sepsis, 206
Endotoxin and endotoxemia
 animal model of gut-liver-lung
   connection, 72, 73
 animal models of inflammation
   and lung injury, 75
 anti-endotoxin immunotherapy, 238–9
 lactate release and, 129
 RANTES and, 69–70
 splanchnic oxygen consumption
   and, 313–14
 ventricular contractility and,
   110, 112
Endotracheal intubation
 airway management and, 100,
   151, 186–9
 blind, 187

chest radiology and, 18
clinical evaluation and indications for, 12–13, 14, 183, 184t
head injury and, 201
hypoventilation and obstruction of, 94t, 95, 96
mechanical ventilation and, 140–1
nosocomial pneumonia and, 255–6, 258–9
Endotracheal suctioning, 190
Energy, and nutritional requirements, 191–2
Enteral nutrition, 192, 193f, 213, 269. *See also* Feeding and feeding tubes; Nutrition
Enterobacteriaceae, 252, 268t
Eosinophilic hyaline membranes, 51f
Ephedrine, and hypotension, 188, 189
Epidemiology, of ARDS. *See also* Mortality
case-fatality rates, 39–40
definition of, 8–9, 29
incidence and, 33–6
multiple system organ failure and, 305–9
risk factors and, 8–9, 29, 31, 33, 36–9
studies documenting, 29, 31–3
Epidermal growth factor (EGF), 290–2
Epinephrine
cardiac output and, 123t
hypotension after intubation and, 188, 189
Erythromycin, 267t
Escherichia coli, 238–9
Esophageal intubation, 18
Esophageal pressure, 98
Esophageal rupture, 203
European Society of Intensive Care Medicine (ESICA), 8, 22, 23t, 29
Euthyroid sick syndrome, 228
Exercise, and survivors of ARDS, 338
Exogenous IL-1ra, 240
Expiratory positive airway pressure (EPAP), 140, 149
Expiratory time, and mechanical ventilation, 145
Extracorporeal carbon dioxide removal (ECCOR) and extracorporeal membrane oxygenation (ECMO), 9, 153–4

Extremities, examination of, 15
Exudative phase, of ARDS, 9, 48–51

FACIT collagens (Fibril-Associated Collagens with Interrupted Triple helices), 285
Fat embolism syndrome, 37t, 39, 197, 204, 235
Feeding and feeding tubes. *See also* Enteral nutrition; Nutrition
hypercapnia and, 154
placement of, 18
Fentanyl, 188, 194
Fibrin and fibrinogen, 282–3
Fibronectin, 283–5
Fibrosing alveolitis, 282–90
Fibrotic phase, of ARDS, 9, 48, 52, 54, 126
Fick's law, 81
FiO₂. *See* Oxygenation
Flail chest, 201, 202
Flow triggering (flow-by), 174
Fluid management, and cardiovascular management of ARDS, 125–7
Fluid resuscitation, 121
Fluoroquinolones, 265
Forced expiratory volume in 1 second (FEV₁), 337
Forced vital capacity (FVC), 337
Fractures, of bone
clinical evaluation and care of ARDS patient, 15, 204
of long bone, 15, 197, 204
pelvic, 15, 204
as risk factor for ARDS, 37t
Free radicals, 241
Fumes, inhalation of, 57–8
Functional residual capacity (FRC), 90, 187
Furosemide, 200

Gag reflex, and intubation, 184
Gamma interferon-inducible protein (IP-10), 68, 69t
Gases, inhalation of, 57–8
Gas exchange
mechanical ventilation and, 150–1, 158, 163–4, 169–70
survivors of ARDS and, 339
Gastric statsis, 213
Gastric tonometry, 130–2, 319
Gastrointestinal system. *See also* Aspiration, of gastric contents
complications of ARDS and, 213–16

infection and pH of, 270–1
liver-lung connection and sepsis, 71–2
microflora of, 254–5
multiple system organ failure and, 211t
Gelatinase B, 288
Gene therapy, and antiproteases, 244
Gentamicin, 267t
Germany, and incidence of ARDS, 35
Glasgow Coma Score (GCS), 14
Glu-Leu-Arg, 68
Glutathione, 241–2
Glycocalyx, 256
Gram-negative bacteremia, 238–9
Gram stain, 22
Granulocyte colony-stimulating factor (G-CSF) and granulocyte-macrophage colony-stimulating factor (GM-CSF), 224
Growth factors, and acute lung injury, 290–4
Guillain-Barré syndrome, 95
Gut ischemia, 131, 132, 214
Gut perfusion, and gastric tonometry, 131

HA-1A (human antibody), 238–9
Head injury, 197, 199–201, 226
Health care system, and costs of ARDS, 1
Heart rate, diastolic filling and right heart failure, 112–13
Hematology
complications of ARDS and, 219–24
organ system failure scoring system (OSF) and, 306t
Hematoma, and tracheostomy, 189–90
Hemodynamics, and right heart failure, 112–13
Hemoglobin, and cardiovascular management, 128–9, 220
Hemorrhagic shock
multiple system organ failure and, 317
oxygen delivery and, 121
resuscitation from, 198, 199t
Hemothorax, and chest tubes, 191, 201, 202
Henderson-Haselbalch equation, 131
Heparin, 221, 223–4, 225f
Hepatocyte growth factor (HGF), 291t, 292–3

Herbicides, 58
High-frequency ventilation (HFV), 147–8
Host factors, and nosocomial pneumonia, 255–6
Human immunodeficiency virus (HIV), and *pneumocystis carinii*, 36
Hyaline membranes, *53f*
Hydrochloric acid, and aspiration of gastric contents, 57
Hydrogen receptor blockers, 132, 213, 270
Hypercapnia
  hypoventilation and, 91–6
  mechanical ventilation and, 154–6
  permissive, 155–6, *157t*
Hyperglycemia, 225–6
Hyperlactatemia, 129, 316–17
Hyperleukocytosis syndrome, 224
Hypertension. *See also* Blood pressure
  as complication of ARDS, 212
  endotracheal suctioning and, 190
  intracranial, 199, 200
  lung injury of ARDS and pulmonary, 11
Hyperthyroidism, 228
Hypoglycemia, 226
Hypokalemia, 226
Hypomagnesemia, *94t*, 95, 227–8
Hyponatremia, 226
Hypophosphatemia, *94t*, 95
Hypotension. *See also* Blood pressure
  causes of in ARDS, *158t*
  clinical evaluation of ARDS patients, 14, 212
  mechanical ventilation and, 150–1, 158
  sepsis-related syndrome and, *207t*
Hypothyroidism, 228
Hypoventilation
  causes of and contributors to, *94t*
  decreased alveolar oxygen pressure, 82
  hypercapnia and, 91–6, 156
  respiratory drive and, 104
Hypovolemia
  fluid resuscitation and, 127
  hypercapnia and, 155
  intubation and correction of, 140
  oxygenation of venous blood, 152

Hypoxemia. *See also* Arterial hypoxemia
  as cause of death, 308
  continuous oximetry and, 86
  intrapulmonary shunting and, 10
  mechanical ventilation and, 152–4, 163–4
Hypoxia
  intubation and, 188
  multiple system organ failure and, 310–11, 312, 314, 315–17, *318f*
  oxygen delivery and, 120

Idiopathic ARDS, 60
Idiopathic interstitial fibrosis, 60
Idiopathic pulmonary fibrosis (IPF), 285
IgM antibodies, 238–9
Imipenem, *209t*, 265
Immune system. *See also* Inflammatory response
  enteral nutrition and, 192, 269
  host factors in nosocomial pneumonia, 255–6
Impaired tissue oxygen extraction, 313
Inception cohort, 30–1
Incidence, of ARDS, 33–6
Incidence density, 33
Increased intracranial pressure (ICP), 199, 200
Infant respiratory distress syndrome (IRDS), 233, 234
Infections. *See also* Inflammatory response; Pneumonia
  computerized tomography scans of chest and, 22
  pathology of ARDS and, 54
  surveillance and control of, 269–70, *271t*
  of wounds, 210
Inflammatory response. *See also* Immune system
  animal models of lung injury and, 74–6
  cell-to-cell communication during, 72–3
  chemokines and, 67–71
  clinical evaluation of ARDS patient and, 14
  cytokines and, 65–6
  gut-liver-lung connection and sepsis, 71–2
  multiple system organ failure and catecholamines, 319–22
  pro- and anti–inflammatory mediators, 66–7

Inhalation. *See also* Smoke inhalation
  of nitric oxide, 234
  of noxious fumes and gases, 57–8
Innovative therapy, for ARDS. *See also* Drugs
  anticytokine agents, 239–41
  anti-endotoxin immunotherapy, 238–9
  antioxidants, 241–2
  antiproteases, 244
  corticosteroids and early stages of, 235–8
  cyclooxygenase inhibitors, 239
  eicosanoids, 242–3
  nitric oxide, 234–5
  pentoxifylline, 243–4
  platelet-activating factor antagonists, 242
  surfactant replacement, 233–4
Inotropes, and cardiac output, 121–2, *123t*
Inspiratory positive airway pressure (IPAP), and mechanical ventilation, 140, 149
Inspiratory time, and mechanical ventilation, 145
Insulin, infusion protocol for, *227f*
Insulin-like growth factor (IGF), 290
Integrative indices, and weaning from mechanical ventilation, 171–3
Interleukin-1 (IL-1)
  acute lung injury and, *291t*, 294
  anticytokine agents and, 240
  initiation and maintenance of inflammatory response, 65–6, 70–1, 74
  sepsis syndrome and, 206, 208
Interleukin-1 receptor antagonist, 66
Interleukin-6, 112, 320
Interleukin-8 (IL-8), 68–9, *71t*, 73
Interleukin-10 (IL-10)
  acute lung injury and, 66
  endotoxin-induced inflammation and, 75–6
  multiple system organ failure and, 320, *321f*
Intermittent hemodialysis, 217
Intermittent mandatory ventilation (IMV), 144, 174–5, 177–9
Intracranial hypertension, management of, 199, 200
Intracranial pressure, and hypercapnia, 156

Intrinsic PEEP, 101–2, *103f. See also* Auto PEEP
Inverse-ratio ventilation (IRV), 144–7, 151
Investigational modes, of mechanical ventilation, 147–8
Ipratropium, 191

Keratinocyte growth factor (KGF), *291t*, 293
Ketamine, 188
Ketoconazole, 243
Kidneys. *See also* Renal failure
complications of ARDS and, 216–18
lactate clearance, 129
prevention and treatment of multiple system organ failure, *211t*
Kreb's cycle, 129
Kupffer cells, 72, 73, 74
Kyphoscoliosis, *94t*, 95

Laboratory assessment, and diagnosis of ARDS, 22–23
Lactate
cardiovascular management and, 129–30
multiple system organ failure and, 315–17, *318f*
Lactic acidosis, 130
Laparotomy, 204
Larynscopy, 186–7, 188
Latency-associated peptide (LAP), 292
Left ventricular pressure-volume relationships, *110f*
Legionella spp., *268t*
Legionnaire's disease, 60
Leukemia, 224
Leukocytes
chemokines and, 67
IL-1 and TNF-dependent cytokine networks, 65–6
as mediators of acute lung injury, 11
multiple system organ failure and, 322
ventricular contractility and, 112
Leukotriene B4, 281
Lidocaine, 188
Limited absorption, of enteral nutrition, 192
Lipids, and enteral nutrition, 192
Lipopolysaccharide (LPS), 72, 74, 206
Liposomal PGE, 243

Liver
disease of and mortality from ARDS, 39
gut-lung connection and sepsis, 71–2
multiple system organ failure and, *211t*
Long bone fractures, 15, 197, 204
Lorazepam, 194
Lower inflection point (LIP), 142–4
Lung, and ARDS. *See also* Acute lung injury
fibrotic phase of, 52, 54
gut-liver connection and sepsis, 71–2
hypoventilation and, *94t*, 96
measures of function and blood oxygenation, 88–9
oxygen transport and, 80–1
proliferative phase of, 51–2
pulmonary pathophysiology and, 80–105
pulmonary wedge pressure and edema, 125–6
surgical or postmortem findings, 48–51
Lung compliance
decrease in and early ARDS, 10
measurement of at bedside, 98–100
Lung injury
animal models for inflammation and, 74–6
contusion of, *37t*, 202–3
inverse ratio ventilation and, 147
scoring systems for, 7–8
tidal volume and, 142
Lung protection strategy, 143–4
Lung volume
inverse ratio ventilation and, *147f*
survivors of ARDS and, 338

Macrophages. *See* Resident macrophages
Magnesium deficiency, 227–8
Mallory's hyaline, 52
Malnutrition. *See also* Nutrition
hypoventilation and, *94t*, 95
nosocomial pneumonia and, 269
respiratory muscle dysfunction and, 165–6
Mannitol, 200
Mask CPAP, 185
Massive hemothorax, 201, 202
Matrix degradation, and pulmonary fibrosis, 288

Maximum compartmental amplitude to VT ratio (MCA/VT), 171
Maximum inspiratory pressure (MIP), 104, 170
Mechanical ventilation
barotrauma and, 145, 146–7, 148, 151, 156–8
choice of mode, 144–8
complications of, 156–8
goals of, 141
hypercapnia and, 154–6
hypoventilation and, 82
hypoxemia and, 152–4
initial ventilator settings, *145t*, 149
initiation of, 139–41
nosocomial pneumonia and, 255, 268–9
oxygen demand and changes in, 119
PEEP levels and, 142–4
principles of, *141t*
primary survey and indications for, 12–13, *140t*
renal failure and, 216
stabilizing of patient, 150–1
tidal volume and, 139, 141–2
transpulmonary pressure and, 98
weaning of patient from, 163–79
Mediastinitis, 203
Medical history, of ARDS patient, 13–14, 340
Meropenem, 265
Mesenchymal cellular changes, and acute lung injury, 288–90
Metabolic acidosis, 93
Metabolic alkalosis, 93, 129
Metabolism
acidosis and alkalosis, 93, 129
complications of ARDS and, 225–8
respiratory muscle pump failure, 154
Methacholine, 338
Methemoglobin, and inhaled nitric oxide, 154
Methicillin-resistant *Staphylococcus aureus* (MRSA), 265–6, *268t*
Methylprednisolone, *236f*, *237f*
Metronidazole, *209t*
Metalloproteinases, 288
Microbial colonization, and nosocomial pneumonia, 253–5
Microbiology, of nosocomial pneumonia, 252

Midazolam, 188, 194
Minute ventilation, 96–7, 170
Misclassification, and definition
    of ARDS, 29
Mixed venous oxygen desatura-
    tion, 84, 85f, 127–8
"Modified sniffing" position, 186
Monobactam, 265
Monokine induced by gamma
    interferon (MIG), 68, 69t
Morbidity, from ARDS, 40–1,
    129. See also Survival and
    survivors
Morphine, 194
Mortality, from ARDS. See also
    Death
    alveolar fluid clearance and,
        278–9
    barotrauma and, 157
    central nervous system dys-
        function and, 16
    complications of ARDS and, 63
    gastric mucosal acidosis and,
        319
    hyperlactatemia and, 129
    multiple system organ failure
        and, 305, 308, 316–17
    new therapeutic approaches
        and, 233
    pneumonia and, 212, 251
    pulmonary angiography and,
        222–3
    rates of, 1, 28, 39–40, 335
    sepsis syndrome and, 205
    supranormal oxygen delivery
        and, 122
Mucociliary clearance and
        mucosal defenses, and infec-
        tion, 256, 257t
Multiple inert gas elimination
        technique (MIGET), 153
Multiple sclerosis, 94t, 95
Multiple system organ failure
        (MSOF), and ARDS
    alternative mechanisms of,
        322–4
    catecholamines and inflamma-
        tion, 319–22
    definitions of, 304–5
    epidemiology of, 305–9
    mortality from, 40, 305, 308,
        316–17
    pathophysiology of, 310–19
    prevention of, 211t
    scoring systems for, 23, 305t,
        306t, 307t
    sepsis and, 11, 207t
Multiple trauma, and ARDS,
        197–9, 201

Muscle relaxants, 195
Muscular dystrophy, 94t, 95
Myasthenia gravis, 94t, 95
Myeloperoxidase (MPO) assay, 75
Myopathy
    as complication of ARDS, 219
    hypoventilation and, 94t, 95
    steroid-induced, 195

N-acetylcysteine (NAC), 242
Narcotics
    hypoventilation and, 93
    intubation and, 141
    for pain control, 194
Nasogastric (NG) tubes, 18, 186
National Institute of Health, Heart
        and Lung Task Force on Res-
        piratory Diseases, 33, 36
Near-drowning, and ARDS, 37t, 57
Nephrotoxins, 216
Neurogenic pulmonary edema,
        15, 199–200
Neurologic failure, and organ sys-
        tem failure scoring system
        (OSF), 306t
Neurologic system. See also Cen-
        tral nervous system; Periph-
        eral nervous system
    clinical evaluation and patient
        care, 15–16, 194–5, 196f
    complications of ARDS and,
        218–19
Neuromuscular blocking agents
    intubation and, 188
    myopathy and prolonged weak-
        ness secondary to use of, 219
    neurologic assessment and
        patient care, 194–5, 196t
Neuromuscular transmission
    hypoventilation and, 94t, 95
    neuromuscular blocking agents,
        188, 194–5, 196t, 219
    weaning from mechanical ven-
        tilation, 164–7
Neutrophil activating protein-2,
        67–8
Neutrophils
    acute lung injury and activa-
        tion or adherence of, 11
    multiple system organ failure,
        323
    neutrophil activating protein-
        2, 67–8
    pathology of ARDS, 68–9
    sepsis syndrome and, 207
NG tube. See Nasogastric tube
Nitric oxide
    gas exchange and mechanical
        ventilation, 153–4

innovative therapy and, 234–5
    myocardial contractility and,
        112
Nitroprusside, 313
Nocodazole, 280
Nomogram-based dosing, of
        heparin, 224, 225f
Noninflammatory cells, and
        chemokines, 70–1
Noninvasive leg studies, 222
Noninvasive positive pressure
        ventilation (NIPPV), 140
Norepinephrine, 122, 123t, 320
Nosocomial pneumonia, and
        ARDS. See also Pneumonia
    antimicrobial therapy for, 263–6
    as complication of ARDS, 190,
        210, 211–12
    diagnosis of, 256–63
    incidence of, 251
    microbiology of, 252
    pathogenesis of, 252–6
    prevention of, 266–72
    sepsis and, 305
Nutrition. See also Enteral nutri-
        tion; Feeding and feeding
        tubes; Malnutrition
    hypercapnia and, 154
    nosocomial pneumonia and, 269
    patient care and, 191–2

Obesity, and hypoventilation, 94t,
        95
Obstetrics, and hyponatremia, 226
Ostructive sleep apnea, 119
Odds ratio, for individual risk fac-
        tors, 38
Ohm's law, 99, 100
Open lung biopsy, 224
Open pneumothorax, 201
Organ failure scoring, 306t, 308–9
Oropharynx
    microflora of, 254
    suctioning of, 190
Orotracheal intubation, 186–7,
        188
Outcome, of ARDS. See also Sur-
        vival and survivors
    medical management after dis-
        charge, 339–41
    mortality and, 335
    pulmonary function test abnor-
        malities and, 337–9
    roentgenographic changes and,
        337
    symptoms and limitations in
        survivors, 336–7
Oxothiazolidine carboxylate
        (OTC), 242

Oxygenation
 hypoventilation, 82
 intubation and, 140, *184t*
 mechnical ventilation, 150
 pulmonary pathophysiology
  and increase of, 87–8
Oxygen consumption
 carbon dioxide production
  and, 97
 hypoxemia and, 152
 oxygen delivery and, 117–20,
  314
 tissue hypoxia and increased
  demand, 313–14
 weaning from mechanical ventilation and, 167–8, *169t*
Oxygen delivery
 cardiac output and, 120–1
 extraction ratio and mixed
  venous oxygen desaturation,
  85f
 hypoxemia and, 152
 multiple system organ failure
  and, 314–15
 oxygen consumption and,
  117–20, 314
 supranormal, 122, 124
 in survivors of ARDS, 11
 tissue hypoxia and, 310–11
Oxygen pressure
 definition of ARDS, 8, 22, *23t*
 lung injury score and, *7t*
 measures of lung function and,
  88–9
Oxygen saturation
 arterial hypoxemia and, 127–8
 measurement of, 87
 target level of in ARDS
  patients, 89–90
Oxygen toxicity, and morbidity
  from ARDS, 40
Oxygen transport
 clinical assessment of, 86–7
 gas transport across alveolar-
  capillary membrane, 81
 measures of lung function and,
  88–9
 review of mechanism of, 80–1

Pain control, 194–5, *196f*
Pancreatis, *37t*, 214
PaO$_2$/FiO$_2$. *See* Oxygenation;
  Oxygen pressure
Paradoxical respiratory move-
  ment, 185
Paralysis, drug-induced, 195. *See
  also* Therapeutic paralysis
Paraquat, 58, *59f*
Pathology, of ARDS, 9

chemical and drug ingestion, 58
classic features of, 48–54
differential diagnosis and, 58, 60
gas and fume inhalation, 57–8
infections and, 54
liquid aspiration and, 57
neutrophils and, 68–9
Patient, total care for ARDS. *See
  also* Clinical evaluation;
  Innovative therapy; Outcome; Positioning, of patient;
  Survival and survivors
 airway management for, 183–91
 complications of ARDS and,
  210–28
 gastrointestinal assessment and
  care of, 191–2, *193f*
 neurologic assessment and care
  of, 194–5, *196f*
 sepsis syndrome and, 205–10
 trauma assessment and care of,
  197–205
Patient history, 13–14, 340
PEEP. *See* Positive end-expiratory
  pressure
Pelvic fractures, 15, 204
Penicillin, 265
Pentothal, 189
Pentoxifylline, 243–4, 321, 322
Perfusion distribution, and multiple system organ failure,
  311–13
Peripheral nervous system, and
  complications of ARDS, 219.
  See also Neurologic system
Peritoneal lavage, 203, 204
Permissive hypercapnia, 155–6,
  157t
Petechial rashes, 218
pH
 of aspirated liquids, 57
 of gastrointestinal system and
  infection, 270–1
 gastric tonometry and, 131–2,
  319
 hypoventilation and, 93
 microflora of stomach and, 254
Phagocytic cell function, and
  infection, 256, *257t*
Phenylephrine, 122, *123t*
Phosphodiesterase inhibitors,
  122, 320–2
Phrenic nerve injury, 164
Physical examination, 14–16, 341
Piperacillin, *209t*, 265, *267t*
Plasminogen-activator inhibitor
  type 1 (PAI-1), 282–3
Platelet-activating factor antagonists, 242

Platelet-derived growth factor
  (PDGF), 285, 290, *291t*
Platelet factor-4, 68, *69t*
Pleural effusions, and computerized tomography scans, 22
Pleural pressure, and lung compliance, 100
Pneumocystis carinii pneumonia,
  36, 235
Pneumomediastinum, 21
Pneumonia, and ARDS. *See also*
  Nosocomial pneumonia
 aspiration of gastric contents
  and, 201
 bacterial, 36, 60, 235
 chest radiographs and diagnosis of, 17
 incidence of, 251
 pathology of ARDS and, 60
 as risk factor for ARDS, 37, 39
 sepsis and, 206, 208
 in survivors of ARDS, 340
 V/Q mismatch and lobar, 83
Pneumopericardium, 21
Pneumoperitoneum, 214–16
Pneumothorax
 chest radiograph and, 18,
  19–21, 22
 chest tubes and, 190–1
 esophageal rupture and, 203
 mechanical ventilation and,
  156–8
 as respiratory complication of
  ARDS, 210–11
Polymicrobial infections, 252
Polymorphonuclear leukocytes
  (PMNs), 323
Polymyositis, *94t*, 95
Polymyxin B, 271
Polyneuropathy, 219
Positioning, of patient
 endotracheal intubation and,
  186
 hypoxemia and mechanical
  ventilation, 152–3
 prevention of nosocomial
  pneumonia and, 267–8
 weaning from mechanical ventilation and, 173–4
Positive end-expiratory pressure
  (PEEP)
 auto PEEP, 145–7, 148, 151,
  155
 cardiac output and, 124–5
 chest tubes and, 157
 hypercapnia and, 155
 hypoxemia and, 152
 intrinsic, 101–2, *103f*
 lung compliance and, 99

Positive end-expiratory pressure
    (*Continued*)
    mechanical ventilation and,
        141, 142–4, 150
    multiple system organ failure
        and, 312
    pathophysiology of ARDS and,
        11
    pulmonary pathophysiology
        and, 90
    studies assessing ARDS ther-
        apy and development of, 64
Preoxygenation, and intubation,
    140, 187
Pressure-control ventilation
    (PCV), 144–5, *146f*
Pressure-cycled modes, of
    mechanical ventilation, 144
Pressure support ventilation
    (PSV), 144, 175–9
Pressure-volume relationships
    measurement of, 98, 101
    mechanical ventilation and,
        142, *143f*
Prevalence, of ARDS, 33
Prevention
    of ARDS, 28
    of hyponatremia, 226
    of multiple system organ failure
        in ARDS, *211t*
    of nosocomial pneumonia,
        266–72
Primary survey, of patient with
    ARDS, 11–13
Prognostic factors, and definition
    of ARDS, 31
Pro-inflammatory mediators,
    66–7, 72
Proliferative phase, of ARDS, 9,
    48, 51–2, 126
Promotional-assist ventilation
    (PAV), 148
Prone position, and hypoxemia,
    152–3
Prophylactic antimicrobials, 271–2
Propofol, 141, 188
Prospective cohort study, *32t*
Prostacyclin (PG-I), 239, 243, 314
Prostaglandin E (PGE), 239,
    242–3, 314
Protected BAL (PBAL), 259, 261
Protected specimen brushing
    (PSB), 259, 260
Protein
    alveolar fluid clearance and,
        278t, 280–1
    nutritional requirements for,
        191, 192
Proteolytic enzymes, 244

Pseudomonas aeruginosa, 208, 252,
    264, 265, *268t*, 281
Psychological problems, and
    weaning from mechanical
    ventilation, 168
Pulmonary angiography, 222–3
Pulmonary artery catheter, 18, 30
Pulmonary contusion, *37t*
Pulmonary edema
    alveolar edema, *278t*
    crystalloid solution and, 127
    neurogenic, 15, 199–200
    pathophysiology of ARDS, 10
    pulmonary wedge pressure,
        125–6
Pulmonary embolus, 17
Pulmonary epithelial cells, and
    lung-derived RANTES, 70
Pulmonary fibrosis, 282, 285
Pulmonary function, in survivors
    of ARDS, 40–1, 337–9, 341
Pulmonary infarction, 17
Pulmonary pathophysiology, in
    ARDS. *See also* Pulmonary
    edema
    airway resistance and, 100
    arterial hypoxemia and, 82–7
    clinical assessment of oxygena-
        tion, 86–7
    direct insults and, 16
    gas transport across alveolar-
        capillary membrane, 81
    hypercapnia and hypoventila-
        tion, 91–6
    lung compliance and, 98–100
    oxygenation and oxygen satu-
        ration, 87–90
    oxygen consumption and car-
        bon dioxide production, 97
    PEEP and, 90, 101–2
    pressure-volume relationships
        and, 101
    respiratory drive and, 104–5
    respiratory mechanics and,
        97–8
    respiratory muscle strength
        and, 103–4
    ventilation measures and, 96–7
Pulmonary thromboembolism
    (PTE), 221–2, 223–4
Pulmonary veins, and arterial
    hypoxemia, 83
Pulmonary wedge pressure, and
    edema formation, 125–6
Pulse oximetry saturation, 150
Pulse and reflectance oximetry, 86
Pulsus paradoxus, and hypoventi-
    lation, 96
Purpura, 218

Pyruvate dehydrogenase (PDH),
    129

Quality of life, for survivors of
    ARDS, 1, 41

Radiographic dye, and renal fail-
    ure, 216
Ramsay Scale of Sedation, *195t*
Randomized control studies, of
    ARDS, 31, *32t*
Random misclassification, 29
RANTES (C-C supergene fam-
    ily), 69–70
Rapid shallow breathing, 170–1,
    172f
Rashes, and drug reactions, 218
Reactive airways disease, *94t*, 96
Reactive oxygen metabolites
    (ROMs), 322–3
Recombinant IL-1ra, 240
Red blood cells, 128–9, 220
Refractory respiratory failure, 308
Refractory septic shock, *207t*
Relative risk, of ARDS, 38
Renal failure. *See also* Kidneys
    hemoglobin concentrations
        and, 128
    mechanical ventilation and, 216
    organ system failure scoring
        system (OSF) for, *306t*
Reperfusion injury, 322–3
Resident macrophages, 70–1, 72–3
Resistance to venous return,
    113–14
Respiratory acidosis
    hypoventilation and, 93, *94t*, 95
    intubation and, 184–5
    mechanical ventilation and,
        155–6, 158, *160t*
    respiratory muscle dysfunction
        and, 165
Respiratory alkalosis, 129
Respiratory arrest, 12
Respiratory burst, 241
Respiratory center output, 164
Respiratory compliance, *7t*
Respiratory drive, 104–5
Respiratory exam, 15
Respiratory failure
    mortality from ARDS and, 39,
        308
    organ system failure scoring
        system (OSF) for, *306t*
Respiratory muscles
    fatigue of, 166–7
    hypoventilation and, *94t*, 95
    pulmonary pathophysiology
        and strength of, 103–4

weaning from mechanical ventilation and, 164–8
Respiratory rate, and measures of
ventilation, 96–7
Respiratory system
complications of ARDS and,
210–2
host factors in nosocomial
pneumonia, 256, 257t
mechanics of and mechanical
ventilation, 159–60
mechanics of and pathophysiology of ARDS, 97–8
support other than ventilation,
190–1
survivors of ARDS and, 336, 340
Resuscitation
fluid, 121
multiple trauma and, 198
of patient with ARDS, 11–13
Retrospective case reports, 31, 32t
Rib cage-abdominal motion, 171
Right heart failure, and hemodynamics, 112–13
Right mainstem intubation, 188
Right ventricular end-diastolic
pressure (RVEDP), 223
Ringer's lactate, 126–7
Risk factors, for ARDS
causality and, 33
definition of, 8–9, 31
epidemiology and, 36–9
misclassification of ARDS and,
29

Salbutamol, 191
San Francisco, and incidence of
ARDS, 35–6
Sedation
mechanical ventilation and,
147, 148, 149, 150, 154
oxygen demand and, 119, 313
patient care and, 194–5, 196f
Selective decontamination of
digestive tract (SDD), 271–2
Sepsis. See also Septic shock
antibiotic regimens for, 209t
assessment of and patient care,
205–10
biologics targeting IL-1 and
TNF, 66
cardiac function curve and
venous return, 116
diagnosis of ARDS and, 22
gut-liver-lung connection and
evolution of, 71–2
hypoventilation and, 94t, 95
impaired tissue oxygen extraction and, 313

lactic acidosis and, 129, 130
mortality from ARDS and, 8,
39, 40
multiple system organ failure
and, 11, 305
polymicrobial-induced, 75–6
as risk factor for ARDS, 36,
37t, 39
ventricular pressure-volume
relationships, 109–12
Septic shock, 14, 207, 209t, 235,
317
Serum lipofuscin, 323
Shock
clinical evaluation of ARDS
patients, 14
esophageal rupture and, 203
hemorrhagic, 121, 198, 199t,
317
hypoventilation and, 94t, 95
intubation and, 184t
mixed venous oxygen desaturation and, 84
oxygen delivery and, 124
pulmonary thromboembolism
and, 221, 223
renal failure and, 216
as risk factor for ARDS, 37t, 38
septic, 14, 207, 209t, 235, 317
splanchnic circulation and,
311, 312
Shunts and shunting, 83, 87–8
Sickle-cell disease, 86
Sickness Impact Profile (SIP), 40,
336–7
Side effects, of medications, 235,
243
Sinusitis, 269
Skeletal muscle atrophy, 166
Sleep apnea, 119
Smoke inhalation, and ARDS,
37t, 58, 204–5
Smoking, of tobacco, 336, 340
Society of Critical Care Medi-
cine, 206
Sodium bicarbonate, 156
Sodium transport, and alveolar
fluid clearance, 276, 277f
Soluble TNF receptors, 240
Spine injury, 199, 201. See also
Cervical spine injury
Spirometry, 337
Splanchnic circulation, and
endotoxic shock, 311, 312
Spontaneous breathing, trials of,
174, 177–9
Squamous metaplasia, 54f
Staphylococcus aureus, 208, 252,
254, 265–6, 268t

Stenotrophomonas maltophilia, 252
Steroid muscle relaxants, 195
Steroid myopathy, 94t, 95, 195
Stevens-Johnson syndrome, 218
Storage lesions, of red blood cells,
220
Streptococcus pneumoniae, 268t
Streptokinase, 223
Stress gastritis, 192
Succinylcholine, 141, 195
Sucralfate, 270
Suctioning catheters, 269
Surfactant replacement, 233–4
Supergene families, of chemotac-
tic peptides, 67
Superoxide dismutase (SOD), 241
Supranormal oxygen delivery,
122, 124
Surgical pulmonary embolectomy,
223
Surveillance, and infection con-
trol, 269–70, 271t
Survival and survivors, of ARDS
medical management after dis-
charge, 339–41
pathophysiology and, 11
pulmonary function testing
and, 337–9, 341
quality of life for, 1, 40–1
roentgenographic changes in,
337
symptoms and limitations in,
336–7
Systemic inflammatory response
syndrome (SIRS), 206, 207t
Systemic vascular resistance
(SVR), 113, 158
Systolic dysfunction, 212

Tachycardia, and mechanical
ventilation, 150–1
Tazobactam, 267t
Temperature, body. See also Cool-
ing
hypercapnia and, 154
oxygenation of venous blood
and, 152
oxygen demand and, 119
Tension pneumothorax, 201,
210–11
Tetanus, 94t, 95
Therapeutic paralysis, and
mechanical ventilation, 147,
148, 149, 152, 154, 314
Thoracotomy, 198–9
Thrombocytopenia, 219
Thrombolytic therapy, 223
Thromboxane, 239, 243
Thyroid hormones, 228

Thyroxine, 228
Tidal breathing, and mechanical ventilation, 139
Tidal volumes
    dead space and, 92
    lung compliance and, 99
    mechanical ventilation and, 96–7, 141–2, 149, 151
    respiratory mechanics and, 98, 104
    rib cage ratio (RC/VT) and, 171
Tissue plasminogen activator, 283
Total lung capacity (TLC), and transpulmonary pressure, 91f
Total parenteral nutrition (TPN), 192
Tracheal gas insufflation (TGI), 148
Tracheal injury, and intubation, 18
Tracheostomy, 189–90
Trial of transfusion in critical care (TRICC), 220
Transforming growth factor-alpha (TGF-alpha), 278, 290–2
Transforming growth factor-beta (TGF-beta), 291t, 292
Transmission oximeters, 86
Transportation, of patient and intubation, 184
Transpulmonary pressure, 91f, 97–8
Trauma. See also Barotrauma; Fractures; Volutrauma
    assessment of and patient care, 197–205
    of chest, 16, 191, 201–3
    as risk factor for ARDS, 36, 37–8, 39
Traumatic air embolism, 201, 202
Tumor necrosis factor-alpha (TNF)
    acute lung injury and, 291t, 293–4
    anticytokine agents and, 240

initiation and maintenance of inflammatory response, 65–6, 70–1, 74, 75–6
multiple system organ failure, 320, 321f
sepsis syndrome and, 206–8
splanchnic blood flow and, 314
systolic contractility and, 112

Ulcers, of gastrointestinal system, 192, 213–14, 215f
United Kingdom, and incidence of ARDS, 35
University of Washington, 8
Upper abdominal surgery, 164
Upper airway burn injury, 204
Upper airways obstruction, 94t, 95
Upper gastrointestinal hemorrhage, 213
Upper inflection point (UIP), 98, 142
Urokinase, 282–3
Utah, and incidence of ARDS, 35

Vancomycin, 209t, 266
Vascular endothelial growth factor (VEGF), 291t, 294
Vascular injury, and sepsis, 207
Vascular permeability, and pathophysiology of ARDS, 9–10
Vasoactive drugs, 152, 313, 322
Vasopressin, 123t
Vasopressors, 121–2, 123t, 189
Vecuronium, 195
Venous catheter, and chest radiograph, 18
Venous return
    cardiac output and, 113–17
    mechanical ventilation and, 150–1
Ventilation. See also Hyperventilation; Hypoventilation; Mechanical ventilation

cardiac output and, 124
intubation and, 184t
measures of, 96–7
Ventilation-perfusion lung scan, 222
Ventilator-induced lung injury, 40
Ventilatory circuit changes, and nosocomial pneumonia, 269
Ventricular preload, in survivors of ARDS, 11
Ventricular pressure-volume relationships, 108–12
Viral pneumonia, 340
Vital capacity, and maximum inspiratory pressure, 104
Vitamin K, 219, 220
Volume-controlled IRV (VC-IRV), 144–5
Volume-cycled modes, of mechanical ventilation, 144
Volutrauma, 151
V/Q mismatch
    hypoxemia and, 83, 87
    measurement of carbon dioxide production, 97

Weakness, muscular, 185, 195, 219. See also Myopathy
Weaning, from mechanical ventilation
    methods of, 173–9
    predicting outcome of, 168–73
    pulmonary gas exchange and, 163–4
West's zone 1 lung, and pulmonary wedge pressure, 126
Wheezing, 191
Whole body oxygen uptake, 118–19
Wound infections, 210

Xanthine oxidase, 322, 323